Molecular Imaging
in Oncology

Springer
*Berlin
Heidelberg
New York
Barcelona
Hong Kong
London
Milan
Paris
Singapore
Tokyo*

E. E. Kim · E. F. Jackson

Molecular Imaging in Oncology

PET, MRI, and MRS

With Contributions by
J. Aoki · H. Baghaei · S. Ilgan · T. Inoue · H. Li · J. Uribe
F. C. L. Wong · W.-H. Wong · D. J. Yang

With 219 Figures in 387 Separate Parts
5 in Full Color

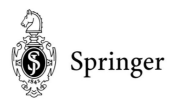

Springer

E. Edmund Kim, M.D., M.S.
Edward F. Jackson, Ph.D.
Division of Diagnostic Imaging
The University of Texas
M.D. Anderson Cancer Center
1515 Holcombe Blvd.
Houston, TX 77030
USA

ISBN 3-540-64101-7 Springer-Verlag Berlin Heidelberg New York

Library of Congress Cataloging-in-Publication Data
Kim, E. Edmund. Molecular imaging in oncology: PET, MRI, and MRS/E.E. Kim and E.F. Jackson. p. cm. Includes bibliographical references and index. ISBN 3-540-64101-7 (alk. paper). 1. Cancer – Imaging. 2. Cancer – Tomography. 3. Cancer – Magnetic resonance imaging. 4. Nuclear magnetic resonance spectroscopy – Diagnostic use. 5. Tomography, Emission. I. Jackson, E.F., (Edward F.), 1961- . II. Title. [DNLM: 1. Neoplasms – diagnosis. 2. Magnetic Resonance Imaging. 3. Nuclear Magnetic Resonance. 4. Tomography, Emission-Computed. QZ 241K49b 1999] RC270.3.D53K54 1999 616.99'40754–dc21 DNLM/DLC for Library of Congress 98-33852

This work is subject to copyright. All rights are reserved, whether the whole or part of the material is concerned, specifically the rights of translation, reprinting, reuse of illustrations, recitation, broadcasting, reproduction on microfilm or in any other way, and storage in data banks. Duplication of this publication or parts thereof is permitted only under the provisions of the German Copyright Law of September 9, 1965, in its current version, and permission for use must always be obtained from Springer-Verlag. Violations are liable for prosecution under the German Copyright Law.

© Springer-Verlag Berlin · Heidelberg 1999
Printed in Germany

The use of general descriptive names, registered names, trademarks, etc. in this publication does not imply, even in the absence of a specific statement, that such names are exempt from the relevant protective laws and regulations and therefore free for general use.

Product liability: The publishers cannot guarantee the accuracy of any information about dosage and application contained in this book. In every individual case the user must check such information by consulting the relevant literature.

Cover design: Anna Deus, Heidelberg
Typesetting: K + V Fotosatz GmbH, Beerfelden
Printing and binding: Konrad Triltsch, Druck- und Verlagsanstalt GmbH, 97070 Würzburg

SPIN 10628559   21/3135-5 4 3 2 1 0 – Printed on acid-free paper

This book is dedicated to

our wives Bo and Sondra
and children
Patrick, Sharon, Matthew
Michelle and Jonathan

Foreword

Medical imaging in oncology mostly has emphasized the relationship of structural changes in the body, as exemplified by detection of "masses". However, recent advances in genetics and molecular biology have led to an interest in mutational changes in cancer that result in alterations in cellular behavior that emphasize "functional" changes on images. This has led to a merging of physics and chemistry that calls for new ways of viewing oncologic diseases. The editors of this book on *Molecular Imaging in Oncology*, a clinician and a physicist, and their colleagues, have taken the challenge of preparing an introductory text to this rapidly growing field.

The emphasis on magnetic resonance imaging (MRI), magnetic resonance spectroscopy (MRS) and positron emission tomography (PET) is appropriate as these are the prototypical technologies used to explore the inner world of the cell by external imaging. Advances in the past decade in instrumentation have been paralleled by radiotracers and contrast materials and are being applied in research directed toward the improvement of diagnosis, treatment selection and disease monitoring. This text will prepare the oncologist, radiologist and nuclear physician to understand current advantages and limitations of these modalities.

The book is divided into two parts. The first part on "basic principles and techniques" is devoted to biologic, chemical and physical subjects along with explanation of techniques. The second part presents current clinical applications in various specific cancers, based both on the experience at the M. D. Anderson Cancer Center and on the literature. As with any medical technology it is important to understand the weaknesses and the strengths of the approach.

As this is a rapidly evolving field, the authors have tried to prepare the reader for what might lie ahead, as well as enlighten the path that has been followed. An honest appraisal would conclude that we have only scratched the surface of this subject. Much exciting territory is yet unexplored. It is to be hoped that readers will be inspired by the progress that has been made to date and will be stimulated to contribute to the field's expansion in the future.

Thomas P. Haynie,
Professor Emeritus of Nuclear Medicine,
UT M.D. Anderson Cancer Center,
Houston, Texas

Preface

The development of molecular biology and genetics over the past two decades has provided medical science with an unprecedented chance to understand the molecular basis of disease. While disease is usually defined as gross structural or histopathological abnormality, it can now be defined on the basis of abnormal deviation from normal regional biochemistry. Cancer is viewed as a failure of multiple chemical processes or genetic disease. Molecular derangements occur at the very beginning of disease processes, and anatomically detectable abnormalities occur much later.

MRI and PET are biochemical or molecular imaging techniques which can be used as probes of molecular and genetic phenomena. MR spectroscopy or spectroscopic imaging can characterize tissues by its metabolic signatures for the tissue diagnosis and evaluation of therapeutic response. PET is the unique method to study both the pharmacokinetics and the pharmacodynamics of new cancer drugs. Tumor or tissue-specific contrast agents for MRI or radiopharmaceuticals will provide a better understanding of tumor receptor systems and metabolic pathways.

The care of cancer patients has become a cooperative multidisciplinary endeavor. If the medical disciplines involved in cancer treatment work well together, they are able to communicate with precision. A multidisciplinary approach in the diagnosis, staging, treatment, and follow-up of cancers takes a great deal of effort, but the rewards to the patient and oncologists are tremendous. It is critical for imaging specialists to embrace and participate in a multidisciplinary environment so that they are considered valued and equal partners. Multidisciplinary participation for the imaging specialist entails routine daily imaging interpretation, multidisciplinary conference, tumor board meeting, and being available for consultation to help oncologists use the most appropriate imaging. Review of outside imaging studies allows oncologists to have all the information necessary to make a therapeutic decision, as well as to fully discuss the treatment plan with the patients.

The major goal of imaging is to answer specific clinical questions. This goal is much easier to accomplish if the questions are known before, rather than after, the examination is performed. Imaging specialists must understand not only the imaging modalities available, but also the clinical problems they present. Familiarity with the natural history and treatment paradigms of cancer and the staging systems is a necessity for successful cancer management.

This book is organized into two parts consisting of eight basic science and nine clinical chapters. Basic science chapters discuss the basic principles of cancer molecular biology, biochemistry, immunology and pathology; imaging strategies and perspectives for cancer diagnosis and monitoring; physical principles of MRI, MRS and PET; radiopharmaceuticals for tumor imaging and MRI contrast agents; MRI receptor imaging and PET technique and artifacts. Clinical chapters deal with basic considerations emphasizing molecular biologic information; pathology, diagnosis, staging; MRI and MRS; and PET of lung, breast, gastrointestinal, gynecologic, urologic, head and neck cancers, musculoskeletal, sarcomas and miscellaneous tumors.

It is our goal and hope that this text will provide the information relevant to molecular or biochemical imaging that is needed by radiologists, nuclear physicians and oncologists dealing with malignant disease.

Acknowledgements

We are very appreciative and indebted to Judy Bunch for her tremendous efforts to make this book the best of its kind by typing and editing materials. We also are deeply grateful to all colleagues whom we often harassed for their timely contributions. We wish to thank Drs. Donald Podoloff and William Murphy for their support of our work. Finally, we wish to thank Dr. Ute Heilmann and her assistants at Springer-Verlag who supported in the creation and editing of this book.

E. E. Kim
E. F. Jackson

Contents

Principles and Technology

1 Principles of Cancer Biology, Biochemistry, Immunology and Pathology 3
E. E. Kim

2 Imaging Strategies and Perspectives in Oncology 13
E. E. Kim

3 Magnetic Resonance Imaging: Physical Principles to Advanced Applications 17
E. F. Jackson

4 Magnetic Resonance Spectroscopy: Physical Principles and Applications 47
E. F. Jackson

5 Principles and Instrumentation of Position Emission Tomography . . 71
W.-H. Wong, J. Uribe, H. Li and H. Baghaei

6 Radiopharmaceuticals for Tumor Imaging and Magnetic Resonance Imaging Contrast Agents 81
D. J. Yang, S. Ilgan and E. E. Kim

7 Receptor Imaging 101
F. C. L. Wong and E. E. Kim

8 Practical Magnetic Resonance Imaging and Positron Emission Tomography Techniques and Their Artifacts 107
E. E. Kim

Clinical Applications of MRI, MRS and PET

9 Lung Cancers 123
T. Inoue, J. Aoki and E. E. Kim

10 Breast Cancer 145
E. E. Kim

11 Gastrointestinal Carcinomas 159
E. E. Kim

12 Urologic Cancers 181
E. E. Kim

13 Gynecologic Cancers 199
   E. E. Kim

14 Brain Tumors 211
   F. C. L. Wong and E. E. Kim

15 Head and Neck Tumors 231
   F. C. L. Wong and E. E. Kim

16 Musculoskeletal Tumors 243
   T. Inoue, J. Aoki and E. E. Kim

17 Melanoma, Lymphoma and Myeloma 271
   E. E. Kim

Subject Index 287

List of Contributors

J. Aoki, M.D.
Department of Surgery, Gunma University School of Medicine, Maebashi, Gunma, 371, Japan

H. Baghaei, Ph.D.
Division of Diagnostic Imaging, The University of Texas,
M.D. Anderson Cancer Center, 1515 Holcombe Blvd, Houston, TX 77030, USA

S. Ilgan, M.D.
Division of Diagnostic Imaging, The University of Texas,
M.D. Anderson Cancer Center, 1515 Holcombe Blvd, Houston, TX 77030, USA

T. Inoue, M.D.
Department of Nuclear Medicine, Gunma University School of Medicine, Maebashi, Gunma, 371, Japan

E. F. Jackson, Ph.D.
Division of Diagnostic Imaging, The University of Texas, M.D. Anderson Cancer Center, 1515 Holcombe Blvd, Houston, TX 77030, USA

E. E. Kim, M.D.
Division of Diagnostic Imaging, The University of Texas,
M.D. Anderson Cancer Center, 1515 Holcombe Blvd, Houston, TX 77030, USA

H. Li, M.D.
Division of Diagnostic Imaging, The University of Texas,
M.D. Anderson Cancer Center, 1515 Holcombe Blvd, Houston, TX 77030, USA

J. Uribe, Ph.D.
Division of Diagnostic Imaging, The University of Texas,
M.D. Anderson Cancer Center, 1515 Holcombe Blvd, Houston, TX 77030, USA

F.C.L. Wong, M.D., Ph.D.
Division of Diagnostic Imaging, The University of Texas,
M.D. Anderson Cancer Center, 1515 Holcombe Blvd, Houston, TX 77030, USA

W.-H. Wong, Ph.D.
Division of Diagnostic Imaging, The University of Texas,
M.D. Anderson Cancer Center, 1515 Holcombe Blvd, Houston, TX 77030, USA

D. J. Yang, Ph.D.
Division of Diagnostic Imaging, The University of Texas,
M.D. Anderson Cancer Center, 1515 Holcombe Blvd, Houston, TX 77030, USA

Principles and Technology

Principles of Cancer Biology, Biochemistry, Immunology, and Pathology

E. E. Kim

Cancer Molecular Biology

Cancer is a cellular or genetic disease. The gene is the basic unit of inheritance and determinant of all phenotypes. The DNA of a normal human cell contains approximately 30 000–40 000 genes, but only a fraction of these are expressed in any particular cell at any given time [1]. A gene exerts its effects by having its DNA transcribed into a messenger RNA (mRNA) which is in turn translated into a protein. Every gene consists of several functional components. However, there are two major functional units: the promoter and coding regions [2]. The promoter region controls when and in what tissue a gene is expressed. The coding region is the part of the gene that dictates the amino acid sequence of the protein encoded by the gene. DNA is a linear polymer of nucleotides which consists of an invariant portion, a five-carbon deoxyribose sugar with a phosphate group, and a variable portion, the base. Of the four bases, two are purines, adenine (A) and guanine (G), and two are pyrimidines, cytosine (C) and thymine (T). Ordinarily, the nucleotide bases of one strand of DNA interact with those of another strand to make double-stranded DNA. This base pairing is specific, so that A interacts with T, and C interacts with G. In every strand of a DNA polymer, the phosphate substitutions are located between the 5′ and 3′ carbons of the ribose molecules. The genetic code reads in the 5′ to 3′ direction. In double-stranded DNA, the strand that carries the translatable code in the 5′ to 3′ direction is called the sense strand, while its complementary partner is the antisense strand. In the nucleus, DNA is not present as naked nucleic acid; rather, DNA is in close association with a number of accessory proteins, such as the histones, to make the structure called chromatin [3]. DNA's double helix is ordinarily twisted on itself to form a super-coiled structure which must unwind partially during DNA replication and transcription [4].

Genes can be cut from total genomic DNA using restriction endonucleases that recognize specific nucleotide sequences [5]. Individual genes can be captured and replicated in bulk for detailed analysis. This process is called cloning and employs bacterial plasmids and viruses (phages) as carriers for the cloned genes [6]. Enzymes called DNA ligases join foreign DNA to plasmid or phage vectors which can then replicate within bacterial cells to create gene libraries [7]. Each colony or plaque represents a different DNA clone. Specific clones containing specific genes can be identified on the basis of their nucleotide sequences, expanded into large-scale cultures and their recombinant DNA isolated. In this way, new genes are cloned.

Cloned gene fragments are called probes because they are used to probe native DNA or RNA for the gene of interest. A gene probe must contain enough nucleotide sequences so that it will recognize the sequences of its corresponding gene. Recognition occurs by a process called nucleic-acid hybridization, in which two pieces of DNA can align themselves by base pairing. Genomic DNA is too large to be analyzed easily in the laboratory, but it can be cut into manageable fragments using restriction endonucleases isolated from bacteria. Electrophoresis through an agarose gel can separate these fragments by size. Pulsed-field gel electrophoresis is a variation of this technique which allows the separation of extremely large DNA molecules. Fragments that carry nucleotide sequences corresponding to a gene of interest can then be detected by Southern blotting [8]. For any given region of DNA, the size and number of restriction fragments may vary among individuals, leading to restriction fragment-length polymorphisms (RFLP), which are exploited both in gene mapping and for cancer diagnostics [9]. If one of the RFLPs present in the heterozygous individual's normal DNA is missing from the tumor cell DNA, the tumor is said to have undergone a reduction to homozygosity. This implies a loss of genetic material from the tumor, specifically the

DNA that includes the missing RFLP. This is the hallmark of a tumor-suppressor gene [10]. Specific nucleotide changes (mutations) that give rise to stable genetic differences can be determined by DNA sequencing. There are two methods used for sequencing DNA: the chemical modification method and the enzymatic chain-termination method. DNA sequencing has been utilized for the analysis of mutated sequences in the tumor-suppressor gene *p53* [11]. By amplifying specific fragments of DNA, the polymerase chain reaction (PCR) technology permits the detection of specific genes in extremely small amounts of tissue or in tissue that has been fixed for histological analysis [12].

Specific nucleotide changes (mutations) that give rise to stable genetic differences can be determined by DNA sequencing. If one of the RFLPs present in the heterozygous individual's normal DNA is missing from the tumor cell DNA, the tumor is said to have undergone a reduction to homozygosity. This implies a loss of genetic material from the tumor, specifically the DNA that includes the missing RFLP, which is the hallmark of a tumor-suppressor gene [10]. The genetic information in DNA is copied or transcribed into mRNA by the enzyme RNA polymerase II. Before being transported to the cytoplasm, primary transcripts in the nucleus are modified by splicing out introns, adding a 5' cap and adding a 3' poly-(A) tract [13]. Cytoplasmic mRNA can be detected by Northern blotting, nuclease-protection assays or by modified PCR. Although nuclease-protection assays are somewhat more technically demanding than Northern blotting, they are more sensitive and can also provide structural information about mRNA transcripts. A retroviral enzyme called reverse transcriptase can make cDNA copies of mRNA transcripts. These cDNAs can be cloned into cDNA libraries, which are useful for isolating and analyzing expressed genes [14].

The genetic information in DNA is transcribed into RNA, and the information in RNA is ultimately translated into protein. Like DNA and RNA, proteins are directional. The amino and carboxy termini of proteins are specified by the 5' and 3' ends, respectively, of the cognate in RNAs. After translation, proteins may require further modification in order to be fully functional. Proteins can be fractionated by size, using electrophoresis through polyacrylamide gels in the presence of the anionic detergent sodium dodecyl sulfate (SDS). SDS-polyacrylamide gel electrophoresis (PAGE) is an integral component of the analytical techniques of immune precipitation and Western blotting [15]. Automated analyzers can directly determine the amino acid sequence of a protein using vanishingly small amounts of material. The mRNA that encodes a protein can be translated in vitro using cellular extracts of rabbit reticulocytes or wheat germ. The DNA that encodes a protein can be transcribed and the RNA translated in vivo using appropriate vector and host-cell combinations in culture [16].

Cancer Biochemistry

The biochemistry of cancer received its real beginning with the work of Otto Warburg, who noted a high production of lactate by tumor slices in the presence of oxygen [17]. It has been pointed out that oxygen, which was consumed by neoplastic cells as effectively as by some normal cells, resulted in an inhibition of the formation of glycolytic end products [18]. The inhibition of glycolysis by oxidative phosphorylation has been called the Pasteur effect. Respiration markedly depends on the availability of intermediates such as adenosine diphosphate (ADP) and inorganic phosphate. Competition for ADP and inorganic phosphate occurs in respiration and glycolysis. Several studies suggested local hypoxia as the underlying cause for the apparent deficiency in respiration of tumors [19]. The hypoglycemic effect may, in part, contribute to the problems associated with cachexia in the tumor-bearing host. Greenstein [20] noted that cancers tended to discard certain enzymes or pathways that were not required for growth processes. The enzymatic profiles of the tumors tended to converge to a common pattern, and the adoption of a similar enzymatic matrix by tumors was a reflection of the increase in growth rate. Van Potter [21] proposed the loss of systems of catabolism as a central feature of tumorigenesis. A number of the enzymatic changes that are observed in tumors resemble those that are found in fetal systems. A tumor may, in fact, represent a dedifferentiation or retrodifferentiation of mature cells. Hexokinases play a vital role in the utilization of glucose, and phosphofructokinase is a key regulatory enzyme in glycolysis. In hepatocarcinogenesis, a progressive reduction in the activity of glucokinase is noted with a concomitant rise in type-I hexokinase [22]. In the normal rapidly proliferating systems, regenerating and fetal liver, as well as hepatomas, type-IV phosphofructokinase was found in much higher amounts than in the normal liver [23]. Terminal deoxynucleotidyltransferase (TdT) catalyzes the linear polymerization of nucleotides onto a suitable template, and TdT+ cells normally appear in the thymus cortex and bone-marrow lymphocytes. TdT+ cells were found in blast cells from patients with acute lymphocytic leukemia [24]. Oncofetal proteins of nonenzyme function are found in a variety of tumors and are often referred to as tumor-specific antigens.

Alpha-fetoprotein (AFP) is the serum protein in early extrauterine development, and elevated serum AFP levels were demonstrated in patients with hepatoma, acute liver toxicity or partial hepatectomy [25]. Carcinoembryonic antigen (CEA) is a serum glycoprotein which is elevated in patients with digestive, lung or genitourinary cancer, as well as colitis, cirrhosis or pancreatitis. The increased CEA level may be the result of its release from the membrane by phospholipase or some defect in the phosphatidylinositol complex [26]. The overproduction of CEA may disrupt the intercellular adhesion forces, resulting in more cell movement, less-ordered architecture, and more dedifferentiation [27]. Although neither AFP nor CEA is specific for tumors, they increase the diagnostic capability and allow for assessing therapeutic efficacy or recurrence of cancer.

Tumors often exhibit bizarre phenotypic expressions that can have profound effects on the patients. A number of nonendocrine cancer cells can manufacture and secrete ectopic substances including hormones and growth factors that enhance bone resorption and lead to increased levels of serum calcium. The exact mechanism underlying these actions is not clear, although enhanced gene expression is involved. Elevated levels of serotonin, antidiuretic hormone calcitonin, adrenocorticotrophic hormone (ACTH), prostaglandin and colony-stimulating-factor osteolytic substance may be observed in certain types of cancer [28].

The growth of tumors is often accompanied by a striking loss of weight, anorexia, asthenia and anemia. Cachexia is a major confounder in the chemotherapy of cancer; an increased gluconeogenesis, enhanced direction of glucose from peripheral tissue to the tumor, increased fat oxidation, decrease in body lipids, great expenditure of energy, increased turnover rate of total body protein and elevation in the catabolism of muscle protein have been observed [29]. Although interleukin 1 (IL-1) has been cast as one of the mediators of cachexia, a greater role falls on the unique polypeptide cachectin or tumor necrosis factor (TNF) [30]. TNF/cachectin is elaborated by tumors and binds to receptors in tissues. The resultant complex causes the suppression of specific mRNA synthesis, which then results in changes in intermediary metabolism to feed tumor cells at the expense of the host.

The naturally-occurring polyamines, putrescine, spermidine and spermine are ubiquitously distributed throughout the eukaryotes. Cell proliferation and differentiation require their biosynthesis [31]. Suppression of tumor growth has been observed when inhibitors of polyamine synthesis were administered [32]. Ornithine decarboxylase (ODC) is a key regulatory enzyme in the biosynthesis of polyamines and undergoes rapid induction upon exposure of cells to stimuli including growth factors, hormones and tumor promoters. Increased ODC was found in skin cancers and familial polyposis, and ODC genes located to chromosome 2 have been reported [33]. Cyclic adenosine monophosphate (cAMP) may play an important role in the differentiation of certain cells and is formed from the catalytic action of adenyl cyclase, a membrane-bound enzyme which utilizes ATP as substrate. cAMP is involved in a number of phosphorylation reactions through the action of cAMP-dependent protein kinase, called A-kinase. cAMP levels are modulated by external stimuli, such as growth factors and prostaglandins, and may regulate the rate of cell proliferation [34]. Poly (ADP-ribose) polymerase or synthetase is a chromatin-bound enzyme involved in cell transformation, cell differentiation, and DNA repair [35]. Poly (ADP-ribosylation) is activated by DNA strand breaks. When the damage to DNA is severe, activation of the polymerase persists, leading to a depletion of the intracellular pool of ATP.

The death of cells is neither always abnormal nor always detrimental. Although necrosis ensues at the sites of massive cellular injury, most cells die through a more subtle, non-inflammatory, energy-dependent form of cell death called apoptosis [36]. Cells undergoing apoptotic cellular suicide rapidly shrink and lose their normal intercellular contacts and, subsequently, exhibit dense chromatin condensation, nuclear fragmentation, cytoplasmic blebbing, and cellular fragmentation into small apoptotic bodies. Necrosis occurs in acute, nonphysiological injury, and necrotic cells swell and lyse, releasing their cytoplasmic and nuclear contents into the intercellular milieu, thus sparking inflammation. Apoptosis is of critical importance both to the pathogenesis of cancers and to their likelihood of resistance to antineoplastic treatments. The protein p53 induces apoptosis by acting as a transcription factor, activating expression of numerous apoptosis-mediating genes. DNA damage causes the p53 protein to turn on genes, the products of which generate free radicals that damage the mitochondria, whose contents, in turn, leak out into the cytoplasm and activate apoptotic caspases [37]. Mutation in genes that lead to reduced apoptosis are generally associated with poor prognosis. New cancer therapies that aim to induce apoptosis specifically in cancer cells are the source of renewed hope for cures. The role of DNA methylation in the production of cancer has been examined [38]. The methylation occurs exclusively in the 5-position of cytosine and, more specifically, when this cytosine is part of the CpG dinucleotide. Less methylation of the CpG sequences in the AFP gene in hepatoma DNA, and hypermethylation of specific regions of human chromosomes in tumor cells have been reported [39]

The production and secretion of proteolytic enzymes by tumors represent old observations. The plasminogen activators are involved in fibrinolysis, tissue remodeling and some stages of malignancy. They are also participants in a number of steps of metastasis [40]. The extracellular matrix (ECM) is a complex medium which is formed from substances that are secreted by cells. The ECM is important in the regulation of cell proliferation and differentiation as well as in determining the metastatic potential of malignant cells. Many cancer cells secrete proteases, glycosidases, heparanases and type-IV collagenase. The ECM is composed of: collagen type I–V, depending on the specific tissue; proteoglycans such as chondroitin sulfate; anchorage proteins such as fibronectin that serve as attachment sites to the matrix; and sometimes elastin. Substantial alterations to the plasma membrane of cells occurs in neoplastic transformation. Cell transformation was shown to alter the gangliosides and neutral glycolipids with a number of tumor systems expressing gangliotriosylceramide (Gg3) [41].

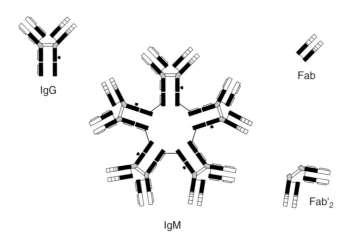

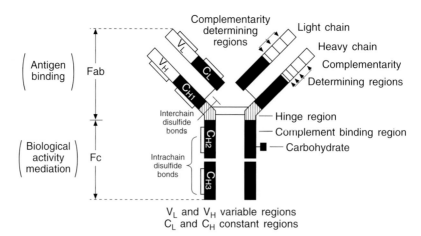

Fig. 1.1. Structure of IgG, IgM and immunoglobulin fragment as well as monomer. IgG consists of one immunoglobulin, but IgM consists of five immunoglobulin monomers linked by disulfide bonds. Fab fragments are generated by cleavage with papain while Fab fragments are generated with pepsin. Ig molecules consist of light and heavy polypeptide chains

Cancer Immunology

The human immune response has evolved to detect and eliminate foreign substances and organisms. This response is mediated by lymphoreticular cells and their products. Bone marrow is the source of both B lymphocytes that produce antibodies and T lymphocytes that mediate cellular immunity [42]. Mature B cells synthesize and express immunoglobulin (Ig) on their cell surface. After interaction with antigen and T-cell products, different clones of B cells differentiate into one or more plasma cells that produce a single antibody which binds noncovalently to a particular antigen. Ig molecules consist of light (L) and heavy (H) polypeptide chains (Fig. 1.1). Each L and H chain can be divided into an amino-terminal variable (V) region and a carboxyl-terminal constant (C) region. The V region of each H and L chain includes three complementarity-determining regions (CDRs), which contribute to the antigen-binding site and which determine the specificity of the antibody. Each H-chain C region (C_H) determines the function and isotype of the antibody. These include IgG1, IgG2, IgG3, IgG4, IgA1, IgA2, IgM, IgD, and IgE. The C_H region permits fixation of complement components, antibody-dependent cell-mediated cytotoxicity, Ig-mediated phagocytosis and transport across the placenta. T lymphocytes arise in bone marrow and differentiate within the thymus [43]. T cells mediate the cellular response, including delayed hypersensitivity, graft rejection and regulation of other T cells, B cells, monocytes and marrow progenitors. The specificity of interactions with different antigens is mediated by a large family of 90-kDa, cell-surface T-cell receptors (TCR) [44]. Different clones of T cells bearing distinctive TCRs recognize different antigenic peptides. T cells mature under the influence of thymic epithelium. Early thymocytes express CD2 and CD7, and common thymocytes acquire CD1, CD4 and CD8. Mature T cells constitute 70–89% of normal peripheral blood lymphocytes, 30–40% of lymph node cells and 20–30% of splenic lymphocytes. B cells are organized in follicular aggregates within lymph nodes, spleen and gut-associated lymphoid tissue. Antibody production can be augmented by T-cell help. A small population of lymphocytes lacks the markers associated with mature B or T cells. Non-T or non-B cells can exert both antibody-dependent cell-mediated cytotoxicity (ADCC) and natural-killer (NK) activity, destroying tumor cells in the presence or absence of specific IgG antibodies. Monocytes, macrophages and dendritic cells can present antigens to lymphocytes and secrete cytokines, such as IL-1, IL-6, TNFα, interferons, prostaglandins and other monokines that can affect the function of both T and B cells. T cells and monocytes produce a large number of factors which mediate intercellular communication and include the interleukins and cytokines. Cytokines can interact synergistically and can stimulate the release of a cascade of secondary factors.

The process of malignant transformation is a series of DNA mutations of cancer-related genes. The immune system has the potential to discriminate between the normal and the aberrant self. Thus, the protein products of these mutated DNA segments are potentially immunogenic. It is likely that human tumors are linked to prolonged exposure to low-dose carcinogens. Cytotoxic T (Tc) cells specific for autologous tumor cells have been cultured from the peripheral blood of melanoma patients or from the tumor-infiltrating lymphocytes [45]. There is increasing evidence that non-immunogenic tumors can stimulate the host immune response by immunological manipulations. T cells are capable of mediating the regression of established tumors when adoptively transferred to the tumor-bearing host [46]. T cells do not recognize a native antigen, but rather interact with peptide fragments derived from protein antigens bound to major histocompatibility complex (MHC) molecules on the cell surface. The two major T-cell subsets recognize short sequences of approximately ten amino acids, presented on the cell surface by an MHC molecule. CD4$^+$ T helper (T_H) cells recognize antigens presented by the MHC class-II molecules on antigen-presenting cells, and CD8$^+$ Tc cells recognize intracellular proteins that are mostly synthesized in the cytoplasm, degraded to small peptides, translocated into the endoplasmic reticulum for insertion into a cleft in the MHC class-I molecule, and transported through the Golgi stack for expression on cell surface [47]. For a tumor to be immunogenic, it needs to present processed antigens as peptides bound to MHC class-I or class-II molecules.

Early studies demonstrated a decreased cell-mediated immunity in cancer patients. It is likely that the immunological deficit does not contribute significantly to the initial tumor progression, especially in patients with solid tumor, but that it reflects a secondary phenomenon. Tumors might arise not because of a general depression in cell-mediated immunity, but because of a specific inability to react effectively against the antigens on the tumor cells. Transfection of MHC class-I genes into murine tumor cells often decreases their ability to grow in immunocompetent hosts [48]. With the exception of hematopoietic cancers, most solid tumors do not express MHC class-II antigens, and they cannot directly activate tumor-specific $CD4^+$ T_H cells. It has become clear that, in addition to T-cell receptor signaling, activation of T cells requires other critical costimulatory signals. Tumor-cell antigen presentation to T cells in the absence of costimulators may induce peripheral tolerance in tumor-specific T-lymphocyte responses. Selective outgrowth of antigen-negative tumor variants under the pressure of tumor-specific T-cell response has been documented in a variety of tumor systems. Antigen-negative immunoselected variants often express fewer immunodominant antigens that can trigger a Tc-cell response [49]. A tumor-bearing host may be immunologically tolerant to some tumor antigens. Tumor cells often express carcinoembryonic antigens (CEA), which are not immunogenic since they are expressed as self proteins during development. However, tolerance to CEA may be broken by immunization with a recombinant vaccinia virus expressing CEA [50]. Tumors can exert local effects that prevent T-cell immune responses from displaying full efficacy. Transforming growth factor β has been known to inhibit IL-2-dependent proliferation of T lymphocytes and a variety of T-cell and macrophage functions. The suppressor T cells have been identified as CD4 cells and appear to need several days to be generated in response to tumor growth. The $CD4^+$ T_H cell population contains two subsets that can be differentiated on the basis of the lymphokines they produce. The T_H 1 cells produce IL-2 and interferon γ (IFN-γ) and induce macrophage activation and delayed-type hypersensitivity responses, whereas T_H 2 cells produce IL-4 and IL-10 and selectively induce B-cell responses. The kinetics of tumor growth may allow for the establishment of progressive tumors before an effective immune response develops. In general, immunologically mediated tumor eradication is at its best when the tumor burden is small.

Both RNA and DNA viruses are implicated in the development of tumors. T-cell immunity against virus-induced tumors follows the rules of antiviral immunity. Any tumor virus protein could serve as a target for T cells, provided that it is processed into peptides and presented by MHC molecules on the surface of antigen-presenting cells. The Epstein-Barr virus is associated with B-cell lymphoma, Hodgkin's lymphoma and nasopharyngeal carcinoma. Human papilloma virus is associated with most human cervical carcinomas. A protective role of the immune system in controlling the growth of DNA virus-induced tumors is suggested by the high frequency of these tumors in immunodeficient individuals.

DNA mutation of cancer-related genes can result in the expression of altered proteins that differ from normal by a single amino acid residue. Somatic mutations of ras oncogenes occur commonly in 90% of pancreatic adenocarcinoma, 50% of colon adenocarcinoma and 30% of hepatocellular carcinoma. Antibodies reactive to ras were detected in 32% of cancer patients but only 3% of people without cancer [51]. The hallmark of chronic myelogenous leukemia is the translocation of the human c-abl proto-oncogene from chromosome 9 to the specific breakpoint (bcr) region on chromosome 22 [52]. A recent report has demonstrated that human Tc cells can be generated against the rearranged bcr–abl fusion peptide, providing hopeful immunotherapy [53]. Some genes, such as MAGE and HER-2/neu, are silent or expressed at low levels in normal tissue. When these genes are deregulated as a consequence of malignant transformation and are expressed inappropriately, they may behave as tumor antigens and evoke immune responses. Patients with HER-2/neu-positive tumors often demonstrate antibody and cellular immunity to HER-2/neu, suggesting that tolerance can be circumvented [54]. A fundamental characteristic of malignant cells is the accumulation of genetic mutations required for malignant transformation or maintenance of malignant phenotype. Missense mutations in the *p53* tumor-suppressor gene are detected in approximately half of human cancers, and p53-derived peptides may represent ideal targets for cellular immunotherapy [55].

Over the years, two approaches have been utilized for cancer immunotherapy: active and passive immunotherapy. In active immunotherapy, attempts have been made to stimulate endogenous antitumor immunity within the host through the administration of bacterial products, chemically defined immunomodulators, cytokines and vaccines. In passive immunotherapy, antibodies or lymphoreticular cells have been given to the host (adoptive immunotherapy), providing exogenous immunity. IFN and IL-2 have been the major cytokines, and their use in melanoma patients has caused some therapeutic response (10–30%) [56]. Unfortunately, toxic effects have been associated with repeated high-dose IL-2 infusions. The secretion of cytokines by gene-modified tumor cells may more closely resemble the physiological mode of lymphokine delivery to antigen-presenting cells or lymphocytes for immune activation. Virtually all described cytokine genes, including IL-1, IL-2, IL-3, IL-4, IL-6, IL-7, IL-12, IFN-γ, TNF-α, granulocytic colony-stimulating factor, and granulocyte-macrophage colony-stimulating factor have been found to be effective in at least some animal tumor models [57]. Using the human melanoma-associated antigen, p97, expressed on murine K1735-M2 cells, it was demonstrated that immunization with transduced tumor cells expressing the costimulation molecule B7 resulted in complete regression of tumors that express the human tumor antigen [58]. The efficacy of cytokine-mediated gene therapy may not necessarily be superior to immunization or immunotherapy. However, combining cytokine gene therapy with other molecules, such as MHC, cell-adhesion protein, tumor or foreign antigen may allow optimizing treatment schemes. The identification of genes that encode tumor cell-surface peptides that are recognized by Tc cells has provided another form of active immunization. Vaccination with antigen-presenting cells expressing tumor proteins and peptides may improve the efficacy of active immunotherapy.

Many variations on the use of passively administered antibodies in cancer therapy have been tried. Antitumor antibodies conjugated to toxic molecules, radioisotopes, and drugs have been tried, but the practical application has proven considerably more difficult than anticipated. Radioimmunodetection of melanoma using monoclonal antibodies has shown a reasonable degree of localization in melanoma nodules [59]; however, there is limited sensitivity as well as specificity. Anti-idiotypic antibodies have been used in the treatment of B-cell lymphomas, but the approach has not proved successful, since surface Ig expression is not functionally related to the malignant transforming property. Some cell-surface antigens expressed by B-cell lymphomas, such as CD19, CD20, CD22, and CD72, are attractive targets for antibody-mediated radioimmunotherapy, and 14 of 28 patients demonstrated a complete remission of a duration exceeding 16 months [60]. Adoptive immunity is the acquisition of immunity in a naive subject as a result of the administration of immunologically activated lymphoid cells. Tumor-reactive lymphoid cells have to be isolated from cancer patients for T-cell therapy to be feasible. This problem was addressed by the discovery of IL-2, a T-cell growth factor. However, early attempts at growing lymphoid cells in IL-2 resulted in the generation of lymphokine-activated killer (LAK) cells [61]. LAK cells have had therapeutic benefit in some patients, but such effector cells frequently lack several of the most attractive qualities of T cells. Use of T cells for tumor treatment is technically more complicated than the use of LAK cells. Potential tumor-reactive T cells isolated from solid tumors of cancer patients, termed tumor-infiltrating lymphocytes (TIL), are specific in their reactivity to tumor cells, and 19 of 56 melanoma patients experienced objected tumor response [62]. Antigen recognition by T cells involves receptor occupancy by antigens and leads to the second step of activation, transmembrane signaling, which is mediated by a protein complex, CD3. Several CD3 proteins have an intracellular polypeptide that is phosphorylated when a T-cell receptor binds with the antigen. Although the reactivity of anti-CD3 to T cells is polyclonal, the antitumor effect mediated by the activated cells is immunologically specific [63]. The method of anti-CD3 IL-2 activation has greatly facilitated the procedure of clinical T-cell immunotherapy because of increased understanding of T-cell responses to human tumors.

Cancer Pathology

A tumor is an abnormal mass of tissue, the growth of which exceeds and is uncoordinated with that of the normal tissues, and persists in the same excessive manner after cessation of the stimuli that evoked the change. Tumors are apparently purposeless; they prey on the host and are virtually autonomous. Solid tumors form a mass that is composed of two compartments: the parenchyma (tumor cells) and the stroma. In epithelial tumors, a basal lamina separates clumps of tumor cells from stroma, which is interposed between malignant cells and normal host tissues, and is essential for tumor growth. Stroma is a product of the host that is induced by tumors. Most tumors require stroma if they are to grow beyond a minimal size of 1–2 mm [64]. Stroma provides a lifeline that is necessary for tumor growth. The bulk of tumor stroma is comprised of interstitial connective tissue. The major components of tumor stroma include: structural proteins; interstitial fluid; proteoglycans and glycosaminoglycans; new blood vessels (produced via angiogenesis); interstitial collagens (type I, III and V); fibron; fibronectin; fibroblasts residing in normal connective tissue; and inflammatory cells derived from the blood.

Tumors differ markedly from each other in stromal content, and these differences are primarily quantitative at times and largely qualitative in other cases. The events of tumor stoma generation closely resemble those of wound healing. The initial event is a local increase in vascular permeability, followed by extravascular clotting, fibrin deposition, fibrin proteolysis, and infiltration by inflammatory and connective tissue cells, leading to the development of granulation tissue and finally of dense fibrous connective tissue (desmoplasia in tumors and scar in healed wounds) [65]. Tumor stroma is generally a disorganized and poorly supportive parody of normal connective tissue. Tumor blood vessels are often poorly differentiated, unevenly spaced; they are unequal to the task of supporting the growth and even the life of rapidly metabolizing tumor cells [66]. The result is irregular blood flow, shifting zones of anoxia, low pH, and coagulative necrosis [67]. The presence of necrosis may be helpful in recognizing malignant tumors and distinguishing them from their benign counterparts. Details of the type and origin of the tumor, its differentiation, level of invasion, the extent of lymph architecture, the presence or absence of hormone receptors, the activity of specific enzymes, ploidy, and frequency of mitosis and cells in S phase may all be relevant in virtually every pathological assessment of tumor. Tumors, not infrequently, generate an extensive inflammatory response, and atypical hyperplasia can be very difficult to distinguish from in situ carcinoma [68].

Tumors of epithelial cell origin are termed adenomas or papillomas when benign and carcinomas when malignant. Carcinomas account for approximately 80% of all malignant tumors. Further classification is often on the basis of the type of epithelium present, e.g., glandular (adenocarcinoma), squamous (squamous cell carcinoma) or transitional (transitional cell carcinoma). Malignant tumors of mesenchymal origin are designated sarcomas, e.g., liposarcoma, fibrosarcoma, leiomyosarcoma. A few tumors contain neoplastic cells of more than a single type. Adenoacanthoma contains both squamous cell carcinoma and adenocarcinoma elements. A few tumors, such as Wilms' tumor, contain neoplastic cells from more than one germ layer. Even within a single organ and within a single type of epithelium, several different types of tumors may arise, each with its own special characteristics, prognosis and response to therapy. The neoplastic cells comprising the benign tumor are usually well-differentiated, closely resembling the corresponding cells of normal tissue. Benign tumors tend to expand uniformly in all directions, and they cause compression atrophy of surrounding normal tissues that results in the formation of a thin rim of fibrous connective tissue. This enveloping connective-tissue rim may serve as a capsule that renders benign tumors discrete, readily palpable, and easily movable. Malignant tumors are characterized primarily by the increased numbers and abnormality of their cells, and commonly exhibit abnormal orientation of both tumor cells and stroma. Cytological features of malignancy include: altered polarity; tumor cell enlargement; increased ratio of nuclear to cytoplasmic area; pleomorphism of tumor cells and their nuclei; clumping of nuclear chromatin and distribution of chromatin along the nuclear membrane; enlarged nucleoli; atypical or bizarre mitoses; and tumor giant cells with one or more nuclei. Malignant tumors invariably lack a capsule and often invade lymphatics and veins. Malignant tumor cells are transported by lymph or blood flow to distant sites [69].

Tumor grading (G) has traditionally referred to a pathologist's judgment as to a tumor's degree of differentiation and growth rate, often on a scale of I to III or IV, where III or IV represents the least-differentiated, fastest-dividing tumors. High-grade tumors are more anaplastic and tend to metastasize sooner. Formal grading systems are less popular today than the early days because of their shortcomings. A different scale is required for each type of tumor, and scoring is not always reproducible. Tumors are typically heterogeneous, and the correlation between histological appearance and biological behavior is seldom perfect. Therefore, many pathologists have abandoned attempts to grade cancers, and have adopted a descriptive terminology [70, 71]. In addition to making an exact histological diagnosis of cancer, it is essential that the clinical stage be determined prior to making a decision regarding therapy. The recognized importance of staging has led to a variety of international and national attempts to standardize the staging.

To date, no single system has been universally accepted. Stage I by the American Joint Committee on Cancer (AJCC) usually indicates a tumor confined to its primary site of origin; stage II indicates metastases to the regional lymph nodes; and stage III, often, and stage IV, always, indicate distant metastatic spread. The TNM system by the Unio Internationale Contra Cankrum (UICC) relies on a statement of tumor extent, in terms of the primary tumor (T), presence or absence of node metastases (N), and the presence or absence of distant metastases (M). Size criteria vary for different tumors, but decreasing prognosis is indicated by increasing numbers after the T for lesions of increasing size. The presence or absence of regional spread is usually indicated by variations in the secondary category under N for nodes. Distant metastasis is indicated by adding subscript 1 following M for metastases. The AJCC recognizes several types of cancer staging schemes. The clinical diagnostic staging represents the extent of the cancer prior to the first definitive treatment. Postsurgical resection-pathological staging provides additional information after operation and is useful in planning adjuvant therapy. Other staging types include surgical-evaluative staging based on surgical exploration, retreatment staging (usually after a cancer-free interval), and autopsy staging when the cancer is first diagnosed at autopsy. One of the great deficiencies of the present staging methods is their inability to indicate subclinical, microscopic, metastatic lesions.

It is necessary to recognize that tumors are not static entities. Progression is a tumor's acquisition of increasingly malignant properties over time, e.g., fast growth rate, anaplasia, loss of hormonal responsiveness, chromosomal aberration, drug resistance and metastatic potential [72]. Progression is thought to depend on clonal evolution. Cancer is associated with genetic and epigenetic plasticity and probably increased mutation rate [73]. Mutant clones have the greatest capacity for proliferation, metastasis and drug resistance. Many tumors develop over time from individual clones of normal stem cell precursors in a series of distinct steps that include dysplasia, carcinoma in situ and frank malignancy. Tumors vary considerably in their capacity for further progression. Tumors of bone marrow and lymphoid origin are most likely to undergo further morphological change. Chronic myelogenous leukemia commonly progresses to blast crisis, and chronic lymphocytic leukemia may proceed to a large-cell phase (Richter's syndrome). Solid tumors are less apt to change morphologically.

References

1. Lewin N (1990) Genes IV, 4th edn. Oxford University Press, Oxford
2. Atchison ML (1988) Enhancers: mechanisms of action and cell specificity. Annu Rev Cell Biol 4:127–137
3. Laskey RA, Earnshaw WC (1980) Nucleosome assembly. Nature 286:763–768
4. Wang JC (1985) DNA topoisomerases. Annu Rev Biochem 54:665–671
5. Smith HO (1979) Nucleotide sequence specificity of restriction endonucleases. Science 205:455–457
6. Cochran BH, Reffel AC, Stiles CD (1983) Molecular cloning of gene sequences regulated by platelet-derived growth factor. Cell 33:939–943
7. Maniatis T, Hardison RC, Lacy E, Lauer J, O'Connell C, Quon D, Sim GK, Efstratiadis A (1978) The isolation of structural genes from libraries of eukaryotic DNA. Cell 15:687–692
8. Southern EM (1975) Detection of specific sequences among DNA fragments separated by gel electrophoresis. J Mol Biol 98:503–508
9. White R, Woodward S, Leppert M, O'Connell P, Hoff M, Herbst J, Laloud JM, Dean M, van de Woude G (1985) A closely linked genetic marker for cystic fibrosis. Nature 318:382–385
10. Knudson AG (1985) Hereditary cancer, oncogenes, and antioncogenes. Cancer Res 45:1437–1442
11. Takahashi T, Nau MM, Chiba I, Birrer MJ, Rosenberg RK, Vinocour M, Levitt M, Pass H, Gazdar A, Minna JD (1989) p53: a frequent target for genetic abnormalities in lung cancer. Science 146:491–493
12. Saiki RK, Gelfand DH, Stoffel S, Scharf SJ, Higuchi R, Horn T, Mullis KB, Erlich HA (1988) Primer-directed enzymatic amplification of DNA with a thermostable DNA polymerase. Science 239:487–489
13. Maniatis T, Reed R (1987) The role of small nuclear ribonucleoprotein particles in pre-mRNA splicing. Nature 325:673–679
14. Efstradiatis A, Kafatos FC, Maniatist (1977) The primary structure of rabbit -globin mRNA as determined from cloned cDNA. Cell 10:571–575
15. Towbin H, Staehelin T, Gordon J (1979) Electrophoretic transfer of proteins from polyacrylamide gels to nitrocellulose sheets: procedure and some applications. Proc Natl Acad Sci U S A 76:4350–4354
16. Derynck R, Remaut E, Saman E, Stanssens P, DeClercq E, Content J, Fiers W (1980) Expression of human fibroblast interferon gene in Escherichia coli. Nature 287:193–195
17. Warburg O (1956) On respiratory impairment in cancer cells. Science 124:269–272
18. Weinhouse S (1955) Oxidative metabolism of neoplastic tissues. Adv Cancer Res 3:269–273
19. Shapot VS (1972) Some biochemical aspects of the relationship between the tumor and the host. Adv Cancer Res 15:253–258
20. Greenstein JP (1956) Some biochemical characteristics of morphologically separable cancers. Cancer Res 16:641–645
21. Potter VR (1982) Biochemistry of cancer. In: Holland JF, Emil Frei III (eds) Cancer medicine, 2nd edn. Lea & Febiger, Philadelphia, pp 133–143
22. Walker PR, Potter VR (1972) Isozyme studies on adult, regenerating precancerous and developing liver in relation to findings in hepatomas. Adv Enzyme Regul 10:339–343
23. Tomaka T, Inamura K, Ann T, Taniuchi K (1972) Multimolecular forms of pyruvate kinase and phosphofructokinase in normal and cancer tissue. Gann Monogr 13:219–224
24. Bollum FJ, Chang LMS (1986) Terminal transferase in normal and leukemic cells. Adv Cancer Res 47:37–41
25. Uriel J (1975) Fetal characteristics of cancer. In: Becker FF (ed) Cancer: a comprehensive treatise, vol. 3. Plenum, New York, pp 21–30
26. Helfta SA, Hefta LJF, Lee TD, Paxton RJ, Shiveley JE (1988) Carcinoembryonic antigen is anchored to membranes by covalent attachment to a glycosylphosphatidylinositol moiety: identification of the ethanolamine linkage site. Proc Natl Acad Sci U S A 85:4648–4652
27. Benchimol S, Fuks A, Jothy S, Beauchemin N, Shirota K, Stamners CP (1989) Carcinoembryonic antigen; a human tumor marker, functions as an intercellular adhesion molecule. Cell 57:327–330
28. Robertson RP, Baylink DJ, Marini JJ, Adkinson HW (1975) Elevated prostaglandins and suppressed parathyroid hormone associated with certain types of cancer. N Engl J Med 293:1278–1281
29. Heber D, Chlebowski RT, Ishibashi DE, Herrold JN, Block JB (1982) Abnormalities in glucose and protein metabolism in noncachectic lung cancer patients. Cancer Res 43:4815–4820
30. Wang AM, Creasey AA, Ladner MB, Lin LS, Strickler J, van Arsdell JN, Yamamoto R, Mark DF (1985) Molecular cloning of the complementary DNA for human tumor necrosis factor. Science 228:149–152
31. Tabor CW, Tabor H (1984) Polyamines. Ann Rev Biochem 53:749–752

32. Luk GD, Baylin SB (1984) ODC as a biologic marker in familial colonic polyposis. N Engl J Med 311:80–83
33. Dice JF (1987) Molecular determinants of protein half-lives in eukaryotic cells. FASEB J 1:349–354
34. Bourne HR, DeFranco AL (1989) Signal transduction and intracellular messengers. In: Weinberg RA (ed) Oncogenes and molecular origins of cancer. Cold Spring Harbor Laboratory, New York, pp 79–84
35. Berger NA (1985) Poly (ADP-ribose) in the cellular response to DNA damage. Radiat Res 101:4–9
36. Hetts SW (1998) To die or not to die. An overview of apoptosis and its role in disease. JAMA 270:300–307
37. Polyak K, Xia Y, Zweier JL, Kinzler KW, Vogelstein B (1997) A model for p53-induced apoptosis. Nature 389:300–305
38. Jones PA, Buckley JD (1990) The role of DNA methylation in cancer. Adv Cancer Res 54:1–6
39. deBustros A, Nelkin BD, Silverman A, Ehrlich G, Poiesz B, Baylin SB (1988) The short arm of chromosome 11 is a hot spot for hypermethylation in human neoplasia. Proc Natl Acad Sci U S A 85:5693–5696
40. Vines RL, Coleman MS, Hutton JJ (1980) Reappearance of terminal deoxynucleotidyl transferase containing cells in rate bone marrow following corticosteroid administration. Blood 56:501–506
41. Itakomori S (1989) Aberrant glycosylation in tumors and tumor-associated carbohydrate antigens. Adv Cancer Res 52:259–261
42. Paul WE (1989) The immune system: an introduction. In: Paul WE (ed) Fundamental immunology, 2nd edn. Raven, New York, pp 3–18
43. Hodes RJ (1989) T-cell-mediated regulation: help and suppression. In: Paul WE (ed) Fundamental immunology, 2nd edn. Raven, New York, pp 587–596
44. Weiss A (1990) Structure and function of the T cell antigen receptor. J Clin Invest 86:1015–1021
45. Celis E, Tsai V, Crimi C (1993) Induction of anti-tumor cytotoxic T lymphocytes in normal humans using primary cultures & synthetic peptide epitopes. Proc Natl Acad Sci U S A 91:2105–2109
46. Shu S, Chou T, Sakai K (1989) Lymphocytes generated by in vivo priming and in vitro sensitization demonstrate therapeutic efficacy against a murine tumor that lacks apparent immunogenicity. J Immunol 143:746–748
47. Miller AR, McBride WH, Hunt K. Economou JS (1994) Cytokine-mediated gene therapy for cancer. Ann Surg Oncol 1:436–450
48. Wallich R, Bulbuc N, Hammerling GJ, Katzar S, Segal S, Feldman M (1985) Abrogation of metastatic properties of tumor cells by de novo expression of H-2 K antigens following H-2 gene transfection. Nature 3125:301–305
49. Dudley ME, Roopenian DC (1996) Loss of a unique tumor antigen by cytotoxic T lymphocyte immunoselection from a 3-methylcholanthrene-induced mouse sarcoma reveals secondary unique and share antigens. J Exp Med 184:441–447
50. McLaughlin JP, Schlom J, Kantor JA, Griener JW (1996) Improved immunotherapy of a recombinant carcinoembryonic antigen vaccinia vaccine when given in combination with interleukin-2. Cancer Res 56:2361–2367
51. Shu S, Plantz GE, Krauss JC, Chang AE (1997) Tumor immunology. JAMA 278:1972–1981
52. Canaani E, Marcelle C, Fainstein E (1991) bcr-abl RNA in chronic myelogenous leukemia and lymphocytic leukemia. In: Deisseroth A, Arlinghaus RB (eds) Chronic myelogenous leukemia: molecular approaches to research and therapy. Part III. Marcel Dekker Inc, New York, pp 217–240
53. Bocchia M, Korontsuit T, Xy Q (1996) Specific human cellular immunity to bcr-abl oncogene-derived peptides. Blood 87:3587–3592
54. Cheever MA, Disis ML, Bernhard H (1995) Immunity to oncogenic proteins. Immunol Rev 145:33–59
55. Houbiers JGA, Nijman HW, van der Burg SH (1993) In vitro induction of human cytotoxic T lymphocyte responses against peptides of mutated and wild type p53. Eur J Immunol 23:2072–2077
56. Rosenberg SA, Lotze M, Yang J (1989) Experience with the use of high-dose interleukin-2 in the treatment of 652 cancer patients. Ann Surg 210:474–484
57. Vieweg J, Gilboa E (1995) Consideration for the use of cytokine-secreting tumor cell preparation for cancer treatment. Cancer Invest 13:193–201
58. Chen L, Ashe S, Brady WA (1992) Costimulation of antitumor immunity by the B7 counter receptor for the T lymphocyte molecule CD 28 and CTLA-4. Cell 71:1093–1102
59. Murrey J, Rosenbaum MG, Sobol RE (1985) Radioimmuno-imaging in malignant melanoma using In-111 labeled monoclonal antibody. Cancer Res 45:2376–2381
60. Kaminski MS, Zasadny RK, Francis IR (1996) Iodine-131 anti-B1 radioimmunotherapy for B-cell lymphoma. J Clin Oncol 14:1974–1981
61. Grimm EA, Robb RJ, Roth JA (1983) Lymphokine-activated killer cell phenomenon, III: evidence that IL-2 is sufficient for direct activation of peripheral blood into lymphokine-activated killer cells. J Exp Med 158:1356–1361
62. Rosenberg SA, Vannelli JR, Yang JC (1994) Treatment of patients with metastatic melanoma with autologous tumor-infiltrating lymphocytes and interleukin-2. J Natl Cancer Inst 86:1159–1166
63. Chang AE, Aruga A, Cameron MJ (1997) Adoptive immunotherapy with vaccine-primed lymph node cells secondarily activated with anti-CD3 and IL-2. J Clin Oncol 15:796–807
64. Folkman J (1985) Tumor angiogenesis. Adv Cancer Res 43:175–180
65. Senger DR, Connolly DT, van de Water L, Feder J, Dvorak HF (1990) Purification and NH_2-terminal amino acid sequence of guinea pig tumor-secreted vascular permeability factor. Cancer Res 50:1774–1779
66. Vaupel P, Kallinowski F, Okunieff P (1989) Blood flow, oxygen and nutrient supply, and metabolic microenvironment of human tumors. A review. Cancer Res 49:6449–6454
67. Tannock IF, Rotin D (1989) Acid pH in tumors and its potential for therapeutic exploitation. Cancer Res 49:4373–4378
68. Dupont WD, Page DL (1985) Risk factors for breast cancer in women with proliferative breast disease. N Engl J Med 312:146–149
69. Schnitt SJ, Silen W, Sadowsky NL, Connoly JL, Harris JR (1988) Ductal carcinoma in situ (intraductal carcinoma) of the breast. N Engl J Med 318:898–902
70. Gleason DF (1988) Histologic grade, clinical stage, and patient age in prostate cancer. Natl Cancer Inst Monogr 7:15–19
71. Elston CW (1984) The assessment of histological differentiation in breast cancer. Aust N Z J Surg 54:11–17
72. Hill RP (1990) Tumor progression: potential role of unstable genomic changes. Cancer Metastasis Rev 9:137–142
73. Nowell PC (1986) Mechanisms of tumor progression. Cancer Res 46:2203–2208

Imaging Strategies and Perspectives in Oncology

E. E. KIM

Basic Considerations

Imaging plays a significant role in the diagnosis, staging, and follow-up of cancer patients. A large percentage of medical imaging is performed in cancer patients. In many patients, more than one imaging study is performed for a specific clinical indication that could have been addressed with one appropriate study. Oncologists must determine which tests are most accurate and economical for a specific clinical indication. A well-designed imaging strategy is an implicit component of the approach to a cancer patient. The primary applications of imaging procedures in cancer patients are in tumor detection, staging and follow-up. The challenge of oncological imaging is complex and varies with each organ site and, often, tumor type. Once the tumor is detected and a specific histological diagnosis has been established, the definition of the T (tumor) lesion is performed.

Imaging Strategies

Film Screening

Of all the common imaging procedures, the film-screen technique provides by far the greatest resolution, often more than can be used. The limiting problems with film radiography in tumor detection are tissue discrimination and resolution of low-contrast objects. Signal-to-noise problems often limit the ability of radionuclide imagings to resolve tumor masses. This is, in part, a deficiency corrected by the tomographic scanning. Radioimmunoimaging using monoclonal antibodies may allow the identification of many tumors at a smaller size than currently is possible. Signal-to-noise problems, suboptimal labeling, and inability to develop tumor-specific antibodies have been the major challenges.

Computed Tomography

In most body imagings, computed tomography (CT) has been the standard, against which other tumor-imaging systems are measured. Image production for CT depends on the physical characteristics of the structure imaged (density, atomic number and number of electrons per gram) and the energy of the X-ray beam. The advantages of CT are better contrast resolution than plain radiographs, the ability to obtain axial images, the ability to guide lesion biopsy and radiotherapy planning, and good depiction of bone detail. CT is superior to magnetic resonance imaging (MRI) in characterizing the margins, periosteal reaction, and matrix of a bone tumor [1]. Disadvantages of CT are the inability to obtain direct coronal or sagittal images of large body parts, inability to image the entire spine in one visit, insensitivity to bone marrow edema and requirement for intravenous injection of the contrast agent.

Magnetic Resonance Imaging

In MRI, a powerful unidirectional magnetic field is used to orient or polarize some of the body's hydrogen atoms in the direction of the magnetic field. Using a computer, the radio-wave emissions from hydrogen atoms within the body can be used to synthesize a three-dimensional volume image.

Image production for MRI depends on the inherent characteristics of the structure imaged (T_1 and T_2 relaxation times), the proton density of the structure, flow effects, and instrument parameters such as repetition time and echo time. The advantages found in the use of MRI include excellent tissue contrast resolution, direct multiplanar imaging, absence of ionizing radiation, ability to image blood flow, increased sensitivity to edema, and very low incidence of reactions to MRI contrast agents. The disadvantages of using MRI can be relatively high cost, poor cortical bone detail, and inherent contraindications with ferromagnetic foreign bodies or implants [2].

With the most commonly used MR imaging technique, known as spin-echo imaging, the T_1-weighted MR images require relatively short repetition and time (T_R and T_E) settings, but T_2-weighted images require long T_R and T_E sequences. Tumors appear relatively dark on T_1-weighted MR images when compared with surrounding normal tissues, and they appear relatively bright on T_2-weighted images. Anatomical detail is somewhat better on T_1-weighted images, whereas tumors and peritumoral edema, as well as reactive tissues, often stand out in better contrast to surrounding normal tissues on T_2-weighted images.

Nuclear Magnetic Resonance

The history of nuclear magnetic resonance (NMR) began with the discovery of the NMR phenomenon that led to the use of NMR as a spectroscopic technique to determine the chemical composition and physical properties of a material and to probe the metabolism of a tissue [3]. Biochemical information relevant to energy status and metabolism can be used to characterize a tumor and indicate response to treatment and progress. It is now possible to do semi-quantitative spectroscopic analyses of metabolites in tissues with MR.

Positron-Emission Tomography

Positron-emission tomography (PET) is recognized as a powerful tool and its clinical applications are increasing, particularly since the introduction of whole-body scanning. The use of positron-emitting tracers is also likely to increase as gamma cameras are adapted with special collimators or coincidence electronics. Like the spectroscopic analyses, PET scanning provides unique information about the metabolic activities of tumors and reveals metabolic changes that may occur with treatment. The short-lived positron-emitting radiopharmaceuticals are used to tag certain normal metabolites or drugs. The rate and intensity of accumulation of radiolabeled metabolites or drugs are analyzed with serial PET scans to evaluate tumor biology and therapeutic response, or to make predictions.

Tumor Size

Tumor size or volume (the T component of the American Joint Committee staging system) has an obvious major impact on both the treatment decision process and patient outcome. Tumor size alone is only a part of the problem, since similarly sized tumors show significantly different behaviors. However, the detection of a cancer at a smaller size or volume that can be effectively treated generally results in a more favorable outcome.

Threshold tumor size is difficult to define. From an imaging standpoint, the limits of resolution of the various imaging systems can be generally characterized. The limitations of detection variables relate to equipment (spatial and contrast resolution), patient and target organ considerations, and interobserver variations. Tumor growth has been shown to be exponential and proceeds along predictable lines until its volume reaches 3–4 mm^3, receiving its nutrition from the extravascular space by diffusion. Subsequent to this growth volume, the cluster of cancer cells induces its own vascular supply, possibly through the elaboration of tumor angiogenesis factor [4]. From this time on, the tumor is able to stimulate new capillaries, acquire nutrients by perfusion, and is capable of metastasizing.

With current imaging techniques, tumor nodules from 5 mm to 1 cm represent the smallest size of detection, and such lesions are biologically advanced. The improved and more sophisticated imaging techniques and procedures have advanced cancer staging through more accurate and specific characterization. The newer techniques also direct more aggressive treatment to both the primary tumor and, occasionally, its metastatic lesions.

Decision Theory Process

The value of cancer screening has been questioned, and random radiographic screening procedures have neither resulted in an improved survival for the cancer patient, nor been justified from the standpoint of cost effectiveness. The exception is the notable yield from mammographic screening. With lung cancers, as well as with most other primary tumor locations, the principal goal of imaging efforts should be tumor definition and staging, not random screening. The decision therapy process has largely been an intuitive one in clinical practice. A clear understanding of the decision theory process must accompany a knowledge of both the disease and the imaging systems being applied to the clinical problem.

Most oncologists are familiar with the common terms of sensitivity, specificity, and positive and negative predictive tests. The more widespread use of computers in medical environments will require oncologists to become more familiar with these terms. The increasingly rigid demands of healthcare reimbursement policies will dictate term use in the prioritization of healthcare services. The sensitivity of a test is a function of the true-positive rate compared with the sum of the true positives and false negatives. The specificity is the relationship of the true-negative yield compared with the sum of true-negative plus false-positive rates. The predictive value is a more important variable of its potential usefulness. The positive predictive value is determined by the true-positive yield compared with the sum of the true- and false-positive rates.

Perspectives

Technological advances have already led to fundamental improvements used to visualize tumors and to assess their metabolic and physical effects on the body. They have not only improved cancer care and lessened patient suffering, but they also may have reduced overall medical expenditures by shortening and simplifying diagnostic procedures, lessening hospitalization requirements and helping to tailor therapeutic approaches more appropriately to individual patient needs [5]. Even with these technological advances, it is necessary to emphasize that imaging studies cannot make a histological diagnosis or pathological grading, and that relevant clinical information is essential for a proper interpretation or consultation. Furthermore, modern ultrasonography, CT and MRI have not replaced most of the standard radiological techniques, but they serve to complement the standard methods. Much research continues on the appropriate uses of diagnostic imaging in cancer management since the current applications of imaging techniques in clinical oncology are still less than optimal. One area of continuing concern is the type and appropriate periodicity of imaging tests for following cancer patients after treatment. A number of new developments in diagnostic imaging have potential impact for the detection, diagnosis, staging and follow-up of cancer patients. Some of the new diagnostic imaging developments include rapid CT and MR imagings, Doppler and endoluminal ultrasound techniques, new contrast and radiopharmaceutical agents, improved PET, single photon-emission tomography (SPECT), and MR spectroscopy or spectroscopic imaging. A plethora of imaging techniques is available, but without sufficient data to use them in the most efficient manner. Accelerating medical costs will force radiologists, nuclear physicians and oncologists to take the difficult steps that are needed to evaluate our existing imaging methods systematically for their contributions to cancer management, and to determine their appropriate places or develop more concerted roles for them.

References

1. Magid D (1993) Two-dimensional and three-dimensional computed tomographic imaging in musculoskeletal tumors. Radiol Clin North Am 31:425–447
2. Shellock FG, Morisoli S, Lanal E (1993) MR procedures and biomedical implants, material and devices: 1993 update. Radiology 189:587–599
3. Negendank WG, Brown TR, Evelhock JL (1992) Proceedings of a National Cancer Institute Workshop: MR spectroscopy and tumor cell biology. Radiology 185:875–883
4. Folkman J, Merler E, Abernathy C, Williams G (1971) Isolation of a tumor factor responsible for angiogenesis. J Exp Med 133:275–288
5. Steckel R, Kagan AR (1990) Pitfalls in the diagnosis of metastatic disease or local tumor extension with modern imaging techniques. Invest Radiol 25:818–824

Magnetic Resonance Imaging: Physical Principles to Advanced Applications

E. F. Jackson

Basic Considerations

The soft tissue contrast provided by magnetic resonance imaging (MRI) frequently makes it the modality of choice in oncological imaging. The excellent sensitivity of MRI for detecting lesions is due to the dependence of the image contrast and signal-to-noise ratio (SNR) on a wide range of both intrinsic and extrinsic parameters. Intrinsic parameters, which depend on the individual tissue characteristics, include the spin-lattice relaxation time (T_1), spin-spin relaxation time (T_2), proton density, and the velocity and local chemical environment of the nuclei of interest. Extrinsic parameters that affect image contrast and SNR are those chosen by the person performing the examination. A partial list of such extrinsic parameters includes the particular type of image acquisition sequence, the echo time (TE), repetition time (TR), field-of-view, slice thickness, acquisition bandwidth, various saturation and inversion pulses, and resolution. By appropriate manipulation of the extrinsic parameters, an incredibly wide range of image contrasts can be obtained and can be tailored to provide excellent visualization of anatomy, pathology, and, in some cases, function. In this chapter, the physical principles of MRI will be briefly introduced, and the current state-of-the-art imaging hardware and acquisition techniques will be reviewed. By necessity, the review of the basics of MR physics will be somewhat brief, and for more detailed discussions the reader is referred to additional introductory references [1–6].

Physical Principles of Magnetic Resonance Imaging

Basic Concepts

There are three major requirements for obtaining images using MRI. The first is the presence of a nucleus with a non-zero nuclear magnetic moment. Such nuclei have an odd number of protons and/or neutrons. Some of the more commonly utilized nuclei in MRI and magnetic resonance spectroscopy are given in Table 3.1. Virtually all clinical imaging studies are based on proton MRI, due to the natural abundance of protons in human tissue.

Nuclei that have non-zero magnetic moments are like very weak bar magnets (Fig. 3.1). However, in the absence of an applied magnetic field, the nuclear magnetic moments point in random directions, so that there is no measurable net magnetization (Fig. 3.1). To generate net magnetization, the nuclear magnetic moments must be polarized. Therefore, given nuclei with non-zero magnetic moments, the second thing required to generate an MR image is a relatively large and highly homogeneous magnetic field, B_0. In clinical imaging studies, the most common magnetic field strengths are in the range of 0.15 Tesla (T) to 2.0 T. However, there are currently a limited number of whole-body scanners with magnetic field strengths in the 3.0–4.7 T range. The magnets are typically resistive or permanent for low field strengths, and are typically superconducting for field strengths of 0.5 T or higher.

The proton is a spin-1/2 nucleus. Therefore, when placed in a magnetic field there are only two allowed states: aligned with the external magnetic field (parallel) or opposed to the magnetic field (antiparallel). If a patient is placed in such a

Table 3.1. Properties of some common nuclei with potential use in magnetic resonance studies

Nucleus	Spin	Gyromagnetic ratio (MHz/T)	Natural isotopic abundance (%)	Sensitivity relative to ^{1}H (%)[a]
^{1}H	1/2	42.57	99.98	100
^{13}C	1/2	10.71	1.11	1.6
^{19}F	1/2	40.06	100	83.4
^{23}Na	3/2	11.26	100	9.3
^{31}P	1/2	17.24	100	6.6

[a] At constant field for equal number of nuclei

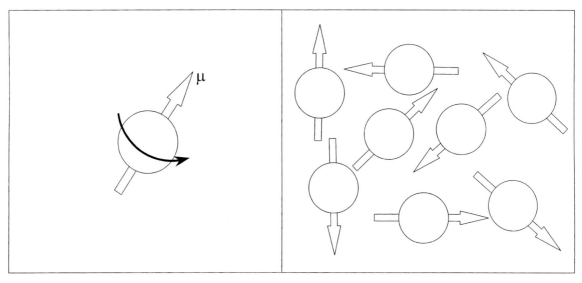

Fig. 3.1. A nucleus with non-zero spin has an associated magnetic moment, μ (*open arrow*), and behaves similar to a very small bar magnet (*left*). A collection of spins in the absence of an applied magnetic field has no net magnetization because the magnetic moments are oriented randomly (*right*)

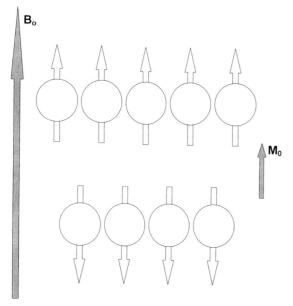

Fig. 3.2. In an applied magnetic field, B_0, there are only two allowed directions of the spin-1/2 magnetic moments: aligned parallel to B_0 or antiparallel to B_0. Since more magnetic moments are aligned parallel to B_0 than antiparallel, there is a net magnetization, M_0, that is the vector sum of all the individual magnetic moments

field, more of the magnetic moments tend to align parallel with the applied magnetic field than antiparallel (Fig. 3.2). The result is a non-zero net magnetization, i.e., an equilibrium magnetization, M_0. However, the population of the nuclei in each of the two states is governed by a Boltzmann distribution [2], and for a sample at room temperature with a 1.5 T magnet, only about ten of a million protons are preferentially aligned with the external field. Therefore, the inherent sensitivity of MRI is quite low; it is fortunate that the human body is predominantly water and fat so that a sufficient number of protons are available to form the image within a reasonable acquisition time.

At this point, there is a net magnetization that is aligned parallel to the applied magnetic field. However, to detect the magnetization requires that it be perpendicular to the magnetic field rather than parallel to it. To accomplish this, an additional magnetic field is applied to the nuclei. This time the applied field, B_1, is time-varying and applied at a frequency proportional to the energy separation of the two allowed states,

$$v_0 = \gamma B_0 \qquad 3.1$$

where γ is the gyromagnetic ratio, a constant for a given nucleus, e.g., 42.57 MHz/T for protons, and B_0 is the applied static magnetic field. This frequency is known as the Larmor frequency, and is a key concept in MRI.

If the radiofrequency (RF) field, B_1, is applied at the Larmor frequency, and perpendicular to the static field, then the net magnetization can be made to rotate by an arbitrary angle with respect to the applied static field. For a rectangular RF pulse, the angle of rotation, commonly called the "flip angle", is given by

$$\theta = \gamma B_1 t_p \qquad 3.2$$

where B_1 is the amplitude of the pulse and t_p is the duration of the pulse. If the values of B_1 and

t_p are chosen such that θ is 90°, the pulse is commonly called a 90° pulse and the net magnetization is perpendicular to the applied static field (in the transverse plane) immediately following the pulse.

The combination of the RF pulse and the precession of spins makes visualizing the result of a 90° pulse on the spins somewhat difficult. However, if one considers the motion of the spins from a frame of reference that is rotating at the precession rate, i.e., the Larmor frequency, then the complication of the precessional motion is removed and the only effect is that due to the applied RF pulse (Fig. 3.3). This choice of reference frame is analogous to choosing to view a child riding on a merry-go-round while standing on the merry-go-round rather than standing on the ground nearby. This frame is known as the rotating frame of reference.

After the pulse is terminated, the net magnetization precesses about the applied static field at the Larmor frequency. The time-varying magnetic field resulting from the precession of the magnetization induces a time-varying voltage, i.e., the free induction decay or FID (Fig. 3.4), in an appropriately tuned and oriented radiofrequency coil, and this is the manner in which the MR signal is measured. In some cases, the RF coil used to produce the B_1 pulse and the RF coil used to detect the MR signal are the same. This is typically true for head and whole-body coils. In other cases, a large RF coil is used to transmit the B_1 pulses and a smaller RF coil is used to detect the signal. In general, to optimize the SNR of the resulting images, the size of the receive coil should be matched as closely as possible to the anatomy of interest. For this reason, a wide variety of RF receive coils, including phased arrays of coils, are available. For further details of RF coil design and integration of the coils in the overall MR scanner hardware, the reader is referred to the reference [7].

Ultimately, the net magnetization returns to the equilibrium condition parallel to the applied static field and, in the process, energy is transferred to the surroundings or, in the solid state physics terminology, to the lattice. The rate at which this occurs is determined by the intrinsic parameter T_1, which is the spin-lattice relaxation time. Fortunately, different tissue types exhibit different T_1 times, and this becomes an important parameter in determining image contrast (Fig. 3.5). At the same time that the net magnetization is recovering, there is a dephasing of the net transverse magnetization due to spin-spin interactions. The rate at which the net transverse magnetization

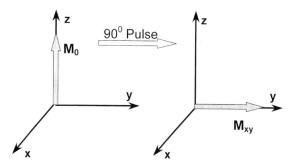

Fig. 3.3. Evolution of the net magnetization, M_0, from the longitudinal (z) direction to the transverse (xy) plane under the influence of a 90° pulse along the x-direction in the rotating frame of reference

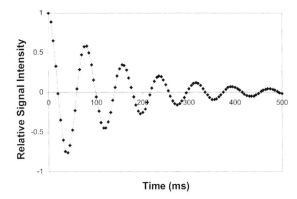

Fig. 3.4. Following the 90° pulse, the net magnetization precesses and the time-varying magnetic field generates a time-varying voltage signal, known as the free induction decay (*FID*), in a receiver coil

Table 3.2. Representative relaxation times [10]

Tissue	T_1 at 0.5 T (ms)	T_1 at 1.5 T (ms)	T_2 (ms)
Gray matter	656	920	101
White matter	539	790	92
Cerebrospinal fluid	>2000	>4000	>4000
Skeletal muscle	600	870	47
Fat	215	260	84
Liver	323	490	47

dephases is determined by the intrinsic parameter T_2, which is the spin-spin relaxation time. As with the T_1 relaxation times, T_2 relaxation times vary with tissue type and can have an important effect on image contrast (Fig. 3.5). Some representative T_1 and T_2 relaxation times are given in Table 3.2. In general, T_1 relaxation times are always greater than T_2 relaxation times, and T_1 and T_2 relaxation times are both long in pure fluids, e.g., the orbits and CSF.

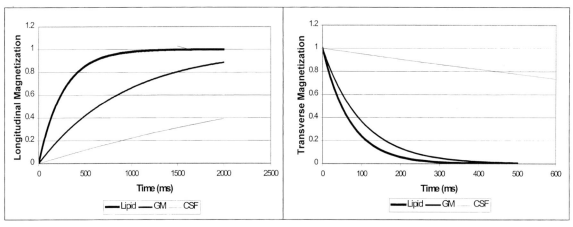

Fig. 3.5. A 90° pulse converts the longitudinal magnetization, M_0, into the measurable transverse magnetization, M_{xy}. Following the pulse, the longitudinal magnetization recovers at a rate determined by the spin-lattice, or T_1, relaxation time (*left*). Independent of the spin-lattice relaxation, the transverse magnetization dephases at a rate determined by the spin-spin, or T_2 relaxation time (*right*). Like the T_1 relaxation times, the T_2 relaxation times vary from tissue to tissue

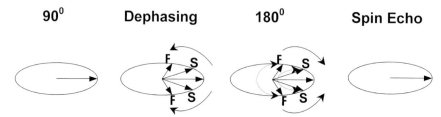

Fig. 3.6. Spin-echo formation. Following the 90° pulse, the transverse magnetization dephases due to both spin–spin interactions and local magnetic field inhomogeneities, with some spins precessing faster (*F*) than others (*S*). Although spin-spin dephasing is irreversible, the dephasing due to the inhomogeneities can be reversed by applying a 180° pulse that "flips" the spins in the transverse plane. Then the faster precessing spins rephase with the slower precessing spins at the echo time, TE, and the effects of the magnetic field inhomogeneities are compensated for

Spin-spin dephasing at a rate determined by T_2 occurs from the moment the net magnetization is flipped into the transverse plane. This dephasing is irreversible, but gives rise to useful image contrast. Unfortunately, there are other contributions to spin dephasing that, uncorrected, yield an overall loss of SNR. With the exception of applications to perfusion imaging and other susceptibility mapping techniques (discussed below), such dephasing phenomena are detrimental to MR imaging. One of the most common sources of dephasing is local magnetic field inhomogeneities due to imperfections in the applied static field homogeneity or, more commonly, due to magnetic susceptibility changes in the human body. These susceptibility changes are most evident at tissue/air or tissue/bone interfaces and give rise to apparent inhomogeneities in the applied field. Such inhomogeneities cause a decrease in the apparent T_2, or T_2^*; the larger the inhomogeneity, the smaller the value of T_2^* and the faster the rate of dephasing, i.e.,

$$\frac{1}{T_2^*} = \frac{1}{T_2} + k\Delta B_0, \qquad 3.3$$

where k is a constant. Fortunately, many of the effects of spin dephasing due to magnetic field inhomogeneities can be reversed using spin echoes. The concept of spin echoes and how they compensate for local field inhomogeneities is illustrated in Fig. 3.6.

Spatial Localization

Thus far, the application of a static field, B_0, and a radiofrequency field, B_1, has resulted in the formation of a net magnetization that can be detected. However, there is as yet no spatial localization of the detected signal. To encode position typically requires the application of three additional spatially varying, or gradient, magnetic fields, each one orthogonal to the other two. For each of the three magnetic gradient fields, the component of the magnetic field parallel to the

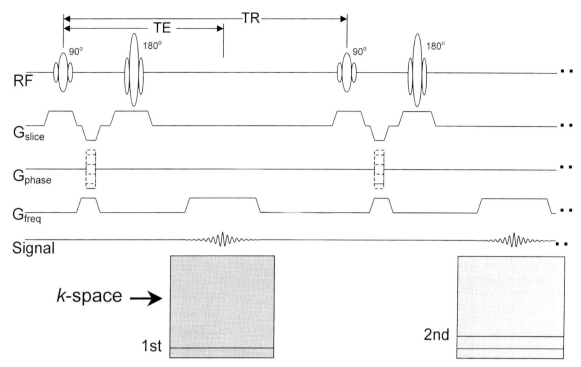

Fig. 3.7. A generic spin-echo pulse sequence timing diagram. *RF* the applied field (B_1) radiofrequency pulses; G_{slice} slice-selection gradient; G_{phase} phase-encoding gradient; G_{freq} frequency-encoding gradient; *Signal* detected spin echo; *TE* echo time; and *TR* repetition time. Two repetitions of the sequence are shown, with each repetition filling in one line of the necessary 128–512 lines of k-space

static field increases linearly with position, i.e., in the x-, y-, or z-direction. Figure 3.7 shows a generic representation of the RF and other fields required to generate a two-dimensional spin-echo (SE) image. Such a diagram is often referred to as a pulse sequence or timing diagram, and generally shows the RF pulses (B_1) and the pulses on the three gradient fields required for spatial localization.

Spatial localization occurs in three steps. For two-dimensional imaging sequences, the MR signal is first localized to a single slice in the patient using a gradient field pulse that is applied simultaneously with a band-limited RF pulse. The thickness of the slice selected by the gradient-RF pulse combination is given by

$$\Delta z = \Delta v_{RF}/\gamma G_{slice} \qquad 3.4$$

where Δv_{RF} is the bandwidth of the RF pulse, and G_{slice} is the amplitude of the slice-selecting gradient field.

The use of the slice-selecting gradient-RF pulse combination localizes the detected MR signal to a slice of thickness Δz. However, assuming there is perfect magnetic field homogeneity within the slice, all of the nuclei resonate at a single frequency, i.e., there is no localization within the slice. To encode position in the remaining two dimensions, two additional gradient pulses are used. The first is known as the frequency-encoding gradient, and is applied at the same time as the MR signal is detected (Fig. 3.7). Under the influence of this additional gradient, assumed for the moment to be applied along the x-direction, the Larmor frequency is modified such that

$$v_{freq} = \gamma(B_0 + xG_{freq}) \qquad 3.5$$

where x is the position along the x-direction, G_{freq} is the amplitude of the frequency-encoding gradient field, and v_{freq} is the Larmor frequency modified by the addition of the gradient field. Equation 3.5 shows there is a linear, one-to-one correspondence between the frequency of precession of the nuclear spins and the position of the spins along the x-direction. Therefore, the action of the frequency-encoding gradient field is to encode position in terms of frequency, and if we can measure the precessional frequencies of the nuclear spins, we can determine their position. Taking the Fourier transform of the detected signal accomplishes this task (Fig. 3.8).

At this point, the signal received from the nuclear spins has been localized to a slice and the location within that slice has been encoded in one

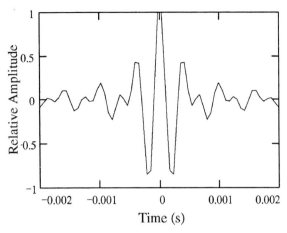 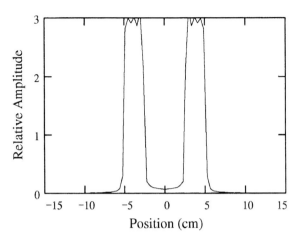

Fig. 3.8. A simulated phantom consisting of four 2.5-cm-diameter tubes centered at (x, y)=(3.75, 3.75), (3.75, −3.75), (−3.75, 3.75), and (−3.75, −3.75) cm. This figure shows the time-domain MR signal that is obtained from the phantom under the influence of only the slice-selection and frequency-encoding gradients (*left*), and the frequency (and therefore position) profiles obtained following the Fourier transformation of the time-domain signal (*right*)

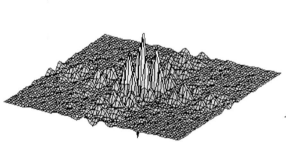 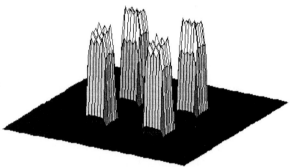

Fig. 3.9. A simulated phantom consisting of four 2.5-cm-diameter tubes centered at (x, y)=(3.75, 3.75), (3.75, −3.75), (−3.75, 3.75), and (−3.75, −3.75) cm. This figure shows the time-domain magnetic resonance (MR) signal that is obtained from the phantom under the influence of the slice-selection, frequency-encoding, and phase-encoding gradients (*left*), and the frequency and phase (and therefore position) profiles obtained following the two-dimensional Fourier transformation of the time-domain signal (*right*)

of the two remaining directions. The location of nuclear spins along the second direction is encoded using a phase-encoding gradient (Fig. 3.7). The phase-encoding gradient is typically applied 128–256 times, once per TR in conventional single-echo spin-echo imaging; at each repetition, the amplitude of the phase-encoding gradient pulse is changed by a fixed amount. The result is that each frequency-encoded echo that is acquired has slightly different phase characteristics than the previous echo. Therefore, there is a one-to-one correspondence of phase to position in a fashion similar to the one-to-one correspondence of frequency to position in the frequency-encoding direction. Taking a second Fourier transform of the detected signal in the phase-encoding direction allows for the complete reconstruction of the image of the anatomy within the slice of thickness Δz (Fig. 3.9).

It should be noted that the gradient magnetic field coil performance has been, and continues to be, the limiting factor in how fast MR images can be obtained. When the gradient coils are activated, the changing magnetic field induces currents, known as eddy currents, in nearby conductors. These induced eddy currents give rise to magnetic fields that oppose the applied gradient fields and generally limit the rate at which the gradient fields can be switched. This, in turn, limits the rate at which images can be acquired. In the last decade, the gradient coil designs and the associated current amplifiers have been optimized for rapid switching, and have allowed commercial scanners with specialized fast receivers and fast gradient subsystems to acquire images in as short a time as 50–100 ms. Such systems are typically characterized by the maximum gradient strength, in millitesla per meter (mT/m), and the slew rate,

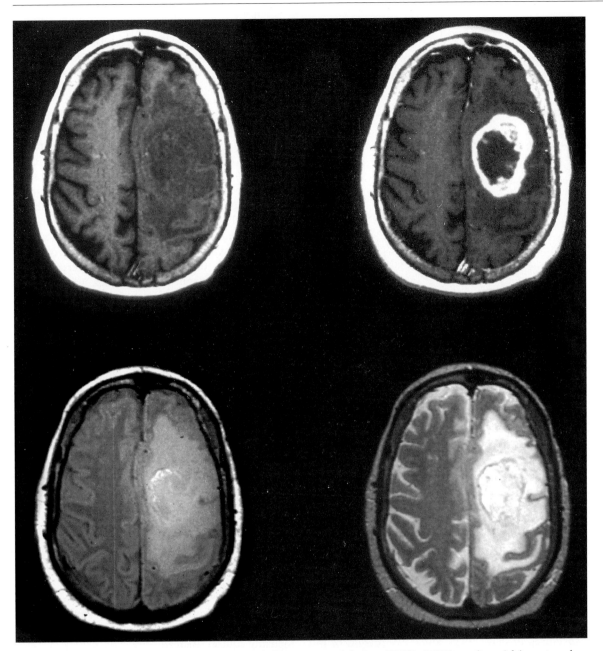

Fig. 3.10. Spin-echo images from a patient with a glioblastoma multiforme: T1-weighted (T1W), echo time (TE)/repetition time (TR)=12/500 ms (*top left*), T1W post-contrast agent infusion, TE/TR=12/500 ms (*top right*), proton density-weighted, TE/TR=30/3000 ms (*bottom left*), and T$_2$-weighted, TE/TR=100/3000 ms (*bottom right*)

in T/m/s. While systems in the early 1990s had slew rates of approximately 10 T/m/s, many systems are currently commercially available with slew rates of 120 T/m/s and above. Such systems are required for ultrafast MRI studies.

Basic Image-Contrast Mechanisms

The advantage of MRI over other modalities used for imaging soft tissue is the wide range of image contrasts that can be obtained by modifying the basic pulse sequence timings or by the use of additional RF pulses. Historically, the three basic types of image contrasts obtained using MRI were proton density-weighted (PDW), T$_1$-weighted (T$_1$W), and T$_2$-weighted (T$_2$W) images. In general, if TE is short such that T$_2$ decay is not significant, and TR is long to allow nearly complete recovery of the longitudinal magnetization, then T$_1$ and T$_2$ processes are not significant and the im-

Table 3.3. Appearance of various substances relative to brain cortex on T1-weighted (T1W), T2-weighted (T2W), and proton density-weighted (PDW) spin-echo images

Substance	T1W	T2W	PDW
Fat and yellow marrow	+++	+	++
Proteinaceous material	++ (Variable)	Variable	Variable
Intracellular methemoglobin	+++	–	–
Extracellular methemoglobin	+++	++	++
Deoxyhemoglobin	–	–	–
Hemosiderin	–	–	–
Melanin	++	–	Isointense
Calcium (some states)	+/–	–	–
Paramagnetic contrast agent	+++	Minimal effect	Minimal effect
Cyst	–	+++	++
Edema	–	+++	++
Vitreous humor	–	++	Isointense
Cerebrospinal fluid	–	+++	Isointense
Multiple sclerosis plaques	–	++	++
Tumors (most)	–	+ (Complex)	+ (Complex)
Abscess	–	+ (Complex)	+ (Complex)
Infarct	–	++	++
Iron (e.g., in globus pallidus)	–	–	–
Air	No signal	No signal	No signal
Cortical bone	No signal	No signal	No signal

age will be PDW. If, however, TE is short such that T_2 decay is minimal and TR is short to enhance differences in T_1 relaxation times (Fig. 3.5), the dominant contributor to image contrast is T1W. Finally, if TE is long such that differences in T_2 relaxation times are emphasized (Fig. 3.5) and TR is long so that all tissues achieve nearly complete recovery of the longitudinal magnetization, the image contrast is primarily determined by T2W. PDW, T1W, and T2W images have been used for many years in MRI. Table 3.3 summarizes the appearance of various tissues and substances in PDW, T1W, and T2W images of the human brain.

In oncological imaging, an additional contrast mechanism is commonly exploited by the administration of contrast agents based on the paramagnetic atom, gadolinium (Gd). Such a paramagnetic substance, if in close proximity to water, will cause a shortening of both the T_1 and T_2 relaxation times, with the shortening of T_1 being the dominant effect. Due to the shortened T_1 relaxation times in areas where Gd is in close proximity to water, these areas become hyperintense on T_1W images compared with identical images made without the administration of Gd. Unfortunately, free Gd is toxic and, therefore, must be tightly chelated to an easily excreted substance. The first Food and Drug Administration (FDA)-approved MR contrast agent used pentetic acid (DTPA) as the chelate, but other chelates are now in clinical use [8, 9].

Gd-based contrast agents do not cross an intact blood-brain barrier (BBB). Therefore, enhancement in T1W images following the infusion of contrast agent demonstrates breakdown of the BBB due to some pathological condition. Brain neoplasms commonly, but not always, cause such a BBB breakdown, as do certain other disease states. Also, neoplasms in other areas of the body may be enhanced following Gd infusion due to lesion-induced increases in permeability and/or vascularity. Other, more organ-specific, contrast agents based on paramagnetic, superparamagnetic, or ferromagnetic substances are currently in clinical trial, and research developing MR contrast agents that are more tumor-specific is underway. Examples of PDW, T1W, T2W, and T1W post-Gd-DTPA infusion images are given in Fig. 3.10.

Other Imaging Sequences

The preceding discussion has been developed around the spin-echo pulse sequence. However, there are several other major classes of pulse sequence that have been introduced primarily to increase the speed of image acquisition. These pulse sequences include gradient-echo and fast spin-echo, as well as the most recent addition to the commercially available fast acquisition techniques, echo-planar sequences.

Gradient-Echo Sequences

Gradient-echo pulse sequences are similar to the spin-echo sequences, but do not use the 180° refocusing pulse. Instead, the MR signal is refocused solely by the use of appropriate gradient pulses. The advantage of the gradient-echo sequences is that the omission of the 180° pulse significantly reduces the image acquisition time and allows for very rapid acquisition of T1W images in particular. Unfortunately for newcomers to MRI, there are several varieties of gradient-echo pulse sequences, and the problem is exacerbated by the fact that each manufacturer has its own lengthy list of names for the sequences. Convenient sources of information for sorting through the alphabet soup of gradient-echo sequences from various manufacturers are found in the references [6, 10].

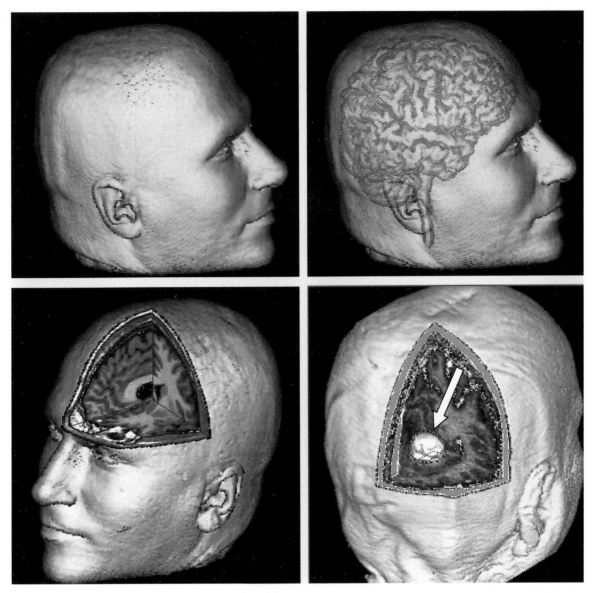

Fig. 3.11. Three-dimensional displays of volume fast-gradient-echo image acquisitions. Shaded-surface display (*top left*), merged shaded-surface displays with semitransparent skin surface overlay (*top right*), shaded-surface display with cut-planes to allow the high-resolution brain image data to be displayed in a user-selected region (*bottom left*), and shaded-surface display with cut planes to allow visualization of an enhancing metastasis (*bottom right*). Also, the volume data can be reformatted in any two-dimensional image plane desired. The fast spoiled gradient-echo data were acquired in 4:08 min using a flip angle of 25°, echo time (TE) of 4.2 ms, repetition time (TR) of 13.4 ms, 124 1.6-mm sections, 30×24-cm field-of-view, and a 256×192 matrix

The most common applications of gradient-echo imaging are in the T1W volume acquisition of (typically) 64–128 1- to 2-mm slices that can be displayed in three-dimensional fashion (Fig. 3.11), in breath-hold abdominal imaging (Fig. 3.12), and in other body imaging applications. Another application of gradient echo-based sequences is in time-of-flight and phase contrast MR angiography (MRA). Although gradient-echo sequences allow for faster image acquisition rates, there are inevitable tradeoffs that come with the omission of the 180° pulse. The primary downside is loss of the compensation for local field inhomogeneities that the spin-echo provides. Therefore, gradient-echo images demonstrate increased artifacts due to dephasing of the MR signal in areas of inhomogeneities, particularly those caused by magnetic susceptibility changes at air/tissue and tissue/bone interfaces [11]. Since the effects of this dephasing become more prominent

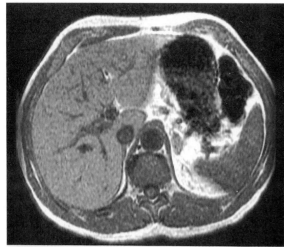

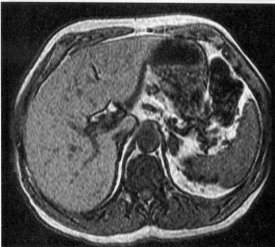

Fig. 3.12. Fast T1-weighted (*T1W*) gradient-echo, breath-hold, abdominal imaging. The in-phase image (*top*) was acquired with an echo time of 4.2 ms so that the fat and water protons were in-phase at the echo time, i.e., the signals from the fat and water added. The out-of-phase image (*bottom*) was acquired with an echo time of 2.1 ms so that the fat and water proton signals were 180° out-of-phase at the echo time, i.e., the fat signal subtracted from the water signal, but only in voxels containing both fat and water. Notice the dark borders of all tissues that are bordered by fat. Such images can be useful in distinguishing fatty infiltration of the liver or adrenal glands. For both images, the flip angle was 80°, the repetition time (TR) was 110 ms, and the images were acquired in a single breath-hold

as TE increases, gradient-echo-based T2W images (more correctly T2*W images) are prone to significant artifacts at such interfaces. Therefore, with a few exceptions, gradient-echo sequences are generally used for T1W imaging and MRA, both of which require short TEs, but not for T2W imaging. Also, gradient-echo sequences are not commonly used to obtain post-contrast T1W images of the brain, even though they are significantly faster than comparably weighted spin-echo images. One reason for this is the decreased conspicuity of enhancing lesions on post-contrast gradient-echo images, compared with spin-echo images [12].

Fast Spin-Echo Sequences

As faster acquisition of T2W images using gradient-echoes was found to be problematic, other imaging techniques were developed that allowed for the acquisition of T2W images of similar quality to spin-echo images, but at a much faster rate. The most commonly used technique is the fast spin-echo (FSE) or turbo spin-echo (TSE) sequence, based on a method originally proposed by Hennig et al. [13]. With this technique, the improved acquisition rate is provided by uniquely phase-encoding several echoes during a given TR interval, rather than encoding a single echo as in the conventional spin-echo sequence shown in Fig. 3.7. The number of echoes phase-encoded in a given TR interval is known as the echo-train length (ETL). For a given ETL, the image acquisition time is theoretically reduced by a factor of ETL compared with the conventional spin-echo sequence. Most commonly, ETLs of 8–16 are used for T2W FSE imaging, although some larger values of ETL may be used for heavily T2W images, such as those used in MR cholangiopancreatography [14–16]. The dramatic savings in acquisition time can be used to improve the SNR, the spatial resolution, or simply to reduce the acquisition time. Of course, there is a practical limit to how large ETL can be without resulting in significant artifacts. This is particularly true for PDW or T1W FSE imaging, for which the use of large values of ETL at short TEs can result in blurring and loss of contrast for small lesions [17, 18]. Fortunately, this blurring issue is much less significant in T2W imaging for which TE values are typically long. Therefore, FSE T2W imaging has become very common in MR imaging.

Although T2W images acquired using FSE are generally similar to those obtained using conventional spin-echo sequences, there are some noticeable differences [17–22]. First, fat is significantly brighter on FSE T2W images than on SE images acquired with the same TE and TR. This is primarily due to decreased J-coupling effects on the signal intensity of fat in the FSE sequence compared with the SE sequence. The increased intensity of fat on FSE T2W images frequently results in the need to use fat suppression techniques (discussed below). A second difference is the increased T2W on FSE images due to the contribution of multiple echoes to the effective TE, rather than a single echo at a well-defined TE as is obtained in the SE sequence. Finally, T2W FSE images typically demonstrate less loss of signal intensity from susceptibility changes secondary to iron or deoxyhemoglobin. Therefore, areas that are hypointense on conventional T2W images because of iron (e.g., globus pallidus and red nucleus) or deoxyhemoglobin are less hypointense on T2W FSE images than similarly weighted SE images.

Echo-Planar Sequences

Currently, the fastest commercially available image acquisition technique is echo-planar imaging (EPI) [23]. The basic idea behind the EPI sequence is similar to the FSE sequence in that multiple phase- and frequency-encoding gradients are applied in a given TR interval, but in EPI this concept is pushed to the extreme limit. In snapshot or single-shot SE EPI acquisitions, for example, every echo is obtained following a single $90°$–$180°$ pulse pair. This results in image acquisition times as short as 50–100 ms, and makes EPI ideal for imaging dynamic processes. The acquisition of snapshot EPI images, however, requires a MR scanner that has very fast acquisition rate capability and extremely good gradient field subsystems. Otherwise, reproducible high quality snapshot EPI images are difficult to obtain. To ease the requirements of single-shot EPI somewhat, multishot or mosaic EPI techniques have also been introduced that are not as fast as single-shot scans, but have decreased geometric distortions and other artifacts. While clinical applications of EPI in routine oncological MRI are currently limited, EPI imaging techniques are commonly used for perfusion, diffusion, and functional MRI research. The continued improvements in scanner hardware will undoubtedly make clinical EPI applications more commonplace in the near future.

MRA Sequences

All current MRA techniques are based on gradient-echo sequences and time-of-flight (TOF), phase contrast (PC), or bolus contrast agent techniques [24, 25]. The physical basis for TOF MRA techniques is known as flow-related enhancement. In TOF MRA, T1W images are acquired with very short TE and TR times. As the images are being acquired from a volume of tissue, the spins in that volume become partially saturated due to the rapidly repeated RF pulses, i.e., the net magnetization never recovers completely during the TR. The signal from the volume of tissue being imaged is decreased due to this partial saturation.

Blood flowing into the imaging volume, however, has not been partially saturated. Therefore, the signal from the blood is typically significantly larger than the signals from the surrounding partially saturated tissues. As a result, the vessels appear bright relative to the surrounding stationary tissue.

The TOF technique works best for relatively rapid flow that is perpendicular to the slices in the imaging volume, as this maximizes the flow-related enhancement. However, it is frequently necessary to spatially saturate the vessels flowing in the direction opposite to the vessels of interest, in order to minimize contribution to the MRA image from these vessels. In this case, to "spatially saturate" means to apply a $90°$ pulse to the blood in the vessels outside of the imaging volume that are to be suppressed. If the saturated blood then flows into the imaging volume and receives a $90°$ pulse (or other large flip angle pulse), the resulting magnetization will be primarily in the longitudinal direction, i.e., parallel to the applied static field. As no signal is detected from magnetization that is parallel or antiparallel to the static field, the signal from the saturated blood will be suppressed. If such spatial saturation techniques are not employed, arterial and venous vessels may both appear in the resulting image and overlap of the two can cause confusion.

The TOF techniques are the most commonly utilized sequences for MRA, particularly for studies of relatively fast flow. They work well with very short TE values, which minimize loss of signal secondary to dephasing of the spins by turbulent flow. Such dephasing can cause significant over-estimation of stenosis as the TE times increase. The MR system improvements that have resulted in increasingly faster imaging, especially the improved gradient subsystems, have also resulted in continuous improvements in the quality of MRA angiography by decreasing acquisition times (which leads to decreased patient motion artifacts, better contrast due to emphasized flow-related enhancement effects, and better throughput) and decreasing TEs (which leads to decreased dephasing and less overestimation of stenosis). Typical TOF MRA examinations of the circle of Willis and carotid arteries are shown in Fig. 3.13.

While TOF techniques currently dominate MRA, PC techniques have some particular benefits. The basic mechanism behind PC MRA is quite different from TOF techniques. Whereas TOF MRA relies on flow-related enhancement and appropriate use of spatial saturation pulses, PC MRA capitalizes on the fact that the signal intensity from nuclear spins can be made to depend on the velocity of the spins. During a PC MRA

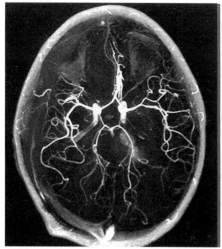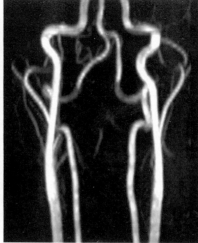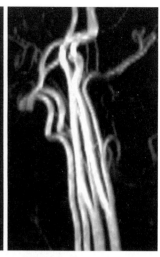

Fig. 3.13. Three-dimensional time-of-flight (TOF) magnetic resonance angiography (MRA) of the circle of Willis presented as an axial plane maximum intensity projection. The data were acquired in 6.53 min using a flip angle of 20° (ramped inferior to superior), echotime (TE)/repetition time (TR)=4.4/31 ms, magnetization transfer saturation pulse, 60 1-mm sections, 22×16-cm field-of-view, 512×256 matrix, 16-kHz bandwidth (*left*). Two views of a two-dimensional TOF MRA of the carotid and vertebral arteries presented as a maximum intensity projection (*center, right*). The data were acquired in 6:05 min using a flip angle of 60°, TE/TR=4.9/23 ms, 80 1.5-mm sections, 18×18-cm field-of-view, superior spatial saturation band, 256×192 matrix, 16-kHz bandwidth

pulse sequence, the moving nuclear spins accrue phase that is directly proportional to their velocity, and this phase can be measured. Therefore, PC MRA can depict the velocity (direction and speed) of the nuclear spins and, if the vessel diameter is also measured, the flow rate. Furthermore, such PC MRA acquisitions can be gated to the cardiac cycle to allow for the display of flow velocity as a function of cardiac cycle to examine multi-directional flow (biphasic or triphasic flow patterns).

Because of the way PC images are formed, they have two main advantages over TOF MRA images. First, PC MRA is more useful when imaging slow flow. This is because the image contrast does not depend on flow-related enhancement, but rather on the actual velocity of the spins. This also means that careful placement of spatial saturation bands to suppress flow opposite to the direction of interest, and preferential placement of the scan plane perpendicular to the direction of the flow, are not necessary. Second, quantitative measures of flow velocities and flow rates can be obtained using PC MRA.

There are, of course, some disadvantages of PC MRA relative to TOF techniques. First, for the same spatial resolution, the image acquisition time for a PC MRA study is typically longer than for a TOF MRA study. Second, the user must specify the expected maximum flow velocity (the VENC, or velocity encoding value) before the scan is initiated. If the actual flow velocity exceeds the specified VENC value, the flow will be aliased in the MRA images, typically resulting in a displayed flow velocity that greatly underestimates the actual flow velocity. On the other hand, if the specified VENC is significantly greater than the actual flow velocity, the signal from the vessel will be small and the SNR in the resulting MR angiogram will be poor. The dependence of the quality of PC MRA on the VENC value sometimes requires the acquisition of quick, low-resolution test scans with a range of VENC values, and then the use of the value that gives optimum SNR for the actual clinical PC MRA data acquisition.

Neither of the MRA techniques discussed requires the infusion of contrast agents, which is one of the chief advantages of MRA. Recently, however, the use of bolus contrast agent infusion immediately prior to the acquisition of very rapid T1W body MRA has substantially improved the visualization of distal and/or small vessels [24, 26]. Recent improvements in gradient subsystems have allowed for the acquisition of three-dimensional bolus contrast agent-enhanced scans of the abdominal vessels in a single breath-hold (Fig. 3.14). In addition to improving the visualization of smaller vessels, the infusion of the contrast agent minimizes the dependence of TOF techniques on flow-related enhancement, and the scan plane can be made independent of flow direction. Unfortunately, the timing of the image acquisition with respect to the initiation of bolus infusion now becomes critical in order to achieve good arterial-phase MRA since spatial saturation bands,

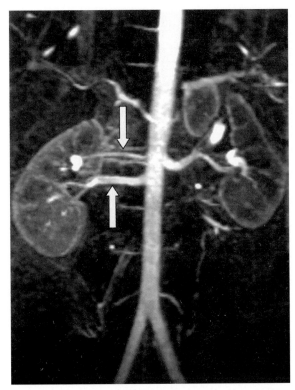

Fig. 3.14. A three-dimensional magnetic resonance angiography (MRA) of the aorta and renal arteries following bolus infusion of gadolinium (Gd)-DTPA presented as a coronal plane maximum intensity projection. Notice the excellent distal coverage of the renal arteries as well as the visualization of the small lumbar arteries. The two renal arteries on the patient's right (*arrows*) were confirmed at surgery. The data were acquired using a fast gradient-echo sequence in a single breath-hold of 22 s. The acquisition parameters were flip angle of 50°, echo time (TE)/repetition time (TR)=1.4/7.3 ms, 28 2-mm sections (with zero-fill interpolation to yield 48 2-mm sections with 1-mm overlap), 32×26-cm field-of-view, 256×128 matrix, 32-kHz bandwidth

used heavily in non-bolus contrast-agent enhanced TOF MRA, are now ineffective in suppressing the venous flow. Due to the short acquisition time, however, several single breath-hold three-dimensional image sets can be acquired following the bolus infusion. This allows the acquisition during various phases of contrast agent distribution, from nearly pure arterial phase to a later venous phase. The use of such bolus contrast agent-enhanced scans has dramatically increased the application of MRA to vascular imaging of the body.

Fat Suppression and Chemical Shift-Specific Imaging Techniques

As mentioned in the discussion of the FSE sequence, to improve the conspicuity of nearby lesions it is sometimes useful to suppress the signal from fat. This is particularly true on FSE T2W images or on some post-contrast T1W images. Currently, the most commonly utilized fat suppression technique is the application of frequency-selective saturation pulses (fat-sat or chem-sat) [6]. Saturation, in this case, refers to the application of a narrow-bandwidth 90° pulse that affects only the fat protons. Fortunately, this is possible since fat and water protons resonate at frequencies that are separated by about 215 Hz (at 1.5 T). If such a pulse is applied to fat protons, and followed immediately by a SE or FSE sequence, the magnetization of the fat protons is left parallel or antiparallel to the applied static field at the TE and is not detected. Water protons, on the other hand, are unaffected (Fig. 3.15). Although this is the most common technique for fat suppression, and does not, ideally, result in a partial loss of water signal the way inversion re-

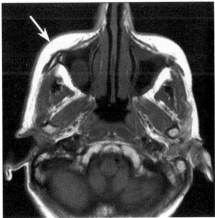 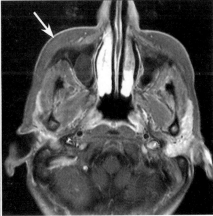

Fig. 3.15. T1-weighted (T1W) spin-echo images (echo time (TE)/repetition time (TR)=9/433 ms, 5/1.5 mm sections, 256×192 matrix, 2 excitations, 16-kHz bandwidth) obtained without (*left*) and with (*right*) frequency-selective saturation of the fat signal (fat-sat pulse). Notice the dramatic suppression of the fat signal in the fat-sat image (*arrows*)

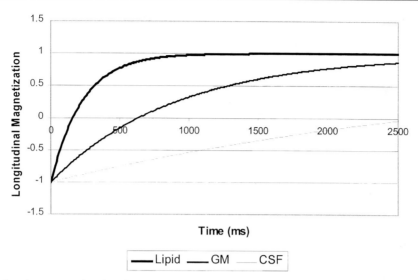

Fig. 3.16. T_1 relaxation curves showing the recovery of the longitudinal magnetization following the application of a 180° inversion pulse. For fat suppression using short TI inversion recovery (STIR) at 1.5 T, a TI of approximately 150 ms is used, as this leaves the net magnetization of the fat protons in the transverse plane when the 90° slice selective pulse is applied, and results in the magnetization from the fat protons being in the longitudinal direction, and hence not detected, when the echo is acquired

covery techniques do, there can be areas of suboptimal fat suppression. This is particularly true for large field-of-view images, for which the variable magnetic field homogeneity can cause shifts of the water and fat resonance frequencies, resulting in uneven suppression of fat within the field-of-view; fat-suppression efficiency decreases as the fat resonance frequency shifts away from the center frequency of the narrow-bandwidth saturation pulse. Other areas of susceptibility-induced inhomogeneities, such as skull base and neck, may also demonstrate variable suppression efficiency.

On large field-of-view scans, for which fat saturation techniques yield suboptimal suppression, inversion recovery (IR) techniques are sometimes used for suppressing the fat signal [1, 6]. The IR sequence is based on a conventional SE sequence, but has a 180° inversion pulse that precedes the 90° slice-selective pulse by an amount of time known as the inversion time, or TI. The inversion pulse rotates the net magnetization by 180° and, immediately after the pulse, the magnetization begins to recover, at a rate determined by the T_1 relaxation time, to the equilibrium position parallel to the applied static magnetic field (Fig. 3.16). If the value of TI is chosen such that the longitudinal magnetization for a given tissue is zero when the 90° pulse of the SE sequence is applied, the magnetization at the time of the spin echo will be in the longitudinal direction and will not be detected. Therefore, one use of IR sequences is to suppress certain tissues of interest by taking advantage of the tissue-dependent T_1 relaxation times. In short tau IR (STIR), a short TI value is used and the value is selected so that the longitudinal magnetization of fat is zero when the 90° pulse is applied. This results in the desired fat suppression in the resulting image. Since the T_1 relaxation times depend on the static magnetic field strength, the value of TI for a given tissue changes with field strength as well. At 1.5 T, the value of TI that yields this suppression is around 150 ms.

The advantage of STIR for fat suppression lies in the fact that the inversion pulse is not frequency-selective like the fat-sat pulse. Therefore, the quality of fat suppression is not as sensitive to magnetic field homogeneities. This is why STIR sequences are sometimes preferred over fat-sat sequences on large field-of-view scans. However, this advantage does not come without a price, which is best understood by considering the magnetization recovery curves shown in Fig. 3.16. If a TI of 150 ms is used for the fat suppression at 1.5 T, the gray matter longitudinal magnetization is only ~70% of its absolute maximal value when the 90° pulse is applied. This yields an unavoidable partial suppression of the water signal in addition to the suppression of the fat signal, with a concomitant decrease in SNR of the resulting image. Therefore, to achieve SNR that is comparable to the fat-sat case, longer image acquisition times (more signal averages) are required. This is com-

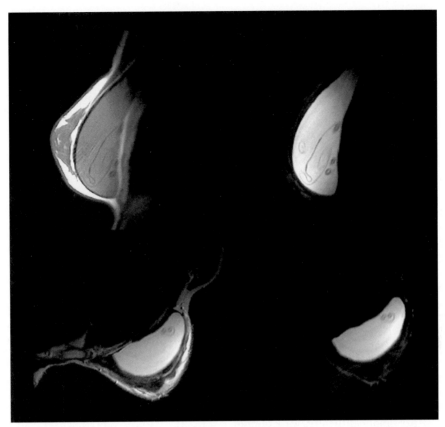

Fig. 3.17. Sagittal T1-weighted (T1W) (*top left*), sagittal fat- and water-suppressed T2-weighted (T2W) (*top right*), axial T2W fast-spin echo (FSE) (*bottom left*), and axial fat- and water-suppressed T2W (*bottom right*) images of the breast and silicone implant. The suppression of water, using chemical saturation techniques, and fat, using fast short TI inversion recovery (STIR) techniques, leaves only the signal from silicone in the images on the right and allows for improved assessment of extracapsular rupture. Notice the presentation of an intracapsular rupture in these images. The silicon-specific images were acquired in 6:55 min using a FSE IR sequence with TI/echo time (TE)/repetition time (TR)=140/68/4316 ms, echo train of 12, 24×24-cm field-of-view, 5/1-mm sections, 256×192 matrix, and three excitations

pounded by the fact that fewer anatomical slices can be acquired per TR in the case of STIR, due to the increased time required to apply the inversion pulse and the increased TI interval compared with the time required to apply the frequency-selective saturation pulse. To capitalize on the benefits of STIR fat suppression, while avoiding unacceptably long acquisition times, IR FSE sequences are typically used instead of IR SE sequences.

There are occasions when the combination of STIR and chem-sat techniques in a single scan is useful and provides a unique means of selectively visualizing anatomy. One such application is in silicone-specific imaging of breast implants. Since the protons in silicone resonate at a frequency that is very close to the resonant frequency of the methylene fat protons, the application of chemical saturation pulses would suppress both fat and silicone. Fortunately, however, the T_1 relaxation time of silicone is significantly different from the T_1 relaxation time for fat. Therefore, in order to visualize the silicone, while maintaining fat suppression, STIR techniques can be used. To further improve the visualization of the silicone, the water signal is also suppressed using a frequency-selective saturation pulse centered on the water resonance. In summary, the fat tissue is suppressed using STIR, and the water is suppressed using the chem-sat technique. Therefore, the only signal contributing to the resulting MR image is that due to the silicone protons. This type of chemical-specific imaging has been very useful in MR examinations of women with silicone implants to evaluate intra- and extra-capsular ruptures (Fig. 3.17).

A final means of fat suppression is the use of the chemical shift-imaging technique. This technique, like the frequency-selective saturation technique, takes advantage of the differing resonance frequencies of fat and water (~215 Hz difference at 1.5 T). Because of this frequency difference, fat protons precess at a faster rate than the water protons. If the water and fat protons are allowed to dephase by exactly 180° at the time the echo is detected, the fat and water signals will partially cancel one another in voxels that contain both fat and water (see Fig. 3.12).

This phenomenon can be used to generate separate images of fat and water using a technique originally proposed by Dixon [27]. With this technique, two SE images are obtained. In the first image, the TE is chosen such that the water and fat protons are in phase at the TE, i.e., $S \sim W+F$, where S is the total signal intensity, F is the fat signal intensity, and W is the water signal intensity. In the second image, the TE of the sequence is modified very slightly such that the fat and water protons are out of phase by 180° at the time the echo is detected, i.e., $S \sim W-F$. If the raw data (real and imaginary channels, not the magnitude data) from the two sets of images are added appropriately, the water image results, i.e., $(W+F)+(W-F)=2W$. However, if they are subtracted, the fat image is obtained, i.e., $(W+F)-(W-F)=2F$. Although conceptually attractive, this technique is not as robust for generating separate fat and water images as it appears to be on theoretical grounds. A primary difficulty, for example, is due to magnetic field inhomogeneities in the field-of-view that modify the resonance frequencies of fat and water in a spatially variant manner.

Current State-of-the-Art Clinical and Research Techniques in Oncology

Historically, PDW, T1W, T2W, and T1W post-contrast images, with or without fat suppression, have formed the primary foundation for oncological imaging using MRI (Fig. 3.10). However, several additional types of image-weighting techniques have recently become increasingly common. This section will introduce some of these techniques.

Fluid-Attenuated Inversion Recovery (FLAIR) Pulse Sequences

FLAIR sequences are based on IR techniques discussed above with respect to fat suppression. However, in FLAIR, the value of TI is chosen such that signals from fluids with long T_1 relaxation times, such as CSF and non-proteinacious cysts, are strongly suppressed, while signals from brain and other tissues with shorter T_1 relaxation times are only minimally affected. A very common use of this technique is in the acquisition of fluid-suppressed T2W images [28, 29]. This can be very beneficial when evaluating, for example, low conspicuity periventricular lesions, e.g., multiple sclerosis plaques, or lesions adjacent to sulci, e.g., cortical infarcts, which can otherwise be masked by the adjacent CSF. An example of the increase in lesion conspicuity in FLAIR T2W images compared with conventional FSE T2W images is

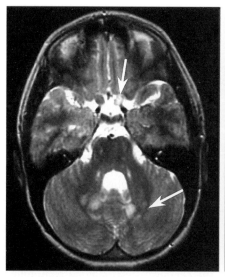
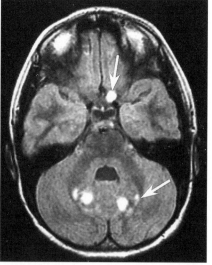

Fig. 3.18. Fast spin-echo T2-weighted (T2W) (*left*) and fast fluid-attenuated inversion recovery (FLAIR) (*right*) images of a patient with neurofibromatosis type-1. Notice the dramatic improvement in lesion conspicuity in the FLAIR images compared with the T2W images (*arrows*). The fast FLAIR images were acquired in 3:40 min with TI/TE/TR=2200/140/10000 ms, a 20×20-cm field-of-view, 4-mm interleaved sections, 256×160 matrix, and two acquisitions

shown in Fig. 3.18. Furthermore, since cysts that do not contain large amounts of proteinacious fluids are usually suppressed, while edema and neoplasms are not, FLAIR images are quite useful in the evaluation of intracranial neoplasms.

The original applications of FLAIR were limited by the very long values of TR and TI (typically 10000–12000 ms and 2200–2500 ms, respectively, at 1.5 T) required to successfully suppress the fluids that have long T_1 relaxation times (see Fig. 3.16). However, the combination of FLAIR and FSE (fast-FLAIR or turbo-FLAIR) allows for the acquisition of high-quality images in as little as 3 min, compared with 20 min or more for conventional SE FLAIR imaging. With such acceptable image acquisition times, and the improved conspicuity of lesions, fast-FLAIR images have replaced the formally ubiquitous PDW images in the evaluation of intracranial lesions at many institutions.

Magnetization Transfer Contrast (MTC) Pulse Sequences

A relatively simple addition of a single RF pulse preceding an SE or gradient-echo sequence adds an additional type of image contrast. In SE MTC imaging, for example, a frequency-selective saturation pulse, similar to that used in fat suppression techniques discussed above, is placed before the conventional SE sequence (Fig. 3.19). The center frequency of the selective pulse is typically offset from the water resonance by about 600–1200 Hz, and ultimately results in the partial suppression of tissues such as brain parenchyma and muscle, thereby improving lesion conspicuity.

To understand how MTC imaging is accomplished, it must be recalled that there are two general types of water protons found in biological systems: those that are bound to macromolecules and those that are bound to free water. However, there is continuous exchange of these protons (Fig. 3.20). Because the bound protons are restricted in their motion, their resonance is very

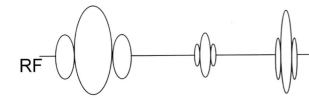

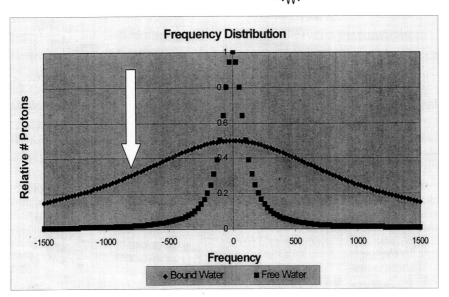

Fig. 3.19. A generic radiofrequency (RF) pulse sequence diagram for spin-echo (SE) magnetization transfer contrast (MTC) acquisitions. In addition to the standard 90° and 180° pulses, there is an additional frequency-selective saturation pulse applied at a frequency removed from the free-water proton resonance frequency (*arrow*). This pulse does not directly affect the free-water protons, but substantially saturates the water protons bound to macromolecules

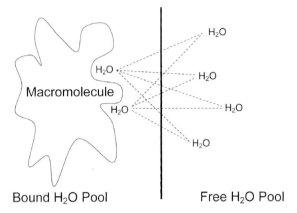

Fig. 3.20. Chemical exchange of water protons bound to macromolecules and those bound to free water results in a transfer of magnetization from the macromolecule-bound water pool to the free-water pool, with the net result being partial saturation of the free-water proton pool

broad. Since the resonance width is inversely proportional to the T_2 relaxation time, this broad resonance corresponds to a short value of T_2, and the signal from these protons decays before the echo is acquired. Therefore, these protons are MR-invisible, and the signal that contributes to the image comes from the free MR-visible water protons. The MTC saturation pulse selectively saturates the bound water protons, and does not directly affect the signal from the free water protons. However, as the bound and free water protons exchange, some of the saturated water protons end up in the free water proton pool, yielding a loss of signal intensity in the resulting image [30–33]. Therefore, the general effect of the MTC saturation pulse is the suppression of signal from tissues that have both bound and free water protons. The degree of suppression depends on several factors, including the frequency at which the saturation pulse is applied.

Both gray and white matter signals are partially suppressed, with the signal from white matter suppressed more than the signal from gray matter. Also, the signal from muscle is partially suppressed. However, the MTC saturation pulse does not significantly affect signals from fat or from pure fluids like CSF. Signals from enhancing lesions are also generally affected rather minimally. Therefore, a common use of MTC imaging is to increase the conspicuity of enhancing lesions on T1W post-contrast agent infusion scans, since the suppression of the brain parenchyma or muscle typically results in increased contrast between these tissues and enhancing lesions (Fig. 3.21) [32, 34–38]. Another common use of MTC is to partially suppress the signal from brain parenchyma in intracranial MRA, thereby improving the conspicuity of the vessels (Fig. 3.13) [39–41]. Finally, some investigators have reported that quantitative assessment of the magnetization transfer rate (MTR) may have diagnostic utility [42], or allow for improved visualization of lesion extent compared with conventional contrast-enhanced T1W imaging [36].

Diffusion-Weighted Pulse Sequences

The addition of appropriate gradient pulses within the TE allows for the generation of image contrast that depends heavily on the rate of diffusion of the nuclear spins [43–48]. In general, T2W images

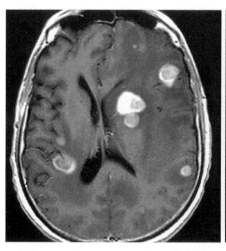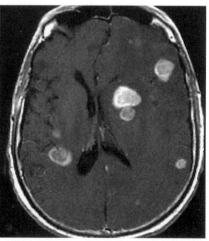

Fig. 3.21. Axial T1-weighted (T1W) spin-echo (SE) images acquired post-contrast agent infusion without (*left*) and with (*right*) the application of a magnetization transfer saturation pulse. The white matter and gray matter both are partially suppressed in the MTC image and generally result in improved conspicuity of the lesions

are acquired with and without diffusion-sensitizing gradient pulses. In the diffusion-sensitized images, tissues with freely diffusing spins are hypointense relative to tissues with spins that have restricted motion. The contrast between the freely diffusing and restricted spins increases as the area of the diffusion-sensitizing gradient pulses increases, and this area is directly related to the often quoted b-factor value [43, 45, 47, 49, 50].

More specifically, the attenuation of the signal from a given tissue in diffusion-weighted images is proportional to e^{-bD}, where b is the b-factor and D is the diffusion coefficient. Therefore, the larger the diffusion coefficient, the greater the signal loss under the influence of diffusion-sensitizing gradients with a given b-factor. Appropriate post-processing of the images also allows the calculation of an apparent diffusion coefficient (ADC) image, in which the pixel intensity is proportional to the diffusion coefficient [43, 45, 47, 49]. In the ADC images, therefore, regions of freely diffusing spins are hyperintense relative to regions where diffusion is restricted. Furthermore, if the diffusion-sensitizing gradients are applied appropriately along the three orthogonal directions, anisotropic diffusion images can be generated in addition to an isotropic diffusion image that is obtained from the trace of the diffusion tensor [51, 52]. There are advantages and disadvantages of each. For example, water diffuses more freely along white matter tracts than it does transverse to the tracts. Therefore, the intensity of normal white matter in anisotropic ADC images depends on the direction of the applied diffusion-sensitizing gradients (Fig. 3.22). This could cause confusion in the characterization of a lesion if the directionality of the white matter tracts is not fully appreciated. Therefore, it is frequently useful to examine the isotropic diffusion-weighted or ADC images, in which the directional information is removed, rather than the anisotropic images. However, the anisotropic images may be quite useful in evaluating disease processes that disrupt the normal white matter tracts, and subtle changes in the tracts may occur before a frank lesion is seen.

Clinical applications of diffusion-weighted images have included the detection and delineation of the extent of acute stroke, separation of tumor core from other components such as cysts, necrosis, and edema, and in evaluating cysts containing high levels of paramagnetic proteins that would otherwise disguise their fluid-like nature and make them more difficult to distinguish from tumors [43, 46–48, 53]. Also, diffusion-weighted imaging has been used for mapping temperature

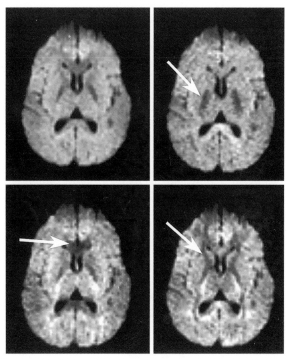

Fig. 3.22. Isotropic and anisotropic diffusion images of normal human brain. The *top left* image is an isotropic diffusion-weighted image acquired using snapshot echo-planar imaging (EPI) with a fluid-attenuated inversion recovery (FLAIR) spin-echo (SE) sequence. The remaining images are diffusion-weighted images with the diffusion-sensitizing gradients applied in the superior-inferior (*top right*), right-left (*bottom left*), and anterior-posterior (*bottom right*) directions. The *arrows* indicate regions of anisotropic diffusion due to the orientation of the white matter tracts. The b-value was 600 s/mm^2 for all images. Fourteen sections were acquired with three sensitizing directions in 1.00 min. (Non-FLAIR diffusion-weighted images with three-axis sensitization can be obtained in 12 s or less)

during hyperthermia induced by radiofrequency or laser applicators [54–56], and for three-dimensional mapping of large white matter tracts in the brain [43].

Practically, high-quality diffusion-weighted images are difficult to obtain using many current MR scanners because the motion due to diffusion is typically quite small compared with gross motion and perfusion. Therefore, diffusion-weighted images are highly susceptible to motion artifacts and typically require very stable gradient subsystems with echo-planar imaging capabilities that allow the acquisition of the diffusion data in times that freeze most other sources of physiological motion. As more snapshot EPI-capable scanners are being installed in clinical sites, and recent FDA approval of several commercial vendor diffusion imaging packages has been obtained, applications of diffusion imaging in oncological radiology should certainly expand.

Perfusion Imaging MR Pulse Sequences

Two major MRI techniques have been proposed for direct mapping of relative cerebral blood volume (rCBV) and relative cerebral blood flow (rCBF). The first technique takes advantage of the transient susceptibility change that occurs when a bolus of paramagnetic contrast agent passes through the capillary beds. Since the susceptibility changes cause enhanced dephasing of nearby spins due to the temporary decrease in T_2^*, this results in a transient decrease in signal intensity on T2W or T2*W images (Fig. 3.23). Therefore, in T2W or T2*W images, areas of increased perfusion will appear hypointense relative to regions of decreased perfusion. Under the assumption that the contrast agent remains intravascular (no BBB breakdown), such images can be used to construct maps of rCBV (Fig. 3.24) and/or rCBF [43, 48, 57]. If, however, the BBB is significantly fenestrated and contrast agent leaks from the vascular space into the interstitial space, the value of rCBV obtained by bolus contrast infusion perfusion mapping will be underestimated. An advantage of this technique, as opposed to other non-bolus techniques, is the favorable SNR of the perfusion images, particularly if double-dose or triple-dose bolus injections of contrast agent are utilized.

It is commonly accepted that tumors frequently induce angiogenesis, and highly vascular tumors are often more malignant than those that do not have increased local vascularity. Treatment-related changes and benign lesions, on the other hand, do not typically exhibit the same level of angiogenesis. Therefore, the ability to assess vascularity should improve the characterization of lesions and bolus-infusion perfusion imaging has been proposed as a tool for aiding the differentiation of tumor versus treatment-related changes and for assessing tumor grade [58–60]. Such quantitative measures of vascularity should also enhance assessment of the efficacy of anti-angiogenesis drug therapy. In addition, although Gd-DTPA does not act as a blood-pool agent in body imaging, perfusion imaging techniques have been used in the evaluation of breast neoplasms, for which strong

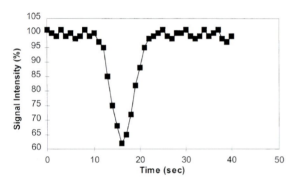

Fig. 3.23. Signal intensity curve obtained from a region of interest on a bolus-contrast infusion perfusion study. Notice the decrease in intensity during the passage of the bolus. The area under the curve is proportional to the relative cerebral blood volume (rCBV)

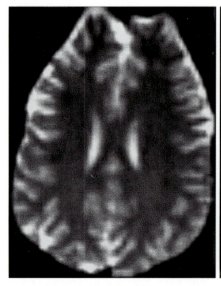 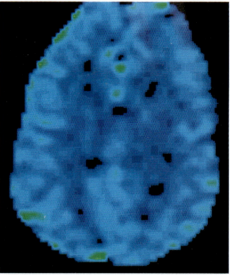

Fig. 3.24. Spin-echo (SE)-echo-planar imaging (EPI) T2-weighted (T2W) image (*left*) and perfusion map (*right*) obtained using the bolus contrast-agent infusion technique (0.1 mmol/kg of Gd-DTPA). Note the expected contrast between gray matter and white matter in the perfusion map. A snapshot SE-EPI sequence was used with echo time (TE)/repetition time (TR)=80/1700 ms, 32-cm field-of-view, 128×128 matrix, 109-kHz bandwidth

susceptibility-mediated signal loss was reported in malignant tumors, but no or only minor effects were noted in fibroadenomas [61]. Finally, the development of Gd-based contrast agents with chelates having larger molecular weights than DTPA provides a means of maintaining a predominantly blood-pool agent, even in body imaging or in the imaging of intracranial lesions with compromised BBBs. Several such agents are in development and preliminary reports of their efficacy for estimating perfusion/vascularity in animal models have been published [62–67].

The second primary means of evaluating perfusion directly is by use of time-of-flight (arterial spin labeling) techniques. Echo-planar MR imaging and signal targeting with alternating radiofrequency (EPISTAR) uses a variation of the inversion recovery technique and requires no injection of contrast agent [68]. However, the SNR, compared with the bolus injection technique, is rather inferior, imaging multiple slices is more difficult, and care must be taken to minimize unwanted magnetization transfer effects. Both means of perfusion mapping, like diffusion-weighted imaging, require high-quality and high-speed gradient subsystems capable of echo-planar imaging.

Dynamic Contrast MRI

While the use of pre- and post-contrast agent-enhanced T1W images is commonplace in oncological imaging, the contrast agent kinetics are generally not considered. The rapid acquisition of T1W images before, during, and after the infusion of a bolus of contrast agent, however, allows for the assessment of the rates of contrast agent uptake and washout from a lesion. In theory, such data allows for the quantitative evaluation of relative vascularity and permeability by two- or three-compartment rate kinetics models. Non-invasive vascularity and permeability information, of course, might be extremely valuable in oncology. The benefit of having a way to assess the local vascularity in a minimally invasive manner was

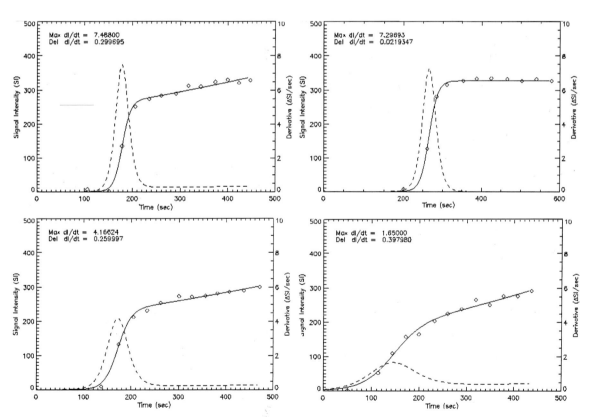

Fig. 3.25. Dynamic magnetic resonance imaging (MRI) contrast agent uptake curves obtained from regions of interest in histopathologically-proven anaplastic astrocytoma (*top left*), meningioma (*top right*), metastatic lesion (*bottom left*), and radiation necrosis (*bottom right*). The *solid lines* are empirical fits to the uptake data using a sigmoidal-exponential fit. The *dashed line* is the derivative of the fitted curve and the peak value of the derivative provides a quantitative measure of the maximal rate of contrast agent uptake. In general, high grade lesions and meningiomas have greater uptake rates than do metastases, and much greater uptake rates than do lesions resulting from treatment-related effects, such as radiation necrosis

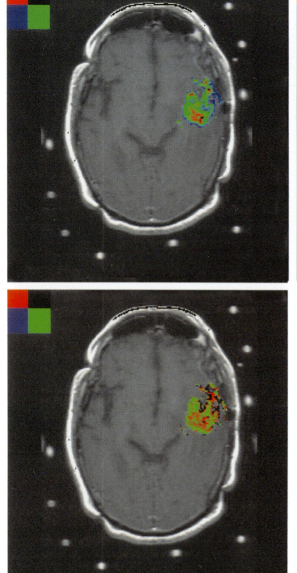

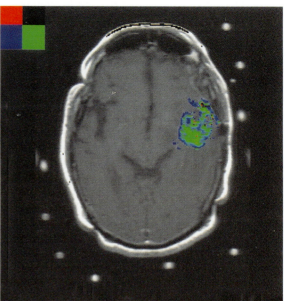

Fig. 3.26. Parametric pharmacokinetic maps obtained by the method proposed by Su et al. [112] in a case of histopathologically proven recurrent malignant astrocytoma. Maps which have pixel color proportional to the degree of vascularity (*top left*), permeability (*top right*), and washout (*bottom left*) are shown. Such studies have been useful in guiding stereotactic biopsies in patients who present with multiple possible biopsy targets, particularly those patients who have received prior therapy

discussed above. In addition, permeability of the capillaries (and/or BBB) to various agents might be highly useful in determining the potential success of chemotherapy. By labeling the therapeutic agent, or an analog, with an MR contrast agent, such as Gd, the rate at which the drug crosses from the vascular space to the interstitial space could be evaluated. Furthermore, quantitative measures of permeability would be highly useful in studies of therapeutic agents, such as receptor-mediated permeabilizers [69], which locally and temporarily increase BBB permeability to allow higher concentrations of chemotherapeutic agent to cross into the interstitial space.

Several reports of qualitative or semi-quantitative applications of dynamic contrast MRI to oncological imaging have been published in cases of breast cancer [61, 70–77], brain tumors [78–81], musculoskeletal tumors [82–89], liver masses [90], colorectal cancer [91, 92], and prostate cancer [93]. As an example of the application of dynamic contrast MRI to the evaluation of intracranial neoplasms, Fig. 3.25 shows typical Gd-DTPA uptake curves from regions of interest in pathologically proven cases of anaplastic astrocytoma, small cell lung cancer metastasis, meningioma, and treatment-related changes. The utility of dynamic contrast MR data in differentiating these types of intracranial lesions was recently reported by Hazle et al. [81], and a correlation between patient outcome and dynamic contrast MRI indices has been reported by Wong et al. [94]. In addition to such qualitative or empirical-model dynamic MRI studies, several quantitative pharmacokinetic studies have been reported that estimate the local permeability and/or vascularity of human brain [95–97], breast [71, 76, 98–101], and cervical [102, 103] neoplasms, as well as multiple sclerosis lesions [104–107] and tumors in animal models [64, 67, 108–114]. In addition to extracting pharmacokinetic data from single or multiple user-defined regions-of-interest (ROIs), several groups have also generated parametric maps that overlay color-coded maps of the pharmacokinetic parameters of interest on a standard high-resolution anatomical image. This decreases the sampling error inherent to ROI techniques, and greatly enhances the assessment of lesion heterogeneity (Fig. 3.26).

As with perfusion and diffusion acquisitions, dynamic contrast MRI requires good temporal resolution, particularly when quantitative assessment of vascularity is required. While some groups have utilized EPI for such studies, many others have optimized the acquisition time of gradient-echo or fast spin-echo sequences for such acquisitions, and comparisons of the spin-echo, gradient-echo, and fast spin-echo sequences for dynamic MRI scanning have been reported [115, 116].

Functional MRI Pulse Sequences

Although MRI has primarily been used clinically for the acquisition of high-resolution anatomic information, two primary techniques exist for acquiring functional MRI (fMRI) data. The underlying physiological principle for both techniques is that neural activation in response to a stimulus, e.g., a motor or vision task, results in local vasodilation and a concomitant increase in CBF and CBV. The first fMRI technique to capitalize on this phenomenon was based on the bolus contrast-agent infusion, or dynamic susceptibility, perfusion mapping technique outlined above [117]. For this technique, two bolus infusions are required. The first bolus is infused during image acquisition in a control state, i.e., without the application of a stimulus. On T2*W or T2W images, the passing bolus of contrast agent causes a loss of signal intensity due to the dynamic susceptibility contrast mechanism. This provides a means of mapping the rCBV in the control state. Following acquisition of the control state data, a second bo-

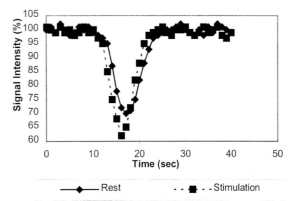

Fig. 3.27. Bolus contrast functional magnetic resonance imaging (fMRI) mapping. The two curves represent the signal intensity in a particular region of interest, with and without task activation. In general, there is up to a ~35% change in the rCBV values in the activated state compared to the rest state

lus is infused during image acquisition in the presence of an applied stimulus, e.g., photic stimulation. In areas of stimulus-induced neuronal activation, there is local vasodilation and subsequent increase in rCBV. Therefore, the dynamic susceptibility contrast near the activated areas is increased relative to the control state, due to the increased local concentration of the contrast agent. Typical signal-intensity curves obtained during the control and activated states are shown in Fig. 3.27.

The advantage of bolus infusion techniques for fMRI is the significant change in signal intensity between the control and activated states (typically ~30% at 1.5 T). The disadvantage, however, is the need for the infusion of contrast agent, which limits the number of times fMRI maps can be acquired during a single session and how soon sessions can be repeated. The second technique for fMRI studies, and currently the most commonly used, eliminates the need for the contrast-agent infusion. This technique is known as blood oxygen level-dependent (BOLD) contrast, and takes advantage of the fact that deoxyhemoglobin is a paramagnetic substance, which causes increased local dephasing of the spins due to T_2^* (susceptibility) effects, while oxyhemoglobin is a diamagnetic substance, which has minimal T_2^* effects.

When neuronal activation occurs, local vasodilation yields a local increase in the concentration of oxyhemoglobin compared with the control (resting) state. PET studies have shown that the rate of oxygen extraction is less than the rate of oxyhemoglobin delivery [118]; thus, there is a local decrease in the deoxyhemoglobin-to-oxyhemoglobin ratio [43, 50, 119]. This results in less T_2^*

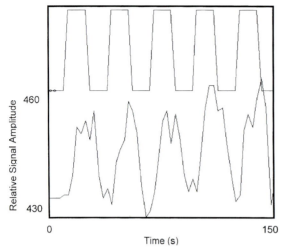

Fig. 3.28. Blood oxygen level-dependent (BOLD) functional magnetic resonance imaging (fMRI) mapping. The signal-intensity curve obtained from a region of interest in the motor strip in a set of images acquired during repeated applications of a simple motor task (tapping fingers to thumb for 15 s followed by 15 s of rest, repeated five times, *bottom trace*). The known stimulus timings are shown on the top trace. Notice the small percentage change in signal intensity (~4%) obtained at 1.5 T. Also notice the latent period between the initiation of the task (*top trace*) and the resulting signal changes (*bottom trace*) due to the fact that the BOLD mapping technique measures the hemodynamic response, not the actual neuronal activation

dephasing in areas near neuronal activation. Therefore, on T2*W images, areas of activation are hyperintense relative to the control state. Unfortunately, this change in signal intensity is relatively small (~1–5% at 1.5 T and ~20% at 4 T, Fig. 3.28) [43, 50, 119], and relatively sophisticated signal analysis must be performed to determine statistically significant regions of activation [120]. However, the BOLD contrast phenomenon does provide a completely non-invasive means of indirectly mapping areas of activation by measuring the hemodynamic response changes secondary to the neuronal activation.

Using the BOLD technique, multiple stimulation paradigms can be applied in a single imaging session, and this generally more than compensates for the lower percentage signal change than the bolus infusion technique. Since the first BOLD studies were published in 1992, a large number have been reported with widely varying applications, including visual stimulation [43, 50, 119, 121–124], auditory stimulation [50, 124–126], memory [127–137], language [126, 138–141], sensory and motor stimulation [43, 50, 124, 140, 142–147], psychiatric disorders [145, 148, 149], and pain research [150, 151]. Examples of BOLD fMRI activation maps are shown in Fig. 3.29 for motor, language, and auditory tasks.

Regardless of the technique used to acquire the fMRI data, the demands on the MRI scanner are extreme in terms of the required acquisition rates. Such studies, for multiple reasons, are best performed using scanners capable of echo-planar imaging [50]. The increased availability of such EPI-capable scanners will undoubtedly continue to drive significant research efforts in fMRI, and the number of clinical applications of fMRI studies should increase dramatically.

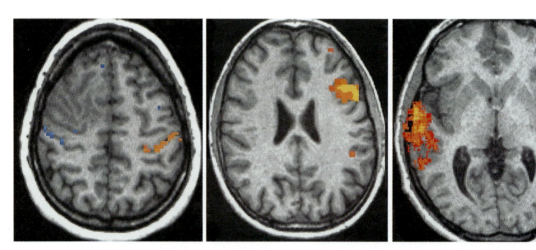

Fig. 3.29. Blood oxygen level-dependent (BOLD) functional magnetic resonance imaging (fMRI) activation maps obtained by cross-correlation of the known stimulus pattern with the signal-intensity time-course on a pixel-by-pixel basis for a bilateral hand mapping task in a patient with a non-enhancing right frontal neoplasm (*left image*, *blue* represents left hand, *yellow* represents right hand), an expressive speech task (*center image*, silent generation of words in response to presented letters alternating with simple motor tasks), and an auditory task (*right image*, verbal presentation of text in addition to the ambient scanner noise alternating with periods of ambient scanner noise)

Interventional MRI

While the capabilities of MRI for visualizing lesions are many, using MRI in an interventional setting to guide therapy has not yet become common. The reasons for this are obvious – the minimal or nonexistent access to the patient while in the scanner, and the potential interaction of the large static magnetic field with the instruments used to perform the procedure. Because of this, the primary application of MRI to therapy was initially the planning of stereotactic neurosurgery procedures, which must be performed with care to avoid unacceptable spatial inaccuracies in the acquired images [152–157]. While this is still a common application, the same advantages that made MRI the modality of choice in visualizing soft tissues are driving the development of interventional MRI devices. Recent reviews have discussed the development and application of interventional MRI [158, 159] and have demonstrated the feasibility of such applications. Applications have ranged from monitoring the delivery of radiofrequency or ultrasound fields used for hyperthermia [158–160] to the guidance of intracranial tumor resection while the patient is in the interventional MRI unit [158]. A recent issue of a leading MR journal was devoted entirely to interventional MRI topics (J Magn Reson Imaging, Volume 8, Issue 1, 1998), and provides a current snapshot of state-of-the-art interventional MRI. With open-access magnet designs now available from several vendors, the application of MRI to oncology will undoubtedly rapidly expand to include numerous novel interventional procedures.

Conclusions

The goals of this chapter have been to briefly introduce the physical principles of MRI, to briefly outline the current state-of-the-art applications of MRI to oncological imaging, and, hopefully, to pique the interest of the reader sufficiently to send him or her to the literature to gain further insight into the rapidly expanding role of MRI in oncology. In the roughly 15-year history of clinical MRI, the number of applications of MRI, and the progress made in discovering and implementing new means of manipulating image contrast based on a wide range of chemical and physiological bases, has been nothing short of astounding. This rate of development does not show any signs of slowing in the near future. Undoubtedly, this will be reflected in the fact that the information presented in this chapter will be quickly outdated, and completely new areas of MRI-based oncological imaging will soon be introduced.

References

1. Weisskoff RM, Edelman RR (1996) Basic principles of MRI. In: Edelman RR, Hesselink JR, Zlatkin MB (eds) Clinical magnetic resonance imaging. Saunders, Philadelphia, pp 3–51
2. Sanders JA (1995) Magnetic resonance imaging. In: Orrison WWJ, Lewine JD, Sanders JA, Hartshorne MF (eds) Functional brain imaging. Mosby, St Louis, pp 145–186
3. Wehrli FW, Haacke EM (1993) Principles of MR imaging. In: Potchen EJ, Haacke EM, Siebert JE, Gottschalk A (eds) Magnetic resonance angiography. Mosby, St. Louis, pp 9–34
4. Wehrli FW (1992) Principles of magnetic resonance. In: Stark DD, Bradley WG (eds) Magnetic resonance imaging. Mosby Year Book, St Louis, pp 3–20
5. Wood ML (1992) Fourier imaging. In: Stark DD, Bradley WG (eds) Magnetic resonance imaging. Mosby Year Book, St. Louis, pp 21–66
6. Elster AD (1994) Questions and answers in magnetic resonance imaging. Mosby, St Louis
7. Matwiyoff NA (1992) Instrumentation. In: Stark DD, Bradley WG (eds) Magnetic resonance imaging. Mosby Year Book, St. Louis, pp 67–87
8. Watson AD, Rocklage SM, Carvlin MJ (1992) Contrast agents. In: Stark DD, Bradley WG (eds) Magnetic resonance imaging. Mosby Year Book, St. Louis, pp 372–437
9. Lauffer RB (1996) MRI contrast agents: basic principles. In: Edelman RR, Hesselink JR, Zlatkin MB (eds) Clinical magnetic resonance imaging. Saunders, Philadelphia, pp 177–191
10. Wood ML, Bronskill MJ, Mulkern RV, Santyr GE (1994) Physical MR desktop data. J Magn Reson Imaging 3S:19–26
11. Wehrli FW (1991) Fast-scan magnetic resonance. Principles and applications. Raven, New York
12. Chappell PM, Pelc NJ, Foo TKF, Glover GH, Haros SP, Enzmann DR (1994) Comparison of lesion enhancement on spin-echo and gradient-echo images. Am J Neuroradiol 15:37–44
13. Hennig J, Nauerth A, Friedburg H (1986) RARE imaging: a fast imaging method for clinical MR. Magn Reson Med 3:823–833
14. Yamashita Y, Abe Y, Tang Y, Urata J, Sumi S, Takahashi M (1997) In vivo and clinical studies of image acquisition in breath-hold MR cholangiopancreatography: single-shot projection techniques versus multislice technique. AJR Am J Roentgenol 168:1449–1454
15. Barish M, Soto J, Yucel E (1996) Magnetic resonance cholangiopancreatography of the biliary ducts: techniques, clinical applications, and limitations. Top Magn Reson Imaging 8:302–311
16. Miyazaki T, Yamashita Y, Tsuchigame T, Yamaoto H, Urata J, Takahashi M (1996) MR cholangiopancreatography using HASTE (half-Fourier acquisition single-shot turbo spin-echo) sequences. AJR Am J Roentgenol 166:1297–1303
17. Constable RT, Gore JC (1992) The loss of small objects in variable TE imaging: implications for FSE, RARE, and EPI. Magn Reson Med 28:9–24
18. Constable RT, Anderson AW, Zhong J, Gore JC (1992) Factors influencing contrast in fast spin-echo MR imaging. Magn Reson Imaging 10:497–511
19. Atlas SW, Hackney DB, Listerud J (1993) Fast spin-echo imaging of the brain and spine. Magn Reson Q 9:61–83

20. Constable RT, Smith RC, Gore JC (1992) Signal-to-noise and contrast in fast spin echo (FSE) and inversion recovery FSE imaging. J Comput Assist Tomogr 16:41–47
21. Henkelman RM, Hardy PA, Bishop JE, Poon CS, Plewes DB (1992) Why fat is bright in RARE and fast spin-echo imaging. J Magn Reson Imaging 2:533–540
22. Norbash AM, Glover GH, Enzmann DR (1992) Intracerebral lesion contrast with spin-echo and fast spin-echo pulse sequences. Radiology 185:661–665
23. Edelman RR, Wielopolski PA (1996) Fast MRI. In: Edelman RR, Hesselink JR, Zlatkin MB (eds) Clinical magnetic resonance imaging. Saunders, Philadelphia, pp 302–352
24. Potchen EJ, Haacke EM, Siebert JE, Gottschalk A (1993) Magnetic resonance angiography. Mosby, St Louis
25. Chien D, Anderson CM, Lee RE (1996) MR angiography: basic principles. In: Edelman RR, Hesselink JR, Zlatkin MB (eds) Clinical magnetic resonance imaging. Saunders, Philadelphia, pp 271–301
26. Prince MR, Grist TM, Debatin JF (1997) 3D contrast MR angiography. Springer-Verlag, Berlin Heidelberg New York
27. Dixon WT (1984) Simple proton spectroscopic imaging. Radiology 153:189–194
28. DeCoene B, Hajnal JV, Gatehouse P (1992) MR of the brain using fluid-attenuated inversion recovery (FLAIR) pulse sequences. AJNR Am J Neuroradiol 13:1555–1564
29. Hajnal JV, DeCoene B, Lewis PD (1992) High signal regions in normal white matter shown by heavily T_2-weighted CSF nulled IR sequences. J Comput Assist Tomogr 16:506–513
30. Wolff SD, Balaban RS (1989) Magnetization transfer contrast (MTC) and tissue water proton relaxation in vivo. Magn Reson Med 10:135–144
31. Wolff SD, Eng J, Balaban RS (1991) Magnetization transfer contrast: Method for improving contrast in gradient-recalled-echo images. Radiology 179:133–137
32. Wolff SD, Balaban RS (1994) Magnetization transfer imaging: practical aspects and clinical applications. Radiology 192:593–599
33. Balaban RS, Ceckler TL (1992) Magnetization transfer contrast in magnetic resonance imaging. Magn Reson Q 8:116–137
34. Hiehle JF, Grossman RI, Ramer KN, Gonzalez-Scarano F, Cohen JA (1995) Magnetization transfer effects in MR-detected multiple sclerosis lesions: comparison with gadolinium-enhanced spin-echo images and nonenhanced T1-weighted images. AJNR Am J Neuroradiol 16:69–77
35. Mehta RC, Pike GB, Haros SP, Enzmann DR (1995) Central nervous system tumor, infection, and infarction: detection with gadolinium-enhanced magnetization transfer MR imaging. Radiology 195:41–46
36. Boorstein JM, Wong KT, Grossman RI, Bolinger L, McGowan JC (1994) Metastatic lesions of the brain: imaging with magnetization transfer. Radiology 191:799–803
37. Elster AD, King JC, Mathews VP, Hamilton CA (1994) Cranial tissues: appearance at gadolinium-enhanced and nonenhanced MR imaging with magnetization transfer contrast. Radiology 190:541–546
38. Finelli DA, Hurst GC, Gullapali RP, Bellon EM (1994) Improved contrast of enhancing brain lesions on postgadolinium, T1-weighted spin-echo images with use of magnetization transfer. Radiology 190:553–559
39. Lin W, Tkach JA, Haacke EM, Masaryk TJ (1993) Intracranial MR angiography: application of magnetization transfer contrast and fat saturation to short gradient-echo velocity-compensated sequences. Radiology 186:753–761
40. Edelman RR, Ahn SS, Chien D et al. (1992) Improved time-of-flight MR angiography of the brain with magnetization transfer contrast. Radiology 184:395–399
41. Pike GB, Hu BS, Glover GH, Enzmann DR (1992) Magnetization transfer time-of-flight magnetic resonance angiography. Magn Reson Med 25:372–379
42. Yousem DM, Montone KT, Sheppard LM, Rao VM, Weinstein GS, Hayden RE (1994) Head and neck neoplasms: magnetization transfer analysis. Radiology 192:703–707
43. Sorenson AG, Rosen BR (1996) Functional MRI of the Brain. In: Atlas SW (ed) Magnetic resonance imaging of the brain and spine. Lippincott-Raven, Philadelphia, pp 1501–1545
44. Le Bihan D, Turner R, Moonen CTW, Pekar J (1991) Imaging of diffusion and microcirculation with gradient sensitization: design, strategy, and significance. J Magn Reson Imaging 1:7–28
45. Le Bihan D, Turner R (1993) Diffusion and perfusion nuclear magnetic resonance imaging. In: Potchen EJ, Haacke EM, Siebert JE, Gottschalk A (eds) Magnetic resonance angiography. Concepts and applications. Mosby-Year Book, Inc, St Louis, pp 323–342
46. Le Bihan D (1993) Clinical intravoxel incoherent motion imaging. In: Potchen EJ, Haacke EM, Siebert JE, Gottschalk A (eds) Magnetic resonance angiography. Concepts and applications. Mosby-Year Book, Inc, St Louis, pp 485–497
47. Le Bihan D, Turner R, Douek P, Patronas N (1992) Diffusion MR imaging: clinical applications. AJR Am J Roentgenol 159:591–599
48. Rosen BR, Aronen HJ, Cohen MS et al. (1993) Diffusion and perfusion fast scanning in brain tumors. In: Leeds NE (ed) Brain tumors. Saunders, Philadelphia, pp 631–648
49. Le Bihan D (1992) Theoretical principles of perfusion imaging. Application to magnetic resonance imaging. Invest Radiol 27:S6-S11
50. Sanders JA, Orrison WWJ (1995) Functional magnetic resonance imaging. In: Orrison WWJ, Lewine JD, Sanders JA, Hartshorne MF (eds) Functional brain imaging. Mosby-Year Book, Inc, St Louis, pp 239–326
51. Moseley ME, Cohen Y, Kucharczyk J et al. (1990) Diffusion-weighted MR imaging of anisotropic water diffusion in cat central nervous system. Radiology 176:439–445
52. van Gelderen P, de Vleeschouwer MHM, Pekar J, van Zijl PCM, DesPres D, Moonen CTW (1993) Diffusion MRI and acute stroke detection: the use of the trace of the diffusion tensor. Book of abstracts, 12th Annual Meeting of the Society of Magnetic Resonance in Medicine, New York:592
53. Conturo T, McKinsrty R, Aronovitz J, Neil J (1995) Diffusion MRI: precision, accuracy, and flow effects. NMR Biomed 8:307–332
54. Delannoy J, Chen C-N, Turner R, Levin RL, Le Bihan D (1991) Noninvasive temperature imaging using diffusion MRI. Magn Reson Med 19:333–339
55. Samulski TV, MacFall J, Zhang Y, Grant W, Charles C (1992) Non-invasive thermometry using magnetic resonance diffusion imaging: potential for application in hyperthermic oncology. Int J Hyperthermia 8:819–829
56. Zhang Y, Samulski TV, Joines WT, Mattiello J, Levin RL, Le Bihan D (1992) On the accuracy on noninvasive thermometry using molecular diffusion magnetic resonance imaging. Int J Hyperthermia 8:263–274
57. Rosen BR, Belliveau JW, Vevea JM, Brady TJ (1990) Perfusion imaging with NMR contrast agents. Magn Reson Med 14:249–265
58. Aronen HJ, Gazit IE, Louis DN et al. (1994) Cerebral blood volume maps of gliomas: comparison with tumor grade and histologic findings. Radiology 191:41–51

59. Aronen HJ, Glass J, Pardo FS et al. (1995) Echo-planar MR cerebral blood volume mapping of gliomas. Clinical utility. Acta Radiologica 36:520–528
60. Aronen HJ, Cohen MS, Belliveau JW, Fordham JA, Rosen BR (1993) Ultrafast imaging of brain tumors. Top Magn Reson Imaging 5:14–24
61. Kuhl C, Bieling H, Gieseke J et al. (1997) Breast neoplasms: T2* susceptibility-contrast, first-pass perfusion MR imaging. Radiology 202:87–95
62. Tacke J, Adam G, Classen H, Muhler A, Prescher A, Gunther R (1997) Dynamic MRI of a hypocascularized liver tumor model: comparison of a new blood pool contrast agent (24-gadolinium-DTPA-cascade-polymer) with gadopentetate dimeglumine. J Magn Reson Imaging 7:678–682
63. Roberts H, Saeed M, Roberts T et al. (1997) Comparison of albumin-(Gd-DTPA)30 and Gd-DTPA-24-cascade-polymer for measurements of normal and abnormal microvascular permeability. J Magn Reson Imaging 7:331–338
64. Su M-Y, Najafi AA, Nalcioglu O (1995) Regional comparison of tumor vascularity and permeability parameters measured by albumin-Gd-DTPA and Gd-DTPA. Magn Reson Med 34:402–411
65. Adam G, Muhler A, Spuntrup E et al. (1996) Differentiation of spontaneous canine breast tumors using dynamic magnetic resonance imaging with 24-gadolinium-DTPA-cascade-polymer, a new blood-pool agent. Preliminary experience. Invest Radiol 31:267–274
66. Vexler V, Clement O, Schmitt-Willich H, Brasch R (1994) Effect of varying the molecular weight of the MR contrast agent Gd-DTPA-polysine on blood pharmacokinetics and enhancement patterns. J Magn Reson Imaging 4:381–388
67. Shames DM, Kuwatsuru R, Vexler V, Mühler A, Brasch RC (1993) Measurement of capillary permeability to macromolecules by dynamic magnetic resonance imaging: a quantitative noninvasive technique. Magn Reson Med 29:616–622
68. Edelman RR, Siewert B, Darby DG et al. (1994) Qualitative mapping of cerebral blood flow and functional localization with echo-planar MR imaging and signal targeting with alternating radio frequency. Radiology 192:513–520
69. Inamura T, Nomura T, Bartus RT, Black KL (1994) Intracarotid infusion of RMP-7, a bradykinin analog: a method for selective drug delivery to tumors. J Neurosurg 81:752–758
70. Perman WH, Heiberg EM, Grunz J, Herrmann VM, Janney CG (1994) A fast 3D-imaging technique for performing dynamic Gd-enhanced MRI of breast lesions. Magn Reson Imaging 12:545–551
71. Tofts PS, Berkowitz B, Schnall MD (1995) Quantitative analysis of dynamic Gd-DTPA enhancement in breast tumors using a permeability model. Magn Reson Med 33:564–568
72. Hulka CA, Smith BL, Sgroi DC et al. (1995) Benign and malignant breast lesions: differentiation with echo-planar MR imaging. Radiology 197:33–38
73. Buadu LD, Maurakami J, Murayama S et al. (1996) Breast lesions: correlation of contrast medium enhancement patterns on MR images with histopatholoic findings and tumor angiogenesis. Radiology 200:639–649
74. Buckley DL, Kerslake RW, Blackband SJ, Horsman A (1994) Quantitative analysis of multi-slice Gd-DTPA enhanced dynamic MR images using an automated simplex minimization procedure. Magn Reson Med 32:646–651
75. Turkat TJ, Klein BD, Polan RL, Richman R (1994) Dynamic MR mammography: a technique for potentially reducing the biopsy rate for benign breast disease. J Magn Reson Imaging 4:563–568
76. Hoffmann U, Brix G, Knopp M, Heß T, Lorenz WJ (1995) Pharmacokinetic mapping of the breast: a new method for dynamic MR mammography. Magn Reson Med 33:506–514
77. Sinha S, Lucas-Quesada FA, DeBruhl ND et al. (1997) Multifeature analysis of Gd-enhanced MR images of breast lesions. J Magn Reson Imaging 7:1016–1026
78. Nägele T, Petersen D, Klose U et al. (1993) Dynamic contrast enhancement of intracranial tumors with snapshot-FLASH MR imaging. AJNR Am J Neuroradiol 14:89–98
79. Gowland P, Mansfield P, Bullock P, Stehling M, Worthington B, Firth J (1992) Dynamic studies of gadolinium uptake in brain tumors using inversion-recovery echo-planar imaging. Magn Reson Med 26:241–258
80. Bullock PR, Mansfield P, Gowland P, Worthington BS, Firth JL (1991) Dynamic imaging of contrast enhancement in brain tumors. Magn Reson Med 19:293–298
81. Hazle JD, Jackson EF, Schomer DF, Leeds NE (1997) Dynamic imaging of intracranial lesions using fast spin-echo imaging: differentiation of brain tumors and treatment effects. J Magn Reson Imaging 7:1084–1093
82. Verstraete KL, Dierick A, De Deene Y et al. (1994) First-pass images of musculoskeletal lesions: a new and useful diagnostic application of dynamic contrast-enhanced MRI. Magn Reson Imaging 12:687–702
83. Mirowitz SA, Totty WG, Lee JKT (1992) Characterization of musculoskeletal masses using dynamic Gd-DTPA enhanced spin-echo MRI. J Comput Assist Tomogr 16:120–125
84. Fletcher BD, Hanna SL, Fairclough D, Gronemeyer SA (1992) Pediatric musculoskeletal tumors: use of dynamic, contrast-enhanced MR imaging to monitor response to chemotherapy. Radiology 184:243–248
85. Erlemann R, Peters PE (1990) Applications of dynamic Gd-DTPA MRI in the investigation of musculoskeletal neoplasms. In: Bydder G, Felix R, Bücheler E, et al. (eds) Contrast media in MRI. International workshop, Berlin. Medicom Europe, Brinklaan, pp 369–379
86. Fletcher BD, Hanna SL (1990) Musculoskeletal neoplasms: dynamic Gd-DTPA-enhanced MR imaging. Radiology 177:287–288
87. Erlemann R (1990) Musculoskeletal neoplasms: dynamic Gd-DTPA-enhanced MR imaging. Radiology 177:288
88. Verstraete KL, De Deene Y, Roels H, Dierick A, Uyttendaele D, Kunnen M (1994) Benign and malignant musculoskeletal lesions: dynamic contrast-enhanced MR imaging – parametric "first-pass" images depict tissue vascularization and perfusion. Radiology 192:835–843
89. Erlemann R, Reiser MF, Peters PE et al. (1989) Musculoskeletal neoplasms: static and dynamic Gd-DTPA-enhanced MR imaging. Radiology 171:767–773
90. Quillin S, Atilla S, Brown J, Borrello J, Yu C, Pilgram T (1997) Characterization of focal hepatic masses by dynamic contrast-enhanced MR imaging: findings in 311 lesions. Magn Reson Imaging 15:275–285
91. Kinkel K, Tardivon A, Soyer P et al. (1996) Dynamic contrast-enhanced subtraction versus T2-weighted spin-echo MR imaging in the follow-up of colorectal neoplasm: a prospective study of 41 patients. Radiology 200:453–458
92. Muller-Schimpfle M, Brix G, Layer G et al. (1993) Recurrent rectal cancer: diagnosis with dynamic MR imaging. Radiology 189:881–889
93. Jager GJ, Ruijter ETG, vd Kaa CA et al. (1997) Dynamic TurboFlash subtraction technique for contrast-enhanced MR imaging of the prostate: correlation with histopathologic results. Radiology 203:645–652
94. Wong ET, Jackson EF, Hess K et al. (1998) Correlations between dynamic MRI and outcome in patients with malignant glioma. Neurology 50:777-781

95. Hawighorst H, Engenhart R, Knopp M et al. (1997) Intracranial meningeomas: time- and dose-dependent effects of irradiation on tumor microcirculation monitored by dynamic MR imaging. Magn Reson Imaging 15:423–432
96. Ott RJ, Brada M, Flower MA, Babich JW, Cherry SR, Deehan BJ (1991) Measurements of blood-brain barrier permeability in patients undergoing radiotherapy and chemotherapy for primary cerebral lymphoma. Eur J Cancer 27:1356–1361
97. Brix G, Semmler W, Port R, Schad LR, Layer G, Lorenz WJ (1991) Pharmacokinetic parameters in CNS Gd-DTPA enhanced MR imaging. J Comput Assist Tomogr 15:621–628
98. Mussurakis S, Buckley D, Horsman A (1997) Dynamic MRI of invasive breast cancer: assessment of three region-of-interest analysis methods. J Comput Assist Tomogr 21:431–438
99. den Boer J, Hoenderop R, Smink J et al. (1997) Pharmacokinetic analysis of Gd-DTPA enhancement in dynamic three-dimensional MRI of breast lesions. J Magn Reson Imaging 7:702–715
100. Mussurakis S, Buckley D, Bowsley S et al. (1995) Dynamic contrast-enhanced magnetic resonance imaging of the breast combined with pharmacokinetic analysis of gadolinium-DTPA uptake in the diagnosis of local recurrence of early stage breast carcinoma. Invest Radiol 30:650–662
101. Knopp M, Brix G, Junkermann H, Sinn H (1994) MR mammography with pharmacokinetic mapping for monitoring of breast cancer treatment during neoadjuvant therapy. Magn Reson Imaging 2:633–658
102. Hawighorst H, Knapstein P, Weikel W et al. (1996) Cervical carcinoma: comparison of standard and pharmacokinetic MR imaging. Radiology 201:531–539
103. Hawighorst H, Knapstein P, Schaeffer U et al. (1996) Pelvic lesions in patients with treated cervical carcinoma: efficacy of pharmacokinetic analysis of dynamic MR images in distinguishing recurrent tumors from benign conditions. AJR Am J Roentgenol 166:401–408
104. Tofts PS (1997) Modeling tracer kinetics in dynamic Gd-DTPA MR imaging. J Magn Reson Imaging 7:91–101
105. Larsson HBW, Tofts PS (1992) Measurement of blood-brain barrier permeability using dynamic Gd-DTPA scanning – a comparison of methods. Magn Reson Med 24:174–176
106. Tofts PS, Kermode AG (1991) Measurement of the blood-brain barrier permeability and leakage space using dynamic MR imaging. 1. Fundamental concepts. Magn Reson Med 17:357–367
107. Larsson HBW, Stubgaard M, Frederiksen JL, Jensen M, Henriksen O, Paulson OB (1990) Quantitation of blood-brain barrier defect by magnetic resonance imaging and gadolinium-DTPA in patients with multiple sclerosis and brain tumors. Magn Reson Med 16:117–131
108. Su M-Y, Jao J-C, Nalcioglu O (1994) Measurement of vascular volume fraction and blood-tissue permeability constants with a pharmacokinetic model: Studies in rat muscle tumors with dynamic Gd-DTPA enhanced MRI. Magn Reson Med 32:714–724
109. Kenney J, Schmiedl U, Maravilla K et al. (1992) Measurement of blood-brain barrier permeability in a tumor model using magnetic resonance imaging with gadolinium-DTPA. Magn Reson Med 27:68–75
110. Schmiedl UP, Kenney J, Maravilla KR (1992) Kinetics of pathologic blood-brain-barrier permeability in an astrocytic glioma using contrast-enhanced MR. AJNR Am J Neuroradiol 13:5–14
111. Schmiedl UP, Kenney J, Maravilla KR (1991) MRI of blood-brain barrier permeability in astrocytic gliomas: application of small and large molecular weight contrast media. Magn Reson Med 22:288–292
112. Su M-Y, Wang Z, Roth GM, Lao X, Samoszuk MK, Nalcioglu O (1996) Pharmacokinetic changes induced by vasomodulators in kidneys, livers, muscles, and implanted tumors in rats as measured by dynamic Gd-DTPA-enhanced MRI. Magn Reson Med 36:868–877
113. Schwarzbauer C, Morrissey SP, Deichmann R et al. (1997) Quantitative magnetic resonance imaging of capillary water permeability and regional blood volume with an intravascular MR contrast agent. Magn Reson Med 37:769–777
114. Griebel J, Mayr N, de Vries A et al. (1997) Assessment of tumor microcirculation: a new role of dynamic contrast MR imaging. J Magn Reson Imaging 7:111–119
115. Jackson E, Hazle J, Reeve D (1996) Dynamic contrast imaging using spin echo, fast spin echo, and fast spoiled gradient echo sequences. Book of abstracts, 4th Annual Meeting of the International Society for Magnetic Resonance in Medicine, New York, pp 1494
116. Jackson EF, Reeve DM, Hazle JD (1998) Image acquisition techniques for dynamic MR imaging of intracranial lesions. Magn Reson Imaging (in press)
117. Belliveau JW, Kennedy DN, McKinstry RC et al. (1991) Functional mapping of the human cortex by magnetic resonance imaging. Science 254:716–719
118. Fox P, Raichle M (1986) Focal physiological uncoupling of cerebral blood flow and oxidative metabolism during somatosensory stimulation in human subjects. Proc Natl Acad Sci U S A 83:1140–1144
119. Kwong KK (1995) Functional magnetic resonance imaging with echo planar imaging. Magn Reson Q 11:1–20
120. Bandettini PA, Jesmanowicz A, Wong EC, Hyde JS (1993) Processing strategies for time-course data sets in functional MRI of the human brain. Magn Reson Med 30:161–173
121. Turner R, Jezzard P, Wen H et al. (1993) Functional mapping of the human visual cortex at 4 and 1.5 Tesla using deoxygenation contrast EPI. Magn Reson Med 29:277–279
122. Menon RS, Ogawa S, Kim S-G et al. (1992) Functional brain mapping using magnetic resonance imaging. Signal changes accompanying visual stimulation. Invest Radiol 27:S47-S53
123. Hathout GM, Kirlew KAT, So GJK et al. (1994) MR imaging signal response to sustained stimulation in human visual cortex. J Magn Reson Imaging 4:537–543
124. DeYoe EA, Bandettini P, Neitz J, Miller D, Winans P (1994) Functional magnetic resonance imaging (FMRI) of the human brain. J Neurosci Methods 54:171–187
125. Calvert GA, Bullmore ET, Brammer MJ et al. (1997) Activation of auditory cortex during silent lipreading. Science 276:593–596
126. FitzGerald DB, Cosgrove GR, Ronner S et al. (1997) Location of language in the cortex: a comparison between functional MR imaging and electrocortical stimulation. AJNR Am J Neuroradiol 18:1529–1539
127. Spitzer M, Kwong KK, Kennedy W, Rosen BR, Belliveau JW (1995) Category-specific brain activation in fMRI during picture naming. Neuroreport 6:2109–2112
128. Gabrieli JDE, Desmond JE, Demb JB et al. (1996) Functional magnetic resonance imaging of semantic memory processes in the frontal lobes. Psychol Sci 7:278–283
129. Busatto G, Howard J, Ha Y et al. (1997) A functional magnetic resonance imaging study of episodic memory. Neuroreport 8:2671–2675

130. Ojemann JG, Buckner RL, Corbetta M, Raichle ME (1997) Imaging studies of memory and attention. Neurosurg Clin North Am 8:307–319
131. Kammer T, Bellemann ME, Guckel F et al. (1997) Functional MR imaging of the prefrontal cortex: specific activation in a working memory task. Magn Reson Imaging 15:879–889
132. D'Esposito M, Detre JA, Alsop DC, Shin RK, Atlas S, Grossman M (1995) The neural basis of the central executive system of working memory. Nature 378:279–281
133. Demb JB, Desmond JE, Wagner AD, Vaidya CJ, Glover GH, Gabrieli JDE (1995) Semantic encoding and retrieval in the left interior prefrontal cortex: a functional MRI study of task difficulty and process specificity. J Neurosci 15:5870–5878
134. McCarthy G, Blamire AM, Puce A et al. (1994) Functional magnetic resonance imaging of human prefrontal cortex activation during a spatial working memory task. Proc Natl Acad Sci U S A 91:8690–8694
135. Gabrieli JDE, Brewer JB, Desmond JE, Glover GH (1997) Separate neural bases of two fundamental memory processes in the human medial temporal lobe. Science 276:264–266
136. Courtney SM, Ungerleider LG, Kell K, Haxby JV (1997) Transient and sustained activity in a distributed neural system for human working memory. Nature 386:608–611
137. Braver TS, Cohen JD, Nystrom LE, Jonides J, Smith EE, Noll DC (1997) A parametric study of prefrontal cortex involvement in human working memory. Neuroimage 5:49–62
138. Benson RR, Logan WJ, Cosgrove GR et al. (1996) Functional MRI localization of language in a 9-year-old child. Can J Neurol Sci 23:213–219
139. Binder JR, Swanson SJ, Hammeke TA et al. (1996) Determination of language dominance using functional MRI: a comparison with the Wada test. Neurology 46:978–984
140. Atlas SW, Howard RSI, Maldjian J et al. (1996) Functional magnetic resonance imaging of regional brain activity in patients with intracerebral gliomas: findings and implications for clinical management. Neurosurgery 38:329–338
141. Hertz-Pannier L, Gaillard WD, Mott SH et al. (1997) Noninvasive assessment of language dominance in children and adolescents with functional MRI: a preliminary study. Neurology 48:1003–1012
142. Biswal B, Yetkin FZ, Haughton VM, Hyde JS (1995) Functional connectivity in the motor cortex of resting human brain using echo-planar MRI. Magn Reson Med 34:537–541
143. Righini A, de Divitiis O, Prinster A et al. (1996) Functional MRI: primary motor cortex localization in patients with brain tumors. J Comput Assist Tomogr 20:702–708
144. Rao SM, Binder JR, Bandettini PA et al. (1993) Functional magnetic resonance imaging of complex human movements. Neurology 43:2311–2318
145. Schröder J, Wenz F, Schad LR, Baudendistel K, Knopp MV (1995) Sensorimotor cortex and supplementary motor area changes in schizophrenia. A study with functional magnetic resonance imaging. Br J Psychiatry 167:197–201
146. Mueller WM, Yetkin FZ, Hammeke TA et al. (1996) Functional magnetic resonance imaging mapping of the motor cortex in patients with cerebral tumors. Neurosurgery 39:515–521
147. Hammeke TA, Yetkin FZ, Mueller WM et al. (1994) Functional magnetic resonance imaging of somatosensory stimulation. Neurosurgery 35:677–681
148. Maddock RJ, Buonocore MH (1997) Activation of left posterior cingulate gyrus by the auditory presentation of threat-related words: an fMRI study. Psychiatry Res 75:1–14
149. Breiter HC, Rauch SL (1996) Functional MRI and the study of OCD: from symptom provocation to cognitive-behavioral probes of cortico-striatal systems and the amygdala. Neuroimage 4:S127-S138
150. Davis KD, Taylor SJ, Crawley AP, Wood ML, Mikulis DJ (1997) Functional MRI of pain- and attention-related activations in the human cingulate cortex. J Neurophysiol 77:3370–3380
151. Rainville P, Duncan GH, Price DD, Carrier B, Bushnell MC (1997) Pain affect encoded in human anterior cingulate but not somatosensory cortex. Science 277:968–971
152. Michiels J, Bosmans H, Pelgrims P et al. (1994) On the problem of geometric distortion in magnetic resonance images for stereotactic neurosurgery. Magn Reson Imaging 12:749–765
153. Rousseau J, Clarysse P, Blond S, Gibon D, Vasseur C, Marchandise X (1991) Validation of a new method for stereotactic localization using MR imaging. J Comput Assist Tomogr 15:291–296
154. Schad L, Lott S, Schmitt F, Strum V, Lorenz JW (1987) Correction of spatial distortion in MR imaging: a prerequisite for accurate sterotaxy. J Comput Assist Tomogr 11:499–505
155. Sumanaweera T, Glover G, Song S, Adler J, Napel S (1994) Quantifying MRI geometric distortion in tissue. Magn Reson Med 31:40–47
156. Sumanaweera TS, Glover GH, Binford TO, Adler JR (1993) MR susceptibility misregistration correction. IEEE Trans Med Imaging 12:251–259
157. Sumanaweera TS, Adler JRJ, Napel S, Glover GH (1994) Characterization of spatial distortion in magnetic resonance imaging and its implication for stereotactic surgery. Neurosurgery 35:696–704
158. Jolesz FA, Blumenfeld SM (1994) Interventional use of magnetic resonance imaging. Magn Reson Q 10:85–96
159. Lufkin RB (1995) Interventional MR imaging. Radiology 197:16–18
160. Cline HE, Hynynen K, Watkins RD et al. (1995) Focused US system for MR imaging-guided tumor ablation. Radiology 194:731–737

Magnetic Resonance Spectroscopy: Physical Principles and Applications

E. F. Jackson

Basic Considerations

While the sensitivity of magnetic resonance imaging (MRI) for detection of soft-tissue lesions is unchallenged, its specificity for characterizing the lesion type or grade is often suboptimal. As a result, it is not uncommon for diagnosis, particularly of lesions that are detected following prior therapy, to be based on tissue biopsies. Longitudinal follow-up of such lesions using repeated biopsies might be tolerable in soft tissue lesions of the extremities, for example. However, multiple repeated biopsies are not really acceptable in the case of intracranial lesions, and are associated with risk and significant discomfort in other anatomical locations. Therefore, any technique that provides information that complements the sensitivity of the MRI exam and increases confidence in a non-invasive diagnosis would clearly be a welcome addition to the diagnostic imaging armamentarium.

Magnetic resonance spectroscopy (MRS) had its beginnings in the 1940s and, with the introduction of pulsed Fourier transform (FT) techniques in 1966 [1], rapidly became, and remains, an indispensable structural analysis tool for analytical chemistry laboratories. Clearly, MRS-based structural determinations were the chief application of the nuclear magnetic resonance (NMR) phenomenon until the advent of clinical MRI in the 1980s. Nevertheless, the chemical applications were not lost on early investigators using whole-body MR scanners that were developed primarily for MRI but adapted to also serve as a platform for performing in vivo MRS exams. The goal of obtaining biochemical information that could complement the exquisite anatomic detail of MRI was, and still is, a powerful stimulus for basic MRS research and, increasingly, for clinical application of in vivo MRS. In essence, by obtaining spectra that might have characteristic patterns specific to a particular type or grade of lesion, the promise of MRS is in obtaining noninvasive biopsies.

Basic Principles of MRS

Many of the important physical principles discussed with regard to MRI (Chap. 3) are also important with regard to MRS. For example, any nucleus with non-zero spin can theoretically be utilized for MRS studies, just as any non-zero spin nucleus can theoretically be used for MRI studies. For in vivo applications, however, only a few nuclei are readily studied; some of the more commonly used nuclei are given in Table 4.1. Although each of these nuclei has its own advantages and disadvantages for in vivo studies, the basic physical principles forming the foundation of the MRS examination is the same.

When a sample is placed in a strong static magnetic field, B_o, more of the nuclear magnetic moments are aligned parallel to the field than antiparallel (see Chap. 3). This gives rise to a net magnetization along the direction of the B_o field, i.e., the longitudinal equilibrium magnetization. Since the longitudinal magnetization is not detected, a short radiofrequency (RF) pulse is applied to tip the net magnetization into the transverse plane where it precesses at the Larmor frequency given by

$$v = \gamma B_{nucleus}, \qquad 4.1$$

where γ is the gyromagnetic ratio and $B_{nucleus}$ is the magnetic field at the nucleus, which is the applied magnetic field B_o modified by the local chemical environment. Therefore, nuclei in differing chemical environments will have slightly different resonant frequencies, depending on the amount of local nuclear shielding [2]. If the nuclear shielding constant is given by σ, then the modified resonant frequency is

$$v = \gamma B_0 (1 - \sigma) \qquad 4.2$$

The local shielding effect, which arises from the electron configuration at the nucleus of interest, results in spectra with multiple peaks for a given nuclear species; the peak positions depend

Table 4.1. Properties of some nuclei useful for in vivo MRS

Nucleus	Resonance frequency at 1.5 T (MHz)	Natural abundance (%)	Sensitivity relative to ^{1}H (%)[a]	Advantages	Disadvantages
^{1}H	63.9	99.98	100	Most abundant and sensitive. Can detect total creatine, choline, lactate, N-acetylaspartate, myo-inositol, citrate, glucose, lipids, and various amino acids	Small chemical shift range (~5 ppm) yields crowded spectra with overlapping spectral peaks. Water signal is extremely large and must be efficiently suppressed in order to detect spectral peaks from biochemicals of interest. Overlapping peaks may require complex spectral editing techniques to resolve peaks of interest
^{31}P	25.9	100	6.6	Simple spectra with moderately large chemical-shift range (~25 ppm). Can detect high-energy compounds such as phosphocreatine and ATP, as well as phosphomonoesters, phosphodiesters, and inorganic phosphate. Allows for non-invasive intracellular pH determinations	Low relative sensitivity results in increased acquisition times relative to ^{1}H MRS. Some compounds, such as ATP, exhibit short T_2 relaxation times and/or significant J-modulation and limits the choices of localization techniques. Good resolution of some resonances requires ^{1}H decoupling
^{19}F	60.1	100	83	Can monitor the uptake and metabolism of fluorinated drugs, such as 5-fluorouracil, and various neuropsychiatric and anesthetic agents	Natural abundance levels are too low to be detected in vivo
^{13}C	16.1	1.1	1.6	Large chemical-shift range (~200 ppm). Useful for studies of metabolism, e.g., TCA cycle and fatty acid metabolism	Very low natural abundance makes in vivo studies quite difficult and acquisition times are long. Studies typically require ^{1}H decoupling

[a] Equivalent number of nuclei at constant field

on the local chemical environment. The position of a given spectral peak is usually given in terms of its chemical shift, δ, with respect to some reference peak. For in vivo applications, the reference peak is commonly chosen to be the water resonance in ^{1}H spectroscopic studies, and the phosphocreatine resonance in ^{31}P studies of tissues, such as muscle, that have a detectable amount of this high-energy substrate. Because the separation between the peaks in a given spectrum increases linearly with the strength of the static magnetic field, the chemical shifts of the spectral peaks in direct frequency units of Hz would require one to specify the static field strength at which the spectrum was acquired. To remove the field-strength dependence of the chemical shifts of the spectral peaks, the shifts are most often reported in terms of parts-per-million (ppm) defined by

$$\delta = \frac{v_{\text{peak}} - v_{\text{reference}}}{v_{\text{reference}}},\qquad 4.3$$

for which v_{peak} and $v_{\text{reference}}$ are the resonance frequencies of the peak of interest and the reference peak, respectively. Defined in this manner, δ is independent of the field strength at which the spectrum was obtained.

Localization

A chemical spectrum from a sample or patient can be obtained by a simple one-dimensional (1D) Fourier transformation of the free-induction decay (FID) that follows a single 90° pulse (see Chap. 3). However, for in vivo spectral data to have any significance, the region from which the spectrum was obtained must be known. Therefore, a localization technique must be utilized that satisfies several basic criteria. First, it should be image based, such that the volume of interest (VOI) from which the spectra are acquired can be selected on a standard MR image. Second, it should be possible to locate the VOI anywhere within the field-of-view of the image while retain-

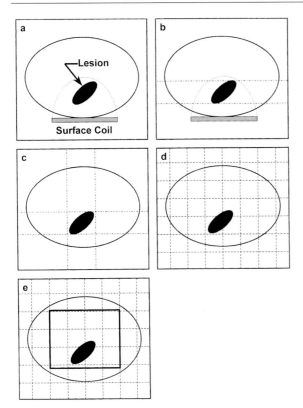

Fig. 4.1a–e. Schematic representations of various techniques of volume localization for in vivo magnetic resonance spectroscopy (MRS) studies. **a** Surface-coil localization. **b** Depth-resolved surface-coil spectroscopy (DRESS) localization. **c** Single-voxel (SV) localization. **d** Spectroscopic imaging (SI) localization. **e** Hybrid SV-SI localization

scribed in Fig. 4.1. The most basic localization technique is the use of a surface coil to define the VOI (Fig. 4.1a). The primary disadvantages of such surface-coil localization methods are the restricted freedom in positioning the VOI within the field-of-view and the rather poorly defined localized volume. The poor localization quality of such a simple technique can be improved by the addition of a slice-selective gradient/RF pulse combination that selects a slice parallel to the plane of the surface coil. The localized volume is then determined by the slice thickness in one direction and by the sensitive volume of the surface coil in the other two directions (Fig. 4.1b). Disadvantages of this technique, typified by the depth-resolved surface-coil spectroscopy (DRESS) sequence [4], are the limited freedom in positioning the VOI and the fact that the localized volume is still rather poorly defined.

To escape the limitations of the surface-coil localization techniques, true image-based techniques were developed that utilize three-dimensional (3D) localization schemes. These techniques can be divided into two basic categories: single-voxel (SV) and spectroscopic-imaging (SI) techniques. In SV techniques, the spectral data are acquired from one VOI at a time, typically by applying three orthogonal slice-selective gradient/RF pulse combinations to define three slabs, the intersection of which defines the VOI (Fig. 4.1c). However, SI techniques (Fig. 4.1d) acquire spectra from a number of VOIs simultaneously [5, 6]. A clear advantage of SV techniques is the ability to optimize the magnetic-field homogeneity within the selected VOI. As the magnetic-field homogeneity is improved, so is the spectral resolution and, in the case of ^{1}H MRS, the degree of water suppression.

Water-Suppression Techniques

While there are numerous techniques for accomplishing the water suppression required for ^{1}H MRS [7], the most commonly utilized technique for in vivo MRS is the application of multiple saturation pulses. These pulses, shown generically in Fig. 4.2, are indicated by WS1–WS3 on all subsequent pulse-sequence diagrams and are most commonly known as chemical shift-selective (CHESS) pulses [8, 9]. They are narrow bandwidth pulses (typically ~50 Hz) that selectively saturate the water resonance in ^{1}H MRS studies. If the water proton magnetization is saturated by these pulses, and the subsequent localization sequence results in the application of an odd number of multiple 90° pulses to the water protons,

ing high-quality localization. Third, to facilitate optimization of the magnetic-field homogeneity within the VOI, it should be possible to obtain a spectrum from the VOI in a single acquisition by automated or interactive shimming, i.e., adjustment of the currents in the magnetic-field correction coils and/or linear gradient coils. Finally, for patient safety and comfort, the localization technique should deposit as little RF power as possible and should require minimal setup and acquisition times. The goal of maintaining short acquisition times is also critical to minimize the deleterious effects of voluntary and/or involuntary patient motion on the spectral quality. In addition to these general requirements, there are also some nucleus-specific requirements. For example, in ^{1}H MRS studies, it is necessary to have a robust and efficient water suppression scheme to detect signals from metabolites of interest that have concentrations approximately 10,000 times less than the concentration of water.

Several localization techniques have been used for in vivo MRS [3] and fall into the classes de-

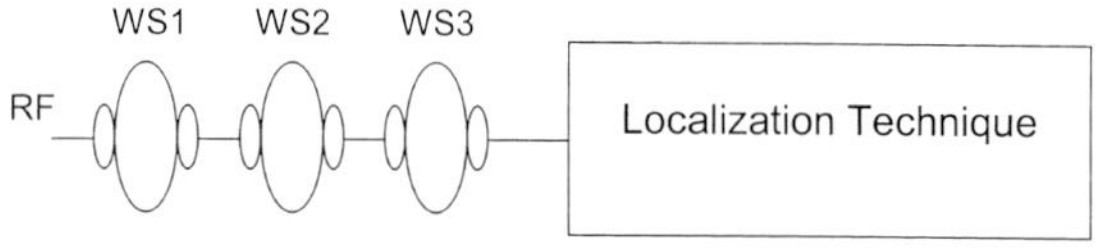

Fig. 4.2. Schematic representation of the basic chemical shift-selective (CHESS) water-suppression technique. *WS1–WS3* are the water-suppression pulses

the water proton magnetization will be in the longitudinal direction during data acquisition and will not be detected. However, the frequency-selective nature of the saturation pulses means that the magnetization due to protons with resonant frequencies that differ from the resonant frequency of water will be minimally affected. This is quite similar to the chem-sat pulse used for suppressing fat in MRI (as discussed in Chap. 3).

The use of three saturation pulses is necessary in the case of in vivo MRS to increase the degree of water-signal suppression. Also, the amplitudes of the three CHESS pulses are not typically chosen to yield exact 90° pulses, but, instead, to result in flip angles (α) greater than or equal to 90°, with $\alpha_{WS1} \geq \alpha_{WS2} \geq \alpha_{WS3}$. The choice of flip angles depends on the T_1 relaxation times of the water signals that are to be suppressed [10]. In addition, each CHESS pulse is followed by a spoiler gradient pulse to destroy the phase coherence of the spins excited by the water suppression pulse, such that no unwanted, non-localized signals arising from the multiple CHESS pulses contribute to the detected echo. The choice of the spoiler gradient amplitudes cannot be made arbitrarily, or unwanted refocusing may occur [11]. With the appropriate flip angles of the CHESS pulses and spoiler-gradient amplitudes, water-suppression factors of 1000 or greater can be obtained in vivo, and are sufficient to allow spectral peaks from several metabolites of interest to be observed.

SV Localization Techniques

For ^{1}H MRS studies, the most commonly used SV techniques are variants of the stimulated-echo acquisition-mode (STEAM) sequence [12–14] and the point-resolved spectroscopy (PRESS) sequence [15]. Both of these sequences have all the characteristics of ideal localization techniques outlined above. For ^{31}P MRS studies, which require minimal T_2-weighting due to the short apparent T_2 relaxation times of the ATP resonances, the image-selected in vivo spectroscopy (ISIS) technique [16] has been commonly used.

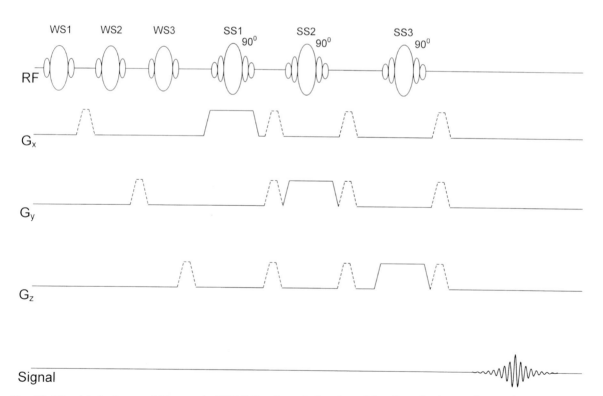

Fig. 4.3. Stimulated-echo acquisition-mode (STEAM) pulse sequence. The *dotted lines* represent spoiler-gradient pulses that are used to destroy any unwanted phase coherences. Refocusing of the slice selection gradient pulses is incorporated with the spoiler gradients

STEAM Sequences

A generic STEAM pulse sequence incorporating water-suppression pulses is shown in Fig. 4.3. There are three orthogonal slice-selecting gradient/RF pulse combinations (SS1–SS3), each acting identically to the slice-selection pulses in an MR imaging sequence (see Chap. 3). The localized VOI is at the intersection of the three orthogonal slices (Fig. 4.1c). The volume of the selected VOI can be set by adjustment of the individual slice thicknesses, and the position of the VOI can be set by appropriate selection of the offset frequencies of the three RF pulses. The three pulses labeled WS1–WS3 are used for suppressing the water signal, as discussed above.

While the slice-selective pulses do generate the desired signal localized to the VOI, it can be shown that three RF pulses actually give rise to a maximum of five echoes [17]. However, in STEAM MRS, only one of the echoes is localized to the VOI, while the others arise from columns of spins rather than from the well-defined 3D VOI. To insure that the unwanted echoes containing information from spins outside the VOI are not detected, spoiler-gradient pulses are applied following each slice-selective RF/gradient pulse (Fig. 4.3). The spoilers destroy unwanted coherences that would otherwise arise from spins outside the VOI and degrade the localization and spectral quality [12, 14, 18]. In addition, if eight or more signal averages are required for adequate signal-to-noise ratio, appropriate phase cycling of the RF pulses and receiver during data acquisition also suppresses the signal from non-localized spins [17]. The high quality of localization obtained with STEAM has made it one of the most frequently utilized SV techniques, despite the fact that only half the available signal from the VOI is obtained in the stimulated echo; the remaining available signal is distributed among the other two- and three-pulse echoes that are not localized completely in the VOI.

PRESS Sequence

A generic PRESS pulse sequence is shown in Fig. 4.4. The sequence differs from the STEAM sequence primarily by the fact that PRESS acquires a localized spin-echo, whereas STEAM acquires a localized stimulated-echo. The primary advantage of PRESS compared with STEAM is the fact that

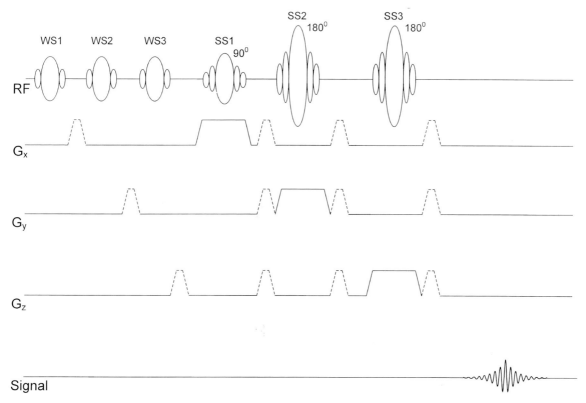

Fig. 4.4. Point-resolved spectroscopy (PRESS) pulse sequence. The *dotted lines* represent spoiler-gradient pulses that are used to destroy any unwanted phase coherences. Refocusing of the slice selection gradient pulses is incorporated with the spoiler gradients

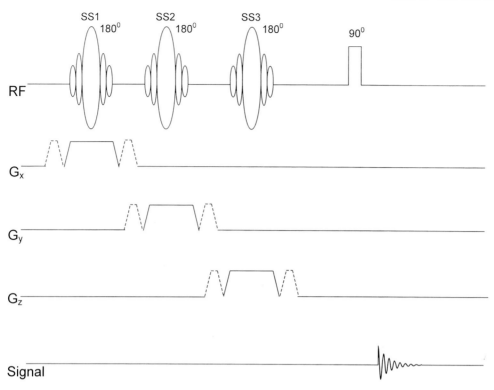

Fig. 4.5. Image-selected in vivo spectroscopy (ISIS) pulse sequence using a FID detection scheme (single 90° readout pulse). The *dotted lines* represent spoiler gradient pulses that are used to destroy any unwanted phase coherences

all available signal from the localized VOI is detected in the form of the spin-echo using PRESS, whereas only 50% of the available signal is detected in the form of the stimulated-echo using STEAM. The primary disadvantage of PRESS relative to STEAM is the lengthened minimum echo time. This can be an important limitation if the metabolites of interest have short T_2 relaxation times. Also, due to the nonlinearity of the spin-system response to the RF pulses, it is more difficult to achieve well-defined slice profiles using 180° slice-selective pulses compared with the 90° slice-selective pulses utilized in the STEAM sequence. More recent designer RF pulses [19], however, have significantly improved the 180° slice-selective pulse profiles.

■ ISIS Sequence

The ISIS pulse-sequence timing diagram is given in Fig. 4.5. There are three slice-selective 180° pulses that are used to localize the VOI, and a 90° pulse (or 90°–180° SE pulse pair) is used to generate the detected transverse magnetization. ISIS does not localize the detected signal to a VOI in a single acquisition, but requires the application of eight unique combinations of the RF and gradient pulses [16]. When the FIDs or echoes from each of these eight combinations are combined appropriately, the signal arising from the VOI is obtained. Therefore, in terms of the characteristics of an ideal localization scheme given above, the ISIS technique is not ideal since it is not a single-shot technique. Because of this, the magnetic-field homogeneity cannot easily be optimized in the VOI by manual shimming of the field. Also, ISIS utilizes subtraction techniques to eliminate the signal from regions outside the VOI. Such subtraction techniques do not efficiently utilize the dynamic range of the MR scanner, and are notoriously unstable if there are instabilities in the MR scanner electronics or if the patient moves.

Despite all of these disadvantages relative to STEAM and PRESS, ISIS does have one distinct advantage: there is very minimal T_2-weighting of the spectra, since magnetization during the localization portion of the sequence is always along the longitudinal direction. This advantage makes ISIS a useful sequence for studies of biochemicals that have resonance peaks corresponding to short T_2 species or species with significant J-coupling modulation, such as the α-, β-, and γ-components of adenosine triphosphate (ATP). Therefore, ISIS is fairly commonly used for in vivo ^{31}P MRS studies, but not for ^1H studies.

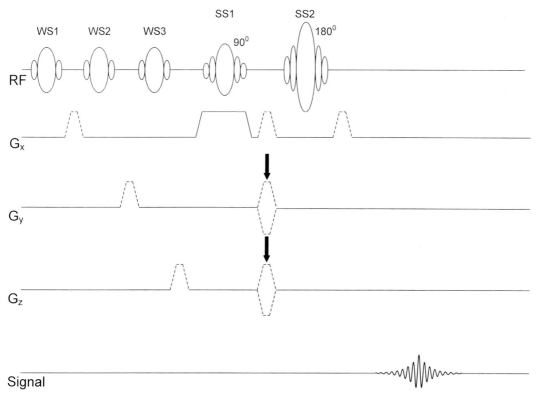

Fig. 4.6. Two-dimensional spectroscopic imaging (SI) pulse sequence. The *arrows* indicate the phase-encoding gradients used to encode the in-plane spatial information. The other *dashed* gradient pulses are spoiler pulses, and refocusing of the slice selection gradient pulse is incorporated with the spoiler gradients. Three-dimensional spectroscopic imaging (SI) sequences are also available in which the slice-selective gradient is not used but rather a third phase-encoding gradient is used as a slice-encoding gradient

Spectroscopic Imaging Techniques

A generic two-dimensional spectroscopic imaging (2D SI) sequence is shown in Fig. 4.6. The 2D SI sequence first uses a slice-selection RF pulse/gradient combination to define the plane of interest. Localization within the plane is then accomplished using phase encoding in a manner that is analogous to phase encoding in 2D imaging (Chap. 3). With this technique, spectra from a number of contiguous VOIs can be acquired simultaneously. This, is a major advantage for in vivo MRS studies, since it allows for the assessment of lesion heterogeneity and, where possible, for the comparison of spectral findings from a lesion with those obtained from contralateral normal-appearing regions. Another advantage is in the acquisition of spectral data from small VOIs. This is primarily due to the phase-encoding localization of the VOIs, compared with the slice-selection localization of the VOI in STEAM, PRESS, and ISIS. Using SV techniques, small voxels are obtained by increasing the amplitude of the slice-selection gradient pulse or by increasing the duration of the gradient/RF pulse combination (and hence, decreasing the RF pulse bandwidth and increasing the area of the gradient pulse). Since increasing the length of the pulses comes at the cost of increased minimum echo time for STEAM and PRESS, the choice is usually made to increase the gradient-pulse amplitude. Large amplitude, rapidly switched gradient fields, however, are associated with the generation of significant eddy currents.

The time-varying magnetic fields induced by eddy currents result in distortions of the ideal gradient fields. The eddy current fields can also be of long enough duration that they result in distortions of the FID or echo signals, and these distortions cannot be easily corrected. However, obtaining small voxel dimensions using phase-encoding techniques, such as those utilized in SI, does not require such large gradient-pulse amplitudes. Therefore, while the typical voxel volumes in SV localization are on the order of 1–10 cm^3, volumes of 0.125 cm^3 or less can be achieved using SI localization, and 1-cm^3 voxel volumes are fairly common.

Another primary advantage of SI- over SV techniques is the ability to reconstruct low-resolution images from the spectral data in which the pixel intensity is proportional to the relative concentrations of the metabolites of interest. Typically, the relative concentration in each voxel is determined by integrating the area under the peak of interest. Such metabolic maps, or met-maps, are quite useful in visually assessing spatial variation in the metabolite concentrations. However, their quality depends strongly on the accuracy of the integration of peak areas, so care should be taken in selecting the limits of integration. In general, while the met-maps provide a quick means of assessing the spatial variations in concentration, the individual spectra should also be inspected, particularly in areas on the met-map that show significant changes in relative concentration (see below).

Disadvantages of SI techniques relative to SV techniques include difficulty in shimming the magnetic field over a large volume of tissue, typically long acquisition times, and the possibility of significant spectral bleed from one voxel to its neighbors [20–22]. The first of these disadvantages is typically the most significant, since inadequate field homogeneity will result in poor resolution of the spectral peaks and unacceptable water suppression. However, the long acquisition times, commonly 15–30 min for ^{1}H 2D SI studies, are also a significant problem, since patient motion during the MRS acquisition will have a deleterious, and uncorrectable, effect on the quality of the spectra. With the recent advances in echo-planar imaging-compatible MR scanners, however, EPI-based SI [23] could dramatically decrease the imaging acquisition times and potentially eliminate this disadvantage relative to SV localization.

The spectral bleed artifacts are also important to consider when acquiring SI MRS data. The result of intervoxel spectral bleed is contamination of the spectrum from a given voxel by the spectral components in neighboring voxels. For example, this can be quite serious in ^{1}H MRS studies of human brain, in which large-amplitude lipid signals from the skull can contaminate voxels located within the brain parenchyma. The false lipid peaks due to the spectral bleed appear in the same chemical-shift range as lactate and true lipid peaks, and can give rise to misleading results. The origin of the spectral-bleed phenomenon is the same as the truncation artifact in MRI; there is insufficient sampling of the k-space data in the phase-encoding directions. The effects are decreased as the number of phase-encoding steps increases, but at the cost of increased scan time and decreased voxel size. Fortunately, the effects can also be reduced during processing of the spectral data (discussed below).

Hybrid SI-SV Methods

In an effort to capitalize upon the advantages of both SI and SV localization methods, while decreasing the impact of the disadvantages of either method, a very common approach to acquiring in vivo MRS data combines SV and SI sequences. The basic idea behind such a hybrid technique is illustrated in Fig. 4.1e. An SV technique is used to localize a relatively large, but well-localized VOI, and phase-encoding gradients are used to subdivide the large VOI into smaller voxels. The advantage of SI localization in obtaining spectra from multiple voxels is retained, while the use of the SV technique to preselect the large VOI greatly minimizes spectral bleed contamination from outside lipid signals. It also allows for improved shimming, with the concomitant improvement in spectral resolution and water suppression. A hybrid SI-SV pulse sequence based on the STEAM SV sequence is shown in Fig. 4.7, and a metabolic map obtained in normal human brain using this technique is shown in Fig. 4.8.

As an alternative to the use of an SV technique to preselect a VOI in order to minimize spectral bleed, multiple spatial saturation bands (see Chap. 3) can be used to saturate the lipid signals outside the true region of interest immediately prior to the application of the SI sequence. This method of outer volume suppression [24–27] tailors the definition of the VOI that will subsequently be subdivided into SI-encoded voxels, i.e., by using multiple spatial saturation bands applied at various angles, the lipid protons in the skull can be suppressed while allowing spectra to be acquired from nearly all of the brain parenchyma.

Spectral Processing

The application of any of the above localization techniques results in one (SV) or more (SI or hybrid SI-SV) averaged echo signals that are typically transformed from the time domain to the frequency domain via Fourier analysis. However, there are several additional steps involved in the actual processing of the raw time-domain data. First, as the MRS data is usually acquired in quadrature, the real and imaginary channels are typically baseline-corrected for any DC offset in the gains of the two data acquisition channels. Also, if the resulting spectra have very broad components that distort the baseline, e.g., residual

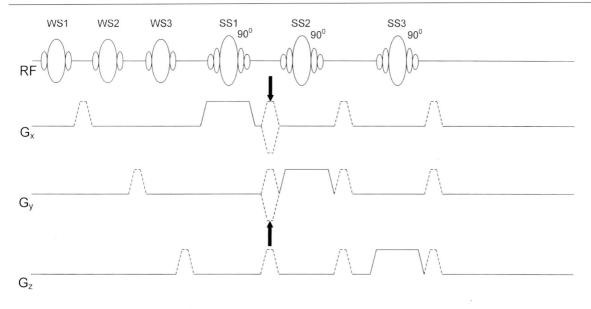

Fig. 4.7. Hybrid spectroscopic imaging (SI)-single-voxel (SV) pulse sequence that combines the stimulated-echo acquisition-mode (STEAM) SV localization of a large volume-of-interest (VOI) and a 2-dimensional SI technique to subdivide the large VOI into smaller voxels. The *arrows* indicate the phase-encoding gradient pulses. The other *dashed* gradient pulses are spoiler pulses, and refocusing of the slice selection gradient pulses is incorporated with the spoiler gradients

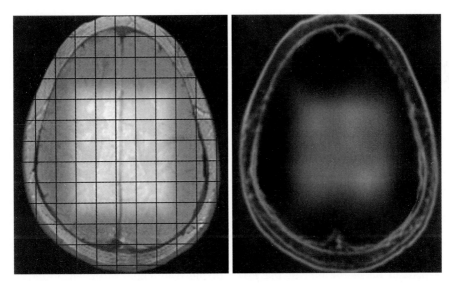

Fig. 4.8. Application of the hybrid spectroscopic imaging (SI)-single-voxel (SV) technique in a normal human brain. The proton density-weighted image with highlighted SV volume-of-interest (VOI) and 2-dimensional SI grid is shown on the *left*. The N-acetylaspartate met-map image is shown on the *right* as an overlay on the outline of the skull

water resonance in ^{1}H spectra or broad resonances in the phosphodiester region of ^{31}P spectra, techniques such as convolution difference processing can improve the baseline quality [28–31].

Following baseline correction, it is not uncommon to apply apodization filters to the time-domain data. These filters are used to improve the spectral resolution of the resulting spectral peaks (line-narrowing filters) and/or improve the signal-

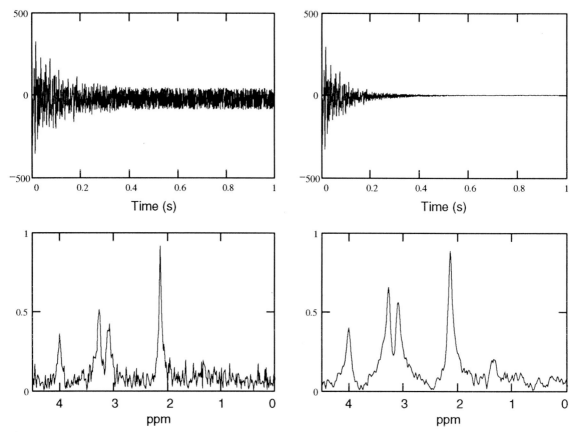

Fig. 4.9. Simulated FID (*top left*), spectrum (*bottom left*), apodized FID (*top right*), and apodized spectrum (*bottom right*). The simulated spectrum is modeled after a spectrum of normal human brain with resonances from total creatine (3.0 and 4.0 ppm), choline (3.2 ppm), N-acetylaspartate (2.0 ppm), and lipids/lactate (1.3 ppm). The apodization function was a decreasing exponential with 5 Hz line-broadening. Notice the significant improvement in signal-to-noise ratio in the filtered spectrum allows the visualization of the peak at 1.3 ppm, which is not easily visualized in the unfiltered spectrum. However, the increase in signal-to-noise ratio is associated with a noticeable decrease in spectral resolution in the filtered spectrum

to-noise ratio of the spectra (line-broadening filters). Common apodization filters include decreasing exponential, Hamming, or Fermi functions to improve signal-to-noise ratio, and increasing exponential, and shifted Gaussian, sine (sine-bell), or sine-squared filters to improve spectral resolution (Fig. 4.9) [29, 32, 33]. Additionally, the resolution of the spectra can be improved by zero filling the time-domain data, e.g., if 2048 data points are acquired in a FID, then 2048 zeros are padded on to the end of the FID before the FT is applied. Because zero filling in the time domain corresponds to interpolation in the frequency domain, this procedure results in an apparent improvement in the resolution of the resulting spectra. Although such apodization filters and interpolation techniques may provide pleasing visual improvements to the spectra, the user should fully understand the side-effects of their application, particularly since many of the filters result in highly non-linear distortions of the spectral peaks as a function of resonance frequency.

Following baseline correction and apodization, the time-domain spectral data are Fourier transformed. In the case of the SV acquisitions, a simple 1D FT is all that is necessary. In the case of SI acquisitions, however, multiple FTs are required. For example, for the 2D SI acquisition illustrated in Fig. 4.1e, three FTs are required: one for each of the two spatial phase-encoding directions, and one for the time-dimension (analogous to SV spectral processing). As a final step in the generation of spectra from the time-domain data, the mode of displaying the spectra must be chosen. Most simply, the real and imaginary data can be combined in quadrature to yield magnitude spectra, but this inevitably leads to broadening of the spectral peaks due to the combination of the absorption and dispersion components of the MR

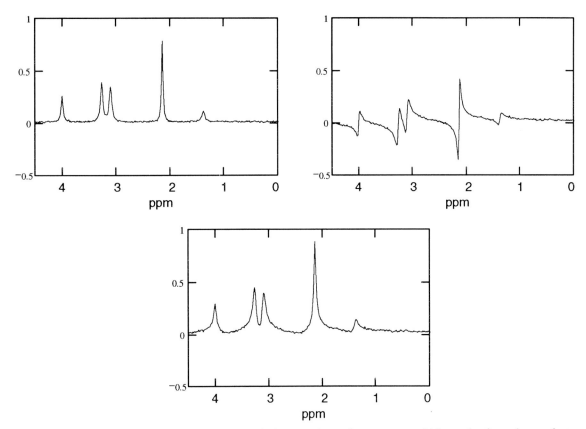

Fig. 4.10. Absorption mode (*top left*), dispersion mode (*top right*), and magnitude mode (*bottom*) simulated brain spectra. Notice the degraded spectral resolution in the magnitude mode spectrum, which results from the quadrature combination of the absorption and dispersion modes, relative to the absorption mode spectrum

signal (Fig. 4.10). Instead of accepting the broadened spectral peaks of the magnitude spectrum, one could display either the real or imaginary component of the spectrum, but, in general, both of these components have distorted spectral peaks that represent neither pure absorption nor pure dispersion. The mixture of the absorption and dispersion terms is a result of phase shifts due primarily to inevitable imperfections in the components of the receiver chain and/or unavoidable delays in the initiation of the digital data acquisition (Fig. 4.11) [29, 33]. Fortunately, such linear phase effects can be corrected. Typically this is done by interactively – or better, automatically – determining the necessary zeroth-order (frequency-independent) and first-order (linearly frequency-dependent) phase-correction terms, and applying them to the data following application of the FT. This yields pure absorption spectra in the real channel of the data [29] and results in spectra with maximum resolution possible within the limits of the magnetic-field homogeneity of the VOI.

Spectral Quantification

Having acquired the localized time-domain data and transformed it into spectral information, the next decision is how to interpret the results. In order of increasing complexity, the most common approaches to spectral quantification are to: (1) visually assess the spectral peaks, (2) compute the relative spectral peak heights, (3) compute the relative spectral peak areas, and (4) compute the absolute metabolite concentrations, based on the peak areas. Option 1 provides little information beyond the assessment of the presence or absence of a particular metabolite, or of a substantial decrease or increase in metabolite concentrations.

Option 2 is more quantitative, but unless extreme care is taken, peak height measurements can be very misleading when comparing multiple spectra. The difficulty with peak height calculations is that the peak height depends on, among other things, the spin-spin relaxation time, which varies from metabolite to metabolite, and the field homogeneity, which typically varies from scan-to-

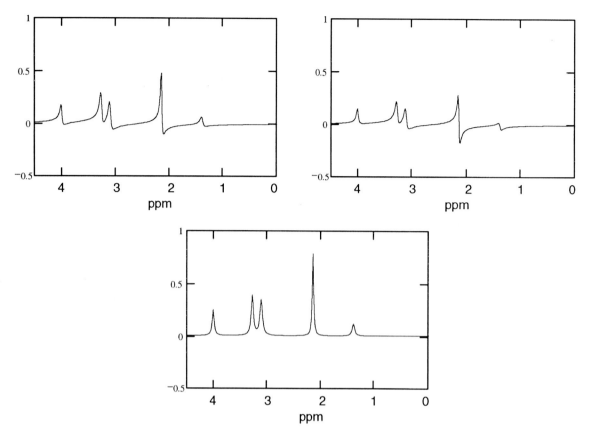

Fig. 4.11. Effects of zero-order (*top left*) and first-order (*top right*) phase shifts on the spectral peaks. The absorption mode spectrum is shown in the *bottom* panel for reference. Notice the zero-order phase distortions of the spectral peaks are independent of frequency, i.e., each peak is similarly distorted. The effects of the first-order phase distortions increase with respect to the frequency offset relative to the resonant frequency of water (4.76 ppm), i.e., the phase distortion of the peak at 4.0 ppm is minimal, while the distortion of the peaks at 2.0 ppm and 1.3 ppm are much more severe. Ideally, appropriate zero- and first-order corrections can be performed to transform the unphased spectra to pure absorption mode spectra

scan (in SV and SI studies) or from voxel-to-voxel (even in a given SI study). This problem is minimized if the spectra are analyzed using option 3, since the peak areas for a given concentration (and acquisition parameters, TE and TR) are independent of the field homogeneity (provided that the resulting spectral resolution is adequate to allow the peaks to be resolved). A problem with both peak height and peak area calculations, however, is that both of these measures will depend on many acquisition parameters, including the TE, TR, number of signal averages, and voxel size.

Of all the options for spectral analysis, option 4 is preferred, since it measures the actual metabolite concentrations independently of the data acquisition parameters. It is, however, the most difficult option, since some reference standard must be used to allow for the calculation of the absolute concentrations. Investigators seeking to obtain absolute concentrations have typically used either an external standard [18, 34–38], such as a vial of known concentration of a standard reagent in the field-of-view, or an internal standard [39–42], such as the assumed concentration of water in the tissue occupying the VOI.

Both means of obtaining the standard reference are fraught with difficulties, and the relative strengths and weaknesses of each have been recently reviewed [43]. For example, the external standard is typically in a location far removed from the VOI, and the magnetic and radiofrequency field homogeneities in such an area are typically significantly different from those in the VOI. If the radiofrequency field homogeneity is poorer in the area of the reference standard, the signal intensity obtained from the sample will be distorted and the absolute measures will be incorrect.

In the case of the internal water-concentration reference method, changes in the assumed normal tissue water concentration due to, for example, large amounts of edema, can lead to inaccurate absolute concentration measurements. Therefore, a very common approach to quantification, which seeks to minimize the dependence of the peak areas or heights on data-acquisition parameters, is to report ratios of peak areas or of peak heights with respect to a chosen standard reference peak. However, care must still be taken in interpreting the results, as changes in the area or height of either spectral peak used in the calculation can change the resulting ratio. Furthermore, the concentrations of some metabolites throughout the brain show regional variations, whereas others are relatively constant (discussed below). This finding reinforces the need for interpreting peak area (or height) ratio values with care.

Finally, it is important to remember that T_1 and T_2 relaxation times vary among the metabolites of interest. Therefore, when comparing peak areas, heights, or even ratios to values in the literature or from previously acquired spectra, it is imperative to remember that individual peak areas and heights change with the TE and TR values used during data acquisition. As a result, comparisons between spectra acquired with differing TE and/or TR times should be performed with caution, and, if there are differences, the peak areas, heights, or ratios must be corrected using known T_1 and T_2 relaxation times of the various metabolites.

Regardless of the technique used to acquire the MRS data or the spectral processing and quantification methodologies used, the reproducibility of MRS results should be carefully validated. Such validation is particularly important if the studies involve longitudinal follow-up scans in a given disease state, or, for example, if they acquire spectra from MRS-difficult regions near sources of local magnetic-field inhomogeneities, such as in areas near the skull base (such as the hippocampus). Because both acquisition and processing variations can affect the quantitative results, reproducibility studies are important for a given site [22, 44] or for multicenter trials [45]. In an effort to provide a common platform for data acquisition and processing of in vivo ^{1}H brain spectra, one vendor has released a Food and Drug Administration (FDA)-approved pulse sequence and spectral processing package known as proton brain exam (PROBE)/SV [45, 46]. The user of PROBE has a choice between STEAM or PRESS localization, and the package incorporates automatic shimming on the VOI and automatic optimization of the water-suppression pulse amplitudes. The spectral processing incorporates residual water peak suppression and resolution-enhancement filters [28, 45], and reports the peak height ratios of N-acetylaspartate (NAA), choline and myo-inositol, with respect to creatine (see below).

Finally, the voxel sizes in in vivo MRS studies are typically rather large and contain a mixture of tissue types. For example, in an MRS exam of intracranial lesions, a voxel may contain a mixture of lesion, white matter, gray matter, and cerebrospinal fluid. This makes comparisons difficult if the relative concentrations of the metabolites are not corrected for the heterogeneous distribution of tissues within the voxel. Several investigators have sought to address this issue by utilizing automated or manual image segmentation techniques to determine the percentage of each tissue in a given voxel and then to correct the relative peak area ratios or heights based on these determinations [47–49].

Clinical Applications of In Vivo MRS

In vivo clinical MRS has a rather long history, nearly as long a clinical MRI. Several review articles and texts have been published that discuss applications of MRS to a variety of normal and pathological conditions [29, 50–60], and the applications presented below were chosen to address more recent studies and those specific to oncology.

^{1}H MRS Studies

Central Nervous System

As a basic consideration for the applications of in vivo MRS to oncology, Fig. 4.12 shows a water-suppressed ^{1}H spectrum acquired from a normal human brain using a STEAM localization sequence. In general, resonances from myo-inositol, total creatine (creatine and phosphocreatine), choline, and NAA are clearly resolved in normal brain spectra acquired at 1.5 T; other, weaker, resonances can also be observed.

The dominant peak at ~2.0 ppm in ^{1}H MR spectra from normal brain is due to NAA. Although the exact biochemical role of NAA has not been fully elucidated [61], it is abundant only in viable mature neurons, and has been widely used as an indicator of neuronal integrity. The concentration of NAA increases during the development of the normal neonate [62, 63] and reaches a concentration of approximately 8–12 mM in adults [18, 38]. In general, most disease processes, including neoplasms [40, 47, 59, 64–80], strokes [81–90], multiple sclerosis [39, 91–

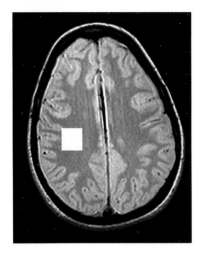 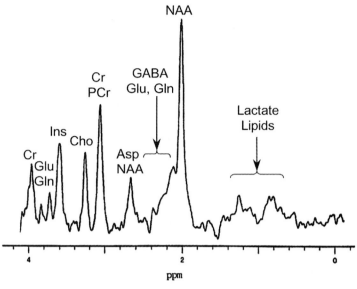

Fig. 4.12. A water-suppressed ¹H spectrum acquired from the highlighted volume in the image of a normal human brain. The spectrum was acquired from a 2×2×2-cm volume-of-interest using the stimulated-echo acquisition mode (STEAM) localization sequence with echo time =20 ms, repetition time =3000 ms, mixing time =7.7 ms. *NAA* N-acetylaspartate; *Cr* creatine; *PCr* phosphocreatine; *Cho* choline compounds; *Glu* glutamate; *Gln* glutamine; *Ins* myo-inositol; *Asp* aspartate; *GABA* γ-aminobutyric acid

99], epilepsy [100–108], dementias [109–113], schizophrenia [114], diabetes mellitus [115], and human immunodeficiency virus (HIV) [116] result in decreased levels of NAA. An increase in NAA compared with controls has been reported only in Canavan's disease [55, 58]. The spatial distributions of NAA and other metabolites have been investigated using both SV and SI techniques [36, 38, 48, 49, 73, 117–120]. NAA, in particular, has been shown to vary depending on tissue type (white versus gray matter) and location within the cranium. Finally, it should be noted that the NAA peak includes contributions from *N*-acetylaspartylglutamate (NAAG) at ~2.05 ppm [55, 58].

The next most prominent spectral peaks in the normal brain spectrum are from total creatine and choline-containing compounds. The total creatine peak at 3.0 ppm has components from creatine and phosphocreatine (PCr). The choline peak at 3.2 ppm has components from compounds associated with membrane synthesis and breakdown, such as phosphorylcholine and glycerophosphorylcholine. Elevated choline levels have been reported in many neoplasms [46, 47, 64, 66, 69, 71, 73, 75, 76, 80, 121–123] and in diabetes mellitus [115]. The most probable explanation for the increase in choline levels in focal and inflammatory processes is the production of choline-containing breakdown products of myelin, but other possible mechanisms have not been fully investigated at this time. Decreased choline levels have been reported in disease states such as hepatic encephalopathy [124, 125] and chronic hyponatremia [126]. Levels of creatine, typically present at concentrations of ~10 mM in normal brain, have been shown to decrease in some neoplasms [46, 47, 64, 69, 71, 73, 75, 76, 80, 123] and in stroke [81, 82, 87, 89, 127, 128].

Even though myelin is rich in lipids, the rigid structure of these lipids makes them MRS invisible in normal brain parenchyma. However, measurable lipid levels have been reported in certain disease states, such as some, but not all, neoplasms [26, 46, 47, 64, 69, 129] and multiple sclerosis lesions [26, 94, 97, 99, 130–132]. It is believed that the lipids and other macromolecules observed in these cases are due to the release of MR-visible lipids and other membrane breakdown products when the normally rigid myelin structure is disrupted. The signals from the lipids and other membrane breakdown products are seen only at short echo times because of their relatively short spin-spin relaxation times and significant J-modulation. Because extracranial lipid signals can contaminate the localized VOI due to poor localization quality or, in the case of SI techniques, due to spectral bleed, one must interpret such signals with care, particularly if the voxel showing significant lipid signals is near the skull.

Lactate is typically maintained at very low levels in the normal brain (<0.5 mM) and is not detected using ¹H MRS. However, in certain patho-

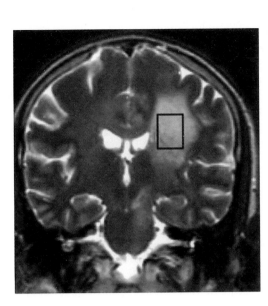
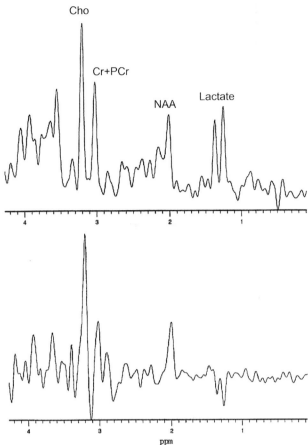

Fig. 4.13. Spectrum acquired using PROBE/single-voxel from the volume-of-interest indicated in the image from a patient with a glioblastoma multiforme. The *top spectrum* was acquired using stimulated-echo acquisition mode (STEAM) with echo time (TE)/mixing time (TM)/repetition time (TR)=30/13.7/2000 ms, while the *bottom spectrum* was acquired using point-resolved spectroscopy (PRESS) with TE/TR=135/2000 ms. Note the inverted lactate doublet in the spectrum acquired with TE=135 ms

logical conditions, such as some, but not all, neoplasms [46, 47, 66–68, 71, 73–77, 133–135], stroke [81–90], and hypoxia/anoxia [55], a doublet resonance from the methyl protons can be observed at 1.35 ppm. A potential difficulty with lactate detection, however, lies in the fact that lactate methyl protons and methylene lipid protons resonate at similar frequencies and can have overlapping peaks. This makes it difficult, if not impossible, to determine whether peaks around 1.3 ppm are due to elevated lactate or lipids.

One common technique used to distinguish lactate from lipids is to acquire spectra at appropriately chosen short and long echo times. The short echo-time spectrum will provide information regarding the lipid and lactate levels, while a judicious choice of longer echo time (~135 ms for 1.5-T systems) will selectively invert the lactate doublet and greatly decrease the contribution of lipid signals, which have short spin-spin relaxation times. An example of this technique is shown in Fig. 4.13.

Other resonances from myo-inositol (3.58 ppm, with additional contributions from inositol monophosphates and glycine), glucose (3.43 and 3.80 ppm), γ-aminobutyric acid (GABA), glutamate/glutamine (2.1–2.5 ppm), and from alanine (doublet at 1.47 ppm) and other amino acids have also been reported [55, 58]. Quantitation of peaks closer to the residual water peak than choline have, until more recently, been exceedingly difficult because of insufficient water suppression. However, improvements in automated field-homogeneity corrections and water-suppression optimization have made quantitative analysis of several peaks in this region possible. Biochemicals with spectral peaks in this region include myo-inositol, glucose, and additional signals from creatine and glutamate/glutamine [55]. Elevated myo-inositol levels have been reported in Alzheimer's dementia

[110–112], in Down's syndrome dementia [113], and in diabetes mellitus [115]. Decreased myo-inositol levels have been reported in some neoplasms [55] and in hepatic encephalopathy [28, 55, 124, 136]. Elevated levels of glutamate/glutamine have also been reported in cases of hepatic encephalopathy [28, 55, 124, 136]. However, because of the large number of overlapping peaks in the glutamate/glutamine region of the spectrum, absolute quantitation is exceedingly difficult without sophisticated spectral editing techniques [137]. Similarly, spectral editing techniques are required for the detection of GABA [138–140] and have been utilized, for example, to monitor the treatment of epilepsy using gabapentin and vigabatrin [141, 142].

In general, the most consistent findings of ^{1}H MRS studies of intracranial neoplasms is that choline levels are elevated, NAA levels are decreased, creatine levels are decreased, lactate may or may not be present, and lipids and other membrane breakdown products may or may not be present. In a multicenter study of 86 brain tumor cases using PRESS localization with TE=135 ms (to allow spectral editing of lactate), Negendank et al. [47] found that choline levels were highest in astrocytomas and anaplastic astrocytomas, creatine levels were lowest in glioblastomas, and NAA levels were decreased in all three tumor grades. However, there was considerable overlap of metabolite levels between the tumor grades, which led the authors to conclude that "the resulting overlaps precluded diagnostic accuracy in the distinction of low- and high-grade tumors". This finding has also been reported in other studies with much smaller numbers of patients. Therefore, it appears that the currently resolved ^{1}H spectral peaks may not be sufficient to allow for diagnostic grading of tumors based solely on the levels of these biochemicals. This conclusion is not surprising, given the degree of heterogeneity found in tumors, particularly those that are large and contain necrotic and active tumor components within the same VOI from which the spectra are acquired. Nevertheless, two groups reported a high specificity of ^{1}H MRS for grading tumor types when more sophisticated pattern recognition [143, 144] or neural network [144, 145] algorithms were applied in the analysis of the spectral peaks. Furthermore, as the spectral resolution improves with the strength of the static magnetic field, the increasing numbers of 3 T and 4 T whole-body scanners may allow for the assessment of additional spectral peaks that are presently insufficiently resolved to allow for quantitative analysis.

Even though the diagnosis of tumor grade might be hampered by the overlap mentioned above, tracking tumor progression or the efficacy of a particular therapeutic modality is possible if the reproducibility of the spectral acquisition and processing techniques are well characterized. For example, there have been reports of the recovery of intratumoral creatine+PCr, choline, and lactate+lipid levels toward normal values during and following radiation therapy [64, 146–148]. However, increased Cho levels have been shown to correlate with malignant degeneration of gliomas [121]. Therefore, in vivo ^{1}H MRS might be useful in the difficult differentiation of tumor recurrence from treatment-related changes. In addition, the effects of radiation therapy on normal brain parenchyma have been reported to include decreased NAA levels without any measurable change in choline or creatine+PCr levels [149, 150]. Therefore, even if the diagnostic accuracy of in vivo ^{1}H MRS is hampered by the suboptimal spectral resolution, and heterogeneity of the tumor yields excessive overlap in the measured levels of the MR-visible metabolites, the evaluation of the efficacy of therapy, the effects of the therapy on normal tissue, and the potential separation of recurrent tumor from treatment-related changes should continue to drive expanded applications of MRS in oncology.

Applications Outside of the Central Nervous System

In general, the ^{1}H spectra acquired from extracranial tissues exhibit relatively few quantifiable spectral peaks, and this has severely limited application outside the central nervous system (CNS). For example, the water-suppressed localized spectrum from human muscle tissue consists primarily of peaks from residual water (~4.7 ppm), choline+carnosine (3.2 ppm), creatine+PCr (3.0 ppm), carnosine (~8 ppm), and lipids (Fig. 4.14). The lipid spectrum itself is rather complex, with resonances due to the following protons: $-CH_3$ (~1.0 ppm), $-CH_2-CH_2-$ (~1.4 ppm), $-CH_2-CH=CH-$ (~2.1 ppm), $=CH=CH-$ (~5.5 ppm). Since the concentrations of water (~45 M) and lipids (~3.5 M in muscle and up to 60 M in adipose tissue and marrow) are quite large relative to the concentrations of other metabolites, either the residual water peak or one or more of the lipid peaks typically masks resonances from other metabolites. Suppression of the lipid resonances using either frequency-selective saturation techniques or inversion recovery techniques usually results in suppression of the signal from many of the metabolites of interest as well.

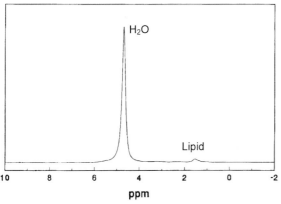
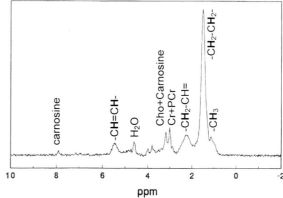

Fig. 4.14. Spectra obtained using stimulated-echo acquisition mode (STEAM) from normal human gastrocnemius muscle without (*left*) and with (*right*) water suppression. In the unsuppressed spectrum, the only peaks are from water (4.76 ppm) and methylene lipids (1.4 ppm). In the water-suppressed spectrum peaks from residual water, choline (Cho)+carnosine, creatine (Cr)+phosphocreatine (PCr), carnosine, and lipids are seen

There have been studies reporting correlations between the muscle lipid levels measured non-invasively with MRS and disease states, such as juvenile dermatomyositis, hypertrophy, other neuromuscular diseases, and exercise-induced changes (see [151] and references therein). In terms of oncological application, some groups have used ^{1}H MRS as a tool to monitor leukemia therapy by observing the lipid level variations in the marrow, and have reported that successful chemotherapy results in a reduction of the water-to-fat ratio in the marrow [152–154]. Lipid signals in bone tumors have also been characterized [155]. Another report summarized the effects of radiation therapy on normal muscle tissue as a dramatic decrease in choline+carnitine and PCr+creatine levels, but only in a single subject [156]. Furthermore, in prostate cancer patients several groups have reported that the level of citrate, which is present in sufficient concentration in the prostate to be detected via in vivo ^{1}H MRS (~70 mM concentration with a multiplet resonance at 2.6 ppm), allows the differentiation between neoplasm and benign prostate hyperplasia (BPH); neoplasms demonstrate consistently lower citrate levels than BPH or normal peripheral zone tissue [157–159]. In general, however, applications of in vivo ^{1}H MRS to oncology in anatomical sites outside the CNS have been quite limited.

^{31}P MRS Studies

Central Nervous System

A ^{31}P spectrum from normal brain (Fig. 4.15) typically demonstrates seven resolved peaks from PCr, inorganic phosphate (Pi), nucleotide triphos-

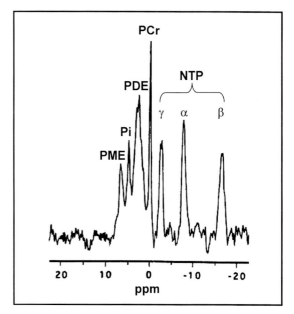

Fig. 4.15. Typical ^{31}P spectrum from normal human brain obtained with image-selected in vivo spectroscopy (ISIS) localization. Major spectral peaks are from phosphomonoesters (PME), phosphodiesters (PDE), inorganic phosphate (Pi), phosphocreatine (PCr), and nucleotide triphosphates (NTP)

phates (NTP; α-, β-, and γ-resonances), phosphomonoesters (PME), and phosphodiesters (PDE). Note that the signals from phosphosotidylcholine and other cell-membrane lipids are not present in ^{31}P spectra from normal brain, because the rigid arrangement of the lipids reduces their mobility to a point at which they are MR-invisible. This is analogous to the MR-invisible myelin lipid signal in ^{1}H MRS studies of normal human brain.

The PME peak is actually composed of resonances from several biochemicals, including: (1) intermediates in carbohydrate metabolism, such as glucose-6-phosphate, glycerol-1-phosphate, and glycerol-3-phosphate, (2) phosphoethanolamine, (3) adenosine monophosphate (AMP), (4) phosphocholine, and (5) 2, 3-diphosphoglycerate (2, 3-DPG) from blood. The PDE peak is also composed of several resonances, including those from glycerophosphoethanolamine and glycerophosphocholine, which are intermediates in phospholipid catabolism. The NTP peaks are due mainly to ATP, but a small percentage are due to guanosine triphosphate and uridine triphosphate. Also, the NTP spectral peaks overlap with peaks from other components, including adenosine diphosphate (ADP) and nicotinamide adenosine dinucleotide (NAD).

One key advantage of ^{31}P MRS lies in the fact that the chemical shift between Pi and PCr is dependent on the intracellular pH. Therefore, in vivo ^{31}P MRS provides a means of obtaining intracellular pH levels in a non-invasive manner. If Δv is the chemical shift between PCr and Pi (in ppm), then the intracellular pH is given by [160]:

$$\text{pH} = 6.75 + \log\left(\frac{\Delta v - 3.3}{5.8 - \Delta v}\right) \qquad 4.4$$

The Pi peak has two components, due to intracellular and extracellular inorganic phosphate, and a split in the spectral peak can be observed in some situations, such as in exercising muscle [160].

Although there are variations observed in ^{31}P MRS studies of intracranial neoplasms, the most consistent findings are elevated PME and PDE levels, increased pH, and decreased PCr. These findings have been reviewed in several reports [51, 54, 55, 59, 60]. In light of the elevated choline and lipid levels observed in many brain neoplasms using ^{1}H MRS, the elevated PME and PDE levels are not surprising. Furthermore, the decrease in PCr reflects the breakdown in oxidative metabolism within the tumor and a probable switch to a more anaerobic metabolism. Because the Pi levels are not consistently elevated, however, it is unlikely that tumor metabolism is purely or even predominantly anaerobic. This is supported by the fact that most tumors have normal or slightly alkaline intracellular pH levels. It is also supported by the inconsistent detection of lactic acid in neoplasms using ^{1}H MRS. Studies of the response of intracranial lesions to radiation and/or chemotherapy have also been reported [59, 60]; successful therapies are typically associated with decreases in PME and/or PDE levels toward more normal values.

As in studies of untreated tumors, there is variability in the results, which might limit the predictive value of ^{31}P MRS for monitoring therapeutic response. A probable cause of such variability is the heterogeneous nature of tumors. Although heterogeneity is also a problem in ^{1}H MRS studies, it is a considerable problem in ^{31}P MRS studies, which typically acquire data from relatively large VOIs (compared with those used in ^{1}H MRS) to maintain a reasonable exam time. As the size of the VOI is increased, however, so is the potential partial volume-averaging of tumor, necrosis, and normal tissue. The use of SI techniques to acquire ^{31}P spectra, of course, should provide improved evaluation of the heterogeneity of brain lesions. One such study was reported by Rutter et al. [161], who demonstrated increased PDE-to-NTP and PME-to-NTP ratios, and normal to increased intracellular pH levels, in glioblastomas and astrocytomas compared with values obtained from normal-appearing brain.

Applications Outside of the CNS

An extensive number of applications of ^{31}P MRS to neoplasms outside of the CNS have been reported in cases of lymphomas [162–166], osteosarcomas and soft-tissue sarcomas [167–172], breast tumors [173–176], and liver lesions [177–180]. Review articles by Cox [52], Negendank [59], and Bottomley [60] discuss several of these studies. As with the ^{31}P studies of intracranial lesions, there is considerable variation in the results. However, some general trends, such as the association of neoplasms with elevated PME and PDE levels and normal to slightly alkaline pH levels, have been demonstrated.

To summarize the current state-of-the-art in clinical MRS at the MR Spectroscopy and Tumor Cell Biology Workshop sponsored by the National Cancer Institute in 1992, Negendank presented a review of 60 publications from 1983 to 1992, in which over 500 patients were studied with ^{31}P MRS [181]. The general findings were that human cancer cells typically have a pH that is normal or slightly alkaline, low PCr levels, high PME levels, and high PDE levels. Some of these characteristics were shown to be statistically significant compared with normal or benign tissues, and some correlated with the response of sarcomas, breast cancers, lymphomas, and other cancers to chemo- or radiation therapy. Clearly, additional highly standardized multicenter trials would be helpful in establishing the feasibility of using ^{31}P MRS as a diagnostic probe and/or as a means of quantitatively assessing the efficacy of therapeutic interventions.

MRS Studies Using Nuclei Other Than ^{1}H and ^{31}P

Although the exceedingly low natural abundance of ^{13}C greatly impedes in vivo studies, a few groups have reported ^{13}C MRS data from skeletal muscle, cardiac muscle, brain, prostate, and liver [182–189]. The studies reported the detection of glycogen, citrate, fatty acids, and glycerol, and none were directly related to oncology. The other nucleus utilized for clinical in vivo MRS studies of cancer is ^{19}F. Although ^{19}F is not sufficiently abundant to be detected using in vivo MRS, it may prove particularly useful for studies of drug metabolism. In particular, several studies have reported the use of ^{19}F MRS in studies of the metabolism of 5-fluorouracil; these studies have been reviewed by Findlay [190, 191].

There has been tremendous interest in the use of in vivo MRS for assessing the biochemical status of normal and pathological tissue. The goal of obtaining non-invasive biopsy information has steadily pushed the development of optimized localization sequences, water-suppression techniques, and advanced spectral editing techniques. Many of these methodologies are now in place, and the next logical step in the evolution of in vivo MRS is a dramatic expansion in the number of carefully controlled and standardized multicenter trials. In addition, the incorporation of techniques aimed at significantly decreasing the time required to obtain high-quality spectra using 2D and 3D SI techniques should provide a tremendous boost to the clinical application of MRS, and would allow improved characterization of heterogeneous lesions. The increased availability of 3 T and even 4 T magnets should further enhance the spectral quality, particularly in ^{1}H studies for which the chemical shift ranges are quite small. In general, although in vivo MRS has developed quite slowly compared with MRI, the potential benefits should continue to drive increased research applications and, most importantly, increased clinical applications.

References

1. Ernst RR, Anderson WA (1966) Application of Fourier transform spectroscopy to magnetic resonance. Rev Sci Instrum 37:93–102
2. Becker ED (1980) High resolution NMR. Theory and chemical applications. Academic Press, New York, Ch4
3. Aue WP (1986) Localization methods for in vivo NMR spectroscopy. Rev Magn Reson Med 1:21–72
4. Bottomley PA, Foster TB, Darrow RD (1984) Depth-resolved surface-coil spectroscopy (DRESS) for in vivo ^{1}H, ^{31}P, and ^{13}C NMR. J Magn Reson 59:338–342
5. Brown TR, Kincaid BM, Ugurbil K (1982) NMR chemical shift imaging in three dimensions. Proc Natl Acad Sci U S A 79:3523–3526
6. Maudsley AA, Hilal SK, Perman WH, Simon HE (1983) Spatially resolved high resolution spectroscopy by "four-dimensional" NMR. J Magn Reson 51:147–152
7. Hore PJ (1989) Solvent suppression. In: Oppenheimer NJ, James TL (eds) Nuclear magnetic resonance part a: spectral techniques and dynamics. Academic Press, New York, pp 64–77
8. Haase A, Frahm J, Hänicke W, Matthei D (1985) ^{1}H NMR chemical shift selective (CHESS) imaging. Phys Med Biol 30:341–344
9. Doddrell DM, Galloway GJ, Brooks WM et al. (1986) Water signal elimination in vivo using "Suppression by mistimed echo and repetitive gradient episodes." J Magn Reson 70:176–180
10. Webb P, Macovski A (1991) Rapid, fully automatic, arbitrary-volume in vivo shimming. Magn Reson Med 20:113–122
11. Moonen CTW, van Zijl PCM (1990) Highly effective water suppression for in vivo proton NMR spectroscopy (DRYSTEAM). J Magn Reson 88:28–41
12. Granot J (1986) Selected volume excitation using stimulated echoes (VEST): application to spatially localized spectroscopy and imaging. J Magn Reson 70:488–492
13. Frahm J, Merboldt K-D, Hänicke W (1987) Localized proton spectroscopy using stimulated echoes. J Magn Reson 72:502–508
14. Kimmich R, Hoepfel D (1987) Volume-selective multipulse spin-echo spectroscopy. J Magn Reson 72:379–384
15. Bottomley PA (1984) Selective volume method for performing localized NMR spectroscopy. U.S. Patent 4, 480, 228
16. Ordidge RJ, Connelly A, Lohman JAB (1986) Image-selected in vivo spectroscopy (ISIS). A new technique for spatially selective NMR spectroscopy. J Magn Reson 66:283–294
17. Fauth J-M, Schweiger A, Braunschweiler L, Forrer J, Ernst RR (1986) Elimination of unwanted echoes and reduction of dead time in three-pulse electron spin-echo spectroscopy. J Magn Reson 66:74–85
18. Frahm J, Bruhn H, Gyngell ML, Merboldt KD, Hänicke W, Sauter R (1989) Localized proton NMR spectroscopy in different regions of the human brain in vivo. Relaxation times and concentrations of cerebral metabolites. Magn Reson Med 11:47–63
19. Pauly J, Le Roux P, Nishimura D, Macovski A (1991) Parameter relations for the Shinnar-Le Roux selective excitation pulse design algorithm. IEEE Trans Med Imaging 10:53–65
20. Jackson EF, Narayana PA, Flamig DP (1990) One-dimensional spectroscopic imaging with stimulated echoes. Phantom and human leg studies. Magn Reson Imaging 8:153–159
21. Moonen CTW, Sobering G, van Zijl PCM, Gillen J, von Kienlin M, Bizzi A (1992) Proton spectroscopic imaging of human brain. J Magn Reson 98:556–575
22. Jackson EF, Doyle TJ, Wolinsky JS, Narayana PA (1994) Short TE hydrogen-1 spectroscopic MR imaging of normal human brain: reproducibility studies. J Magn Reson Imaging 4:545–551
23. Posse S, Tedeschi G, Risinger R, Ogg R, Le Bihan D (1995) High speed ^{1}H spectroscopic imaging in human brain by echo planar spatial-spectral encoding. Magn Reson Med 33:34–40
24. de Crespigny AJS, Carpenter TA, Hall LD (1989) Region-of-interest selection by outer-volume saturation. J Magn Reson 85:595–603
25. Dunn JH, Matson GB, Maudsley AA, Weiner MW (1992) 3D phase encoding ^{1}H spectroscopic imaging of human brain. Magn Reson Imaging 10:315–319

26. Posse S, Schuknecht B, Smith ME, van Zijl PCM, Herschkowitz N, Moonen CTW (1993) Short echo time proton MR spectroscopic imaging. J Comput Assist Tomogr 17:1-14
27. Shungu DC, Glickson JD (1993) Sensitivity and localization enhancement in multinuclear in vivo NMR spectroscopy by outer volume presaturation. Magn Reson Med 30:661-671
28. Kreis R, Farrow N, Ross BD (1991) Localized ^{1}H NMR spectroscopy in patients with chronic hepatic encephalopathy. Analysis of changes in cerebral glutamine, choline and inositols. NMR Biomed 4:109-116
29. Cady EB (1990) Clinical magnetic resonance spectroscopy. Plenum, New York
30. Marion D, Ikura M, Bax A (1989) Improved solvent suppression in one- and two-dimensional NMR spectra by convolution of time-domain data. J Magn Reson 84:425-430
31. Kuroda Y, Wada A, Yamazaki T, Nagayama K (1989) Postacquisition data processing method for suppression of the solvent signal. J Magn Reson 84:604-610
32. Sanders JKM, Hunter BK (1993) Modern NMR spectroscopy. A guide for chemists. Oxford University Press, New York, Chap. 1
33. Fukushima E, Roeder SBW (1981) Experimental pulse NMR. A nuts and bolts approach. Addison-Wesley, Reading, Chap. 2
34. Soher BJ, van Zijl PCM, Duyn JH, Barker PB (1996) Quantitative proton MR spectroscopic imaging of the human brain. Magn Reson Med 35:356-363
35. Husted CA, Duijn JH, Matson GB, Maudsley AA, Weiner MW (1994) Molar quantitation of in vivo proton metabolites in human brain with 3D magnetic resonance spectroscopy imaging. Magn Reson Imaging 12:661-667
36. Michaelis T, Merboldt K-D, Bruhn H, Hänicke W, Frahm J (1993) Absolute concentration of metabolites in the adult human brain in vivo: quantification of localized proton MR spectra. Radiology 187:219-227
37. Kreis R, Ernst T, Ross BD (1993) Development of the human brain: in vivo quantification of metabolite and water content with proton magnetic resonance spectroscopy. Magn Reson Med 30:424-437
38. Narayana PA, Fotedar LK, Jackson EF, Bohan TP, Butler IJ, Wolinsky JS (1989) Regional in vivo proton magnetic resonance spectroscopy of brain. J Magn Reson 83:44-52
39. Davie CA, Barker GJ, Webb S et al. (1995) Persistent functional deficit in multiple sclerosis and autosomal dominant cerebellar ataxia is associated with axon loss. Brain 118:1583-1592
40. Usenius J-PR, Kauppinen RA, Vainio PA et al. (1994) Quantitative metabolite patterns of human brain tumors: detection by ^{1}H NMR spectroscopy in vivo and in vitro. J Comput Assist Tomogr 18:705-713
41. Christiansen P, Henriksen O, Stubgaard M, Gideon P, Larsson HBW (1993) In vivo quantification of brain metabolites by ^{1}H-MRS using water as an internal standard. Magn Reson Imaging 11:107-118
42. Pan JW, Hetherington HP, Hamm JR, Shulman RG (1991) Quantitation of metabolites by ^{1}H NMR. Magn Reson Med 20:48-56
43. Danielsen ER, Michaelis T, Ross BD (1995) Three methods of calibration in quantitative proton MR spectroscopy. J Magn Reson Ser B 106:287-291
44. Charles HC, Lazeyras F, Tupler LA, Krishnan RR (1996) Reproducibility of high spatial resolution proton magnetic resonance spectroscopic imaging of the human brain. Magn Reson Med 35:606-610
45. Webb PG, Sailasuta N, Kohler SJ, Raidy T, Moats RA, Hurd RE (1994) Automated single-voxel proton MRS: technical development and multisite verification. Magn Reson Med 31:365-373
46. Tien RD, Lai PH, Smith JS, Lazeyras F (1996) Single-voxel proton brain spectroscopy exam (PROBE/SV) in patients with primary brain tumors. AJR Am J Roentgenol 167:201-209
47. Negendank WG, Sauter R, Brown TR et al. (1996) Proton magnetic resonance spectroscopy in patients with glial tumors: a multicenter study. J Neurosurg 84:449-458
48. Doyle TJ, Bedell BJ, Narayana PA (1995) Relative concentrations of proton MR visible neurochemicals in gray and white matter in human brain. Magn Reson Med 33:755-759
49. Hetherington HP, Pan JW, Mason GF et al. (1996) Quantitative ^{1}H spectroscopic imaging of human brain at 4.1 T using imaging segmentation. Magn Reson Med 36:21-29
50. Jackson EF, Meyers CA (1997) Basic considerations to hippocampal spectroscopy. In: Tien RD (ed) Neuroimaging clinics of north America. Saunders, Philadelphia, pp 143-154
51. Ross B, Michaelis T (1996) MR spectroscopy of the brain: neurospectroscopy. In: Edelman RR, Hesselink JR, Zlatkin MB (eds) Clinical magnetic resonance imaging. Saunders, Philadelphia, pp 928-981
52. Cox IJ (1996) Development and applications of in vivo clinical magnetic resonance spectroscopy. Prog Biophys Mol Biol 65:45-81
53. Falini A, Calabrese G, Origgi D et al. (1996) Proton magnetic resonance spectroscopy and intracranial tumors: clinical perspectives. J Neurol 243:706-714
54. Vion-Dury J, Meyerhoff DJ, Cozzone PJ, Weiner MW (1994) What might be the impact on neurology of the analysis of brain metabolism by in vivo magnetic resonance spectroscopy? J Neurol 241:354-371
55. Ross B, Michaelis T (1994) Clinical applications of magnetic resonance spectroscopy. Magn Reson Q 10:191-247
56. Leach MO (1994) Magnetic resonance spectroscopy applied to clinical oncology. Tech Health Care 2:235-246
57. Barker PB, Glickson JD, Bryan RN (1993) In vivo magnetic resonance spectroscopy of human brain tumors. Top Magn Reson Imaging 5:32-45
58. Howe FA, Maxwell RJ, Saunders DE, Brown MM, Griffiths JR (1993) Proton spectroscopy in vivo. Magn Reson Q 9:31-59
59. Negendank W (1992) Studies of human tumors by MRS: a review. NMR Biomed 5:303-324
60. Bottomley PA (1989) Human in vivo NMR spectroscopy in diagnostic medicine: clinical tool or research probe? Radiology 170:1-15
61. Birken DL, Oldendorf WH (1989) N-acetyl-L-aspartic acid: a literature review of a compound prominent in ^{1}H-NMR spectroscopic studies of brain. Neurosci Biobehav Rev 13:23-31
62. Kreis R, Ernst T, Ross BD (1993) Development of the human brain: in vivo quantification of metabolite and water content with ^{1}H-MRS. Society of Magnetic Resonance in Medicine, New York, pp 126
63. van der Knaap MS, van der Grond J, van Rijen PC, Faber JA, Valk J, Willemse K (1990) Age-dependent changes in localized proton and phosphorus MR spectroscopy of the brain. Radiology 176:509-15
64. Bizzi A, Movsas B, Tedeschi G et al. (1995) Response of non-Hodgkin lymphoma to radiation therapy: early and long-term assessment with H-1 MR spectroscopic imaging. Radiology 194:271-276
65. Sijens PE, Knopp MV, Brunetti A et al. (1995) ^{1}H MR spectroscopy in patients with metastatic brain tumors: a multicenter study. Magn Reson Med 33:818-826
66. McBride DQ, Miller BL, Nikas DL et al. (1995) Analysis of brain tumors using ^{1}H magnetic resonance spectroscopy. Surg Neurol 44:137-144
67. Kugel H, Heindel W, Bunke J, Du Mesnil R, Friedmann G (1994) Human brain tumors: spectral patterns de-

tected with localized H-1 MR spectroscopy. Radiology 183:701–709
68. Yamagata NT, Miller BL, McBride D et al. (1994) In vivo proton spectroscopy of intracranial infections and neoplasms. J Neuroimaging 4:23–28
69. Ott D, Hennig J, Ernst T (1993) Human brain tumors: assessment with in vivo proton MR spectroscopy. Radiology 186:745–752
70. Sutton LN, Wang Z, Gusnard D et al. (1992) Proton magnetic resonance spectroscopy of pediatric brain tumors. Neurosurgery 31:195–202
71. Fulham MJ, Bizzi A, Dietz MJ et al. (1992) Mapping of brain tumor metabolites with proton MR spectroscopic imaging: clinical relevance. Radiology 185:675–686
72. Demaerel P, Johannik K, van Hecke P et al. (1991) Localized ^{1}H NMR spectroscopy in fifty cases of newly diagnosed intracranial tumors. J Comput Assist Tomogr 15:67–76
73. Frahm J, Bruhn H, Hänicke W, Merboldt K-D, Mursch K, Markakis E (1991) Localized proton NMR spectroscopy of brain tumors using short-echo time STEAM sequences. J Comput Assist Tomogr 15:915–922
74. Henriksen O, Wieslander S, Gjerris F, Jensen KM (1991) In vivo ^{1}H spectroscopy of human intracranial tumors at 1.5 T. Acta Radiol 32:95–99
75. Alger JR, Frank JA, Bizzi A et al. (1990) Metabolism of human gliomas: Assessment with H-1 MR spectroscopy and F-18 fluorodeoxyglucose PET. Radiology 177:633–641
76. Gill SS, Thomas DG, van Bruggen N et al. (1990) Proton MR spectroscopy of intracranial tumors: in vivo and in vitro studies. J Comput Assist Tomogr 14:497–504
77. Luyten PR, Marien AJH, Heindel W et al. (1990) Metabolic imaging of patients with intracranial tumors: H-1 MR spectroscopic imaging and PET. Radiology 176:791–799
78. Segebarth CM, Baleriaux DF, Luyten PR, den-Hollander JA (1990) Detection of metabolic heterogeneity of human intracranial tumors in vivo by ^{1}H NMR spectroscopic imaging. Magn Reson Med 13:62–76
79. Arnold DL, Shoubridge EA, Emrich J, Feindel W, Villemure JG (1989) Early metabolic changes following chemotherapy of human gliomas in vivo demonstrated by phosphorus magnetic resonance spectroscopy. Invest Radiol 24:958–961
80. Bruhn H, Frahm J, Gyngell ML et al. (1989) Noninvasive differentiation of tumors with use of localized H-1 MR spectroscopy in vivo: initial experience in patients with cerebral tumors. Radiology 172:541–548
81. Bruhn H, Frahm J, Gyngell ML, Merboldt KD, Hänicke W, Sauter R (1989) Cerebral metabolism in man after acute stroke: new observations using localized proton NMR spectroscopy. Magn Reson Med 9:126–131
82. Fenstermacher MJ, Narayana PA (1990) Serial proton magnetic resonance spectroscopy of ischemic brain injury in humans. Invest Radiol 25:1034–1039
83. Gideon P, Sperling B, Arlien-Soborg P, Olsen TS, Henriksen O (1994) Long-term follow-up of cerebral infarction patients with proton magnetic resonance spectroscopy. Stroke 25:967–973
84. Graham GD, Blamire AM, Howseman AM et al. (1992) Proton magnetic resonance spectroscopy of cerebral lactate and other metabolites in stroke patients. Stroke 23:333–340
85. Graham GD, Kalvach P, Blamire AM, Brass LM, Fayad PB, Prichard JW (1995) Clinical correlates of proton magnetic resonance spectroscopy findings after acute cerebral infarction. Stroke 26:225–229
86. Graham GD, Blamire AM, Rothman DL et al. (1993) Early temporal variation of cerebral metabolites after human stroke. A proton magnetic resonance study. Stroke 24:1891–1896
87. Mathews VP, Barker PB, Bryan RN (1992) Magnetic resonance evaluation of stroke. Magn Reson Q 8:245–263
88. Mathews VP, Barker PB, Blackband SJ, Chatham JC, Bryan RN (1995) Cerebral metabolites in patients with acute and subacute strokes: concentrations determined by quantitative proton MR spectroscopy. AJR Am J Roentgenol 165:633–638
89. Sappey-Marinier D, Calabrese G, Hetherington H et al. (1992) Proton magnetic resonance spectroscopy of human brain: applications to normal white matter, chronic infarction, and MRI white matter signal hyperintensities. Magn Reson Med 26:313–327
90. Saunders DE, Howe FA, van den Boogaart A, McLean MA, Griffiths JR, Brown MM (1995) Continuing ischemic damage after acute middle cerebral artery infarction in humans demonstrated by short-echo proton spectroscopy. Stroke 26:1007–1013
91. Arnold DL, Matthews PM, Francis G, Antel J (1990) Proton magnetic resonance spectroscopy of human brain in vivo in the evaluation of multiple sclerosis: assessment of the load of disease. Magn Reson Med 14:154–159
92. Arnold DL, Matthews PM, Francis GS, O'Connor J, Antel JP (1992) Proton magnetic resonance spectroscopic imaging for metabolic characterization of demyelinating plaques. Ann Neurol 31:235–241
93. Hagberg G, Burlina AP, Mader I, Roser W, Radue EW, Seelig J (1995) In vivo proton MR spectroscopy of human gliomas: definition of metabolic coordinates for multi-dimensional classification. Magn Reson Med 34: 242–252
94. Larsson HBW, Christiansen P, Jensen M et al. (1991) Localized in vivo proton spectroscopy in the brain of patients with multiple sclerosis. Magn Reson Med 22:23–31
95. Hiehle JF, Lenkinski RE, Grossman RI et al. (1994) Correlation of spectroscopy and magnetization transfer imaging in the evaluation of demyelinating lesions and normal appearing white matter in multiple sclerosis. Magn Reson Med 32:285–293
96. Husted CA, Goodin DS, Hugg JW et al. (1994) Biochemical alterations in multiple sclerosis lesions and normal-appearing white matter detected by in vivo ^{31}P and ^{1}H spectroscopic imaging. Ann Neurol 36:157–165
97. Narayana PA, Wolinsky JS, Jackson EF, McCarthy M (1992) Proton MR spectroscopy of gadolinium-enhanced multiple sclerosis plaques. J Magn Reson Imaging 2:263–270
98. Pan JW, Hetherington HP, Vaughan JT, Mitchell G, Pohost GM, Whitaker JN (1996) Evaluation of multiple sclerosis by ^{1}H spectroscopic imaging at 4.1 T. Magn Reson Med 36:72–77
99. Wolinsky JS, Narayana PA, Fenstermacher MJ (1990) Proton magnetic resonance spectroscopy in multiple sclerosis. Neurology 40:1764–1769
100. Vainio P, Usenius JP, Vapalahati M et al. (1994) Reduced N-acetylaspartate concentration in temporal lobe epilepsy by quantitative ^{1}H MRS in vivo. Neuroreport 5:1733–1736
101. Breiter SN, Arroyo S, Mathews VP, Lesser RP, Bryan RN, Barker PB (1994) Proton MR spectroscopy in patients with seizure disorders. AJNR Am J Neuroradiol 15:373–384
102. Cendes F, Andermann F, Preul MC, Arnold DL (1994) Lateralization of temporal lobe epilepsy based on regional metabolic abnormalities in proton magnetic resonance spectroscopic images. Ann Neurol 35:211–216
103. Cross JH, Connelly A, Jackson GD, Johnson CL, Neville BG, Gadian DG (1996) Proton magnetic resonance spectroscopy in children with temporal lobe epilepsy. Ann Neurol 39:107–113

104. Gadian DG, Isaacs EB, Cross JH et al. (1996) Lateralization of brain function in childhood revealed by magnetic resonance spectroscopy. Neurology 46:974–977
105. Hugg JW, Laxer KD, Matson GB, Maudsley AA, Weiner MW (1993) Neuron loss localizes human temporal lobe epilepsy by in vivo proton magnetic resonance spectroscopic imaging. Ann Neurol 34:788–794
106. Incisa della Rocchetta A, Gadian DG, Connelly A et al. (1995) Verbal memory impairment after right temporal lobe surgery: role of contralateral damage as revealed by ^{1}H magnetic resonance spectroscopy and T_2 relaxometry. Neurology 45:797–802
107. Matthews PM, Andermann F, Arnold DL (1990) A proton magnetic resonance spectroscopy study of focal epilepsy in humans. Neurology 40:985–989
108. Strauss WL, Tsuruda JS, Richards TL (1995) Partial volume effects in volume-localized phased-array proton spectroscopy of the temporal lobe. J Magn Reson Imaging 5:433–436
109. Sostman HD, Charles HC (1990) Noninvasive differentiation of tumors with use of localized H-1 spectroscopy in vivo: initial experience in patients with cerebral tumors. Invest Radiol 25:1047–1050
110. Miller BL, Moats RA, Shonk T, Ernst T, Woolley S, Ross BD (1993) Alzheimer disease: depiction of increased cerebral myo-inositol with proton MR spectroscopy. Radiology 187:433–7
111. Moats RA, Ernst T, Shonk TK, Ross BD (1994) Abnormal cerebral metabolite concentrations in patients with probable Alzheimer disease. Magn Reson Med 32:110–115
112. Shonk TK, Moats RA, Gifford P et al. (1995) Probable Alzheimer disease: diagnosis with proton MR spectroscopy. Radiology 195:65–72
113. Shonk T, Ross BD (1995) Role of increased cerebral myo-inositol in the dementia of Down syndrome. Magn Reson Med 33:858–861
114. Nasrallah HA, Skinner TE, Schmalbrock P, Robitaille PM (1994) Proton magnetic resonance spectroscopy (^{1}H MRS) of the hippocampal formation in schizophrenia: a pilot study. Br J Psychiatry 165:481–485
115. Kreis R, Ross BD (1992) Cerebral metabolic disturbances in patients with subacute and chronic diabetes mellitus: detection with proton MR spectroscopy. Radiology 184:123–130
116. Meyerhoff DJ, MacKay S, Poole N, Dillon WP, Weiner MW, Fein G (1994) N-acetylaspartate reductions measured by ^{1}H MRSI in cognitively impaired HIV-seropositive individuals. Magn Reson Imaging 12:654–659
117. Tedeschi G, Bertolino A, Campbell G et al. (1995) Brain regional distribution pattern of metabolite signal intensities in young adults by proton magnetic resonance spectroscopic imaging. Neurology 45:1384–1391
118. Tedeschi G, Righini A, Bizzi A, Barnett AS, Alger J (1995) Cerebral white matter in the centrum semiovale exhibits a larger N-acetyl signal than does gray matter in long echo time ^{1}H-magnetic resonance spectroscopic imaging. Magn Reson Med 33:127–133
119. Hetherington HP, Mason GF, Pan JW et al. (1994) Evaluation of cerebral gray and white matter metabolite differences by spectroscopic imaging at 4.1 T. Magn Reson Med 32:565–571
120. Narayana PA, Johnston D, Flamig DP (1991) In vivo proton magnetic resonance spectroscopy studies of human brain. Magn Reson Imaging 9:303–308
121. Tedeschi G, Lundbom N, Raman R et al. (1997) Increased choline signal coinciding with malignant degeneration of cerebral gliomas: a serial proton magnetic resonance spectroscopy imaging study. J Neurosurg 87:516–524
122. Miller BL, Chang L, Booth R et al. (1996) In vivo ^{1}H MRS choline: correlation with in vitro chemistry/histology. Life Sci 58:1929–1935
123. Tzika AA, Ball WS, Vigneron DB, Dunn RS, Kirks DR (1993) Clinical proton MR spectroscopy of neurodegenerative disease in childhood. AJNR Am J Neuroradiol 14:1267–1281
124. Kreis R, Ross BD, Farrow NA, Ackerman Z (1992) Metabolic disorders of the brain in chronic hepatic encephalopathy detected with H-1 MR spectroscopy. Radiology 182:19–27
125. Ross BD, Jacobson S, Villamil F et al. (1994) Subclinical hepatic encephalopathy: proton MR spectroscopic abnormalities. Radiology 193:457–463
126. Videen JS, Michaelis T, Pinto P, Ross BD (1995) Human cerebral osmolytes during chronic hyponatremia. A proton magnetic resonance spectroscopy study. J Clin Invest 95:788–793
127. Gideon P, Henriksen O (1992) In vivo relaxation of N-acetyl-aspartate, creatine plus phosphocreatine, and choline containing compounds during the course of brain infarction: a proton MRS study. Magn Reson Imaging 10:983–988
128. Henriksen O, Gideon P, Sperling B, Olsen TS, Jørgensen HS, Arlien-Søborg P (1992) Cerebral lactate production and blood flow in acute stroke. J Magn Reson Imaging 2:511–517
129. Tzika AA, Vigneron DB, Ball WSJ, Dunn RS, Kirks DR (1993) Localized proton MR spectroscopy of the brain in children. J Magn Reson Imaging 3:719–729
130. Davie CA, Hawkins CP, Barker GJ et al. (1994) Serial proton magnetic resonance spectroscopy in acute multiple sclerosis lesions. Brain 117:49–58
131. Davie CA, Hawkins CP, Barker GJ et al. (1993) Detection of myelin breakdown products by proton magnetic resonance spectroscopy. Lancet 341:630–631
132. Koopmans RA, Li DKB, Zhu G, Allen PS, Penn A, Paty DW (1993) Magnetic resonance spectroscopy of multiple sclerosis: in-vivo detection of myelin breakdown products. Lancet 841:631–632
133. Poptani H, Gupta RK, Jain VK, Roy R, Pandey R (1995) Cystic intracranial mass lesions: possible role of in vivo MR spectroscopy in its differential diagnosis. Magn Reson Imaging 13:1019–1029
134. Chang L, McBride D, Miller BL et al. (1995) Localized in vivo ^{1}H magnetic-resonance spectroscopy and in vitro analysis of heterogeneous brain tumors. J Neuroimaging 5:157–163
135. Arnold DL, Shoubridge EA, Villemure JG, Feindel W (1990) Proton and phosphorus magnetic resonance spectroscopy of human astrocytomas in vivo. Preliminary observations on tumor grading. NMR Biomed 3:184–189
136. Kreis R, Farrow N, Ross BD (1990) Diagnosis of hepatic encephalopathy by proton magnetic resonance spectroscopy. Lancet 336:635–636
137. Pan JW, Mason GF, Pohost GM, Hetherington HP (1996) Spectroscopic imaging of human brain glutamate by water-suppressed J-refocused coherence transfer at 4.1 T. Magn Reson Med 36:7–12
138. Keltner JR, Wald LL, Frederick BdB, Renshaw PF (1997) In vivo detection of GABA in human brain using a localized double-quantum filter technique. Magn Reson Med 37:366–371
139. Keltner JR, Wald LL, Christensen JD et al. (1996) A technique for detecting GABA in the human brain with PRESS localization and optimized refocusing spectral editing radiofrequency pulses. Magn Reson Med 36:458–461
140. Rothman DL, Petroff OA, Behar KL, Mattson RH (1993) Localized ^{1}H NMR measurements of gamma-aminobutyric acid in human brain in vivo. Proc Natl Acad Sci U S A 90:5662–5666

141. Mattson RH, Petroff O, Rothman D, Behar K (1994) Vigabatrin: Effects on human brain GABA levels by nuclear magnetic resonance spectroscopy. Epilepsia 35:S29-S32
142. Petroff OA, Rothman DL, Behar KL, Lamoureux D, Mattson RH (1996) The effect of gabapentin on brain gamma-aminobutyric acid in patients with epilepsy. Ann Neurol 39:95-99
143. Pruel MC, Caramanos Z, Collins DL et al. (1996) Accurate, noninvasive diagnosis of human brain tumors by using proton magnetic resonance spectroscopy. Nat Med 2:323-325
144. Somorjai RL, Dolenko B, Nikulin AK et al. (1996) Classification of ^{1}H MR spectra of human brain neoplasms: the influence of preprocessing and computerized consensus diagnosis of classification accuracy. J Magn Reson Imaging 6:437-444
145. Usenius J-P, Tuohimetsa S, Vainio P, Ala-Korpela M, Hiltunen Y, Kauppinen RA (1996) Automated classification of human brain tumours by neural network analysis using in vivo ^{1}H magnetic resonance spectroscopic metabolite phenotypes. Neuroreport 7:1597-1600
146. Tomoi M, Kimura H, Yoshida M et al. (1997) Alterations of lactate (+lipid) concentration in brain tumors with in vivo hydrogen magnetic resonance spectroscopy during radiotherapy. Invest Radiol 32:288-296
147. Sijens PE, Vecht CJ, Levendag PC, Dijk PV, Oudkerk M (1995) Hydrogen magnetic resonance spectroscopy follow-up after radiation therapy of human brain cancer. Invest Radiol 30:738-744
148. Heesters M, Kamman R, Mooyaart E, Go K (1993) Localized proton spectroscopy of inoperable brain gliomas. Response to radiation therapy. J Neurooncol 17:27-35
149. Usenius T, Usenius J-P, Tenhunen M et al. (1995) Radiation-induced changes in human brain metabolites as studied by ^{1}H nuclear magnetic resonance spectroscopy in vivo. Int J Radiat Oncol Biol Phys 33:710-724
150. Szigety SK, Allen PS, Huyser-Wierenga D, Urtasun RC (1993) The effect of radiation on normal human CNS as detected by NMR spectroscopy. Int J Radiat Oncol Biol Phys 25:695-701
151. Narayana PA, Jackson EF, Butler IJ (1996) ^{1}H-MRS of muscle physiology and pathophysiology. In: Fleckenstein JL, Crues JVI, Reimers CD (eds) Muscle imaging in health and disease. Springer-Verlag, Berlin Heidelberg New York, pp 133-147
152. Schick F, Einsele H, Kost R et al. (1994) Hematopoietic reconstitution after bone marrow transplantation: assessment with MR imaging and H-1 localized spectroscopy. J Magn Reson Imaging 4:71-78
153. Schick F, Bongers H, Jung W-I, Skalej M, Lutz O, Claussen CD (1992) Volume-selective proton MRS in vertebral bodies. Magn Reson Med 26:207-217
154. Jensen KE, Jensen M, Grundtvig P, Thomsen C, Karle H, Henriksen O (1990) Localized in vivo proton spectroscopy of the bone marrow in patients with leukemia. Magn Reson Imaging 8:779-789
155. Schick F, Duda SH, Lutz O, Claussen CD (1996) Lipids in bone tumors assessed by magnetic resonance: chemical shift imaging and proton spectroscopy in vivo. Anticancer Res 16:1569-1574
156. Bongers H, Schick F, Skalej M, Jung W-I, Stevens A (1992) Localized in vivo ^{1}H spectroscopy of human skeletal muscle: normal and pathologic findings. Magn Reson Imaging 10:957-964
157. Heerschap A, Jager GJ, van der Graaf M et al. (1997) In vivo proton MR spectroscopy reveals altered metabolite content in malignant prostate tissue. Anticancer Res 17:1455-1460
158. Kurhanewicz J, Vigneron DB, Nelson SJ et al. (1993) In vivo citrate levels in the normal and pathologic human prostate. Society of Magnetic Resonance in Medicine, New York, pp 212
159. Sanders JA, Sillerud LO (1993) Proton STEAM spectroscopy of the human prostate in vivo. Society of Magnetic Resonance in Medicine, New York, pp 1029
160. Bolinger L, Insko EK (1996) Spectroscopy: basic principles and techniques. In: Edelman RR, Hesselink JR, Zlatkin MB (eds) Clinical magnetic resonance imaging. Saunders, Philadelphia, pp 353-379
161. Rutter A, Hugenholtz H, Saunders JK, Smith ICP (1995) One-dimensional phosphorus-31 chemical shift imaging of human brain tumors. Invest Radiol 30:359-366
162. Negendank WG, Padavic-Shaller KA, Li C-W et al. (1995) Metabolic characterization of human non-Hodgkin's lymphomas in vivo with the use of proton-decoupled phosphorus magnetic resonance spectroscopy. Cancer Res 55:3286-3294
163. Redmond OM, Stack JP, O'Connor NG et al. (1992) ^{31}P MRS as an early prognostic indicator of patient response to chemotherapy. Magn Reson Med 25:30-44
164. Smith SR, Martin PA, Edwards RHT (1991) Tumour pH and response to chemotherapy: an in vivo ^{31}P magnetic resonance spectroscopy study in non-Hodgkin's lymphoma. Br J Radiol 64:923-928
165. Bryant DJ, Bydder GM, Case HA et al. (1988) Use of phosphorus-31 MR spectroscopy to monitor response to chemotherapy in non-Hodgkin lymphoma. J Comput Assist Tomogr 12:770-774
166. Ng TC, Vijayakumar S, Majors AW, Thomas FJ, Meaney TF, Baldwin NJ (1987) Response of non-Hodgkin lymphoma to ^{60}Co therapy monitored by ^{31}P MRS in situ. Int J Radiat Oncol 13:1545-1551
167. Li C-W, Kuesel AC, Padavic-Shaller KA et al. (1996) Metabolic characterization of human soft tissue sarcomas in vivo and in vitro using proton-decoupled phosphorus magnetic resonance spectroscopy. Cancer Res 56:2964-2972
168. Sostman HD, Prescott DM, Dewhirst MW et al. (1994) MR imaging and spectroscopy for prognostic evaluation in soft-tissue sarcomas. Radiology 190:269-275
169. Hoekstra HJ, Boeve WJ, Kamman RL, Mooyaart EL (1994) Clinical applicability of human in vivo localized phosphorus-31 magnetic resonance spectroscopy of bone and soft tissue tumors. Ann Surg Oncol 1:504-511
170. Redmond OM, Bell E, Stack JP et al. (1992) Tissue characterization and assessment of preoperative chemotherapeutic response in musculoskeletal tumors by in vivo ^{31}P magnetic resonance spectroscopy. Magn Reson Med 27:226-237
171. Redmond OM, Stack JP, Dervan PA, Hurson BJ, Carney DN, Ennis JT (1989) Osteosarcoma: use of MR imaging and MR spectroscopy in clinical decision making. Radiology 172:811-815
172. Ross B, Helsper JT, Cox IJ, Young IR, Kempt R, Makepeace A, Pennock J (1987) Osteosarcoma and other neoplasms of bone. Magnetic resonance spectroscopy to monitor therapy. Arch Surg 122:1464-1469
173. Twelves CJ, Lowry M, Porter DA et al. (1994) Phosphorus-31 metabolism of human breast - an in vivo magnetic resonance spectroscopic study at 1.5 Tesla. Br J Radiol 67:36-45
174. Kalra R, Wade KE, Hands L et al. (1993) Phosphomonoester is associated with proliferation in human breast cancer: a ^{31}P MRS study. Br J Cancer 67:1145-1153
175. Lowry M, Porter DA, Twelves CJ, et al (1992) Visibility of phopholipids in ^{31}P NMR spectra of human breast tumors in vivo. NMR Biomed 5:37-42

176. Redmond OM, Stack JP, O'Connor NG, et al. (1991) In vivo phosphorus-31 magnetic resonance spectroscopy of normal and pathological breast tissues. Br J Radiol 64:210–216
177. Brinkmann G, Melchert UH, Lalk G et al. (1997) The total entropy for evaluating ^{31}P-magnetic resonance spectra of the liver in healthy volunteers and patients with metastases. Invest Radiol 32:100–104
178. Jalan R, Taylor-Robinson SD, Hodgson HJ (1996) In vivo hepatic magnetic resonance spectroscopy: clinical or research tool? J Hepatol 25:414–424
179. Brinkmann G, Melchert UH, Emde L et al. (1995) In vivo P-31-MR-spectroscopy of focal hepatic lesions. Effectiveness of tumor detection in clinical practice and experimental studies of surface coil characteristics and localization technique. Invest Radiol 30:56–63
180. Cox IJ, Sargentini J, Calam J, Bryant DJ, Iles RA (1988) Four dimensional phosphorus-31 chemical shift imaging of carcinoid metastases in the liver. NMR Biomed 1:56–60
181. Negendank WG, Brown TR, Evelhoch JL et al. (1992) Proceedings of a National Cancer Institute workshop: MR spectroscopy and tumor cell biology. Radiology 185:8875–883
182. Mason GF, Behar KL, Lai JC (1996) The ^{13}C isotope and nuclear magnetic resonance: unique tools for the study of brain metabolism. Metabol Brain Dis 11:283–313
183. Beckmann N, Fried R, Turkalj I, Seelig J, Keller U, Stalder G (1993) Noninvasive observation of hepatic glycogen formation in man by ^{13}C MRS after oral and intraveneous glucose adminstration. Magn Reson Med 29:583–590
184. Beckmann N, Brocard J-J, Keller U, Seelig J (1992) Relationship between the degree of unsaturation of dietary fatty acids and adipose tissue fatty acids assessed by natural-abundance ^{13}C magnetic resonance spectroscopy in man. Magn Reson Med 27:97–106
185. Price TB, Rothman DL, Avison MJ, Buonamico P, Shulman RG (1991) ^{13}C-NMR measurements of muscle glycogen during low-intensity exercise. J Appl Physiol 70:1836–1844
186. Beckmann N, Müller S (1991) Natural abundance ^{13}C spectroscopic imaging applied to humans. J Magn Reson 93:186–194
187. Bottomley PA, Hardy CJ, Roemer PB, Mueller OM (1989) Proton-decoupled, Overhauser-enhanced, spatially localized carbon-13 spectroscopy in humans. Magn Reson Med 12:348–363
188. Sillerud LO, Halliday KR, Griffey RH, Fenoglio-Preiser C, Sheppard S (1988) In vivo ^{13}C NMR spectroscopy of the human prostate. Magn Reson Med 8:224–230
189. Jue T, Lohman JAB, Ordidge RJ, Shulman RG (1987) Natural abundance ^{13}C NMR spectrum of glycogen in humans. Magn Reson Med 5:377–379
190. Findlay MPN, Leach MO (1994) In vivo monitoring of fluoropyrimidine metabolites: magnetic resonance spectroscopy in the evaluation of 5-fluorouracil. Anti-Cancer Drugs 5:260–280
191. Findlay MPN, Raynaud F, Cunningham D, Iveson A, Collins DJ, Leach MO (1996) Measurement of plasma 5-fluorouracil by high-performance liquid chromatography with comparison of results to tissue drug levels observed using in vivo ^{19}F magnetic resonance spectroscopy in patients on a protracted venous infusion with or without interferon-α. Ann Oncol 7:47–53

Principles and Instrumentation of Positron Emission Tomography

W.-H. Wong, J. Uribe, H. Li, H. Baghaei

Basic Principles of Positron Emission Tomography

Positron-emitting tracers are used for imaging because of their unique tomographic capability and their group of metabolically important radionuclides. The unique tomographic capability comes from the simultaneous emission of two back-to-back, 511-KeV gamma rays from a positron-labeled molecule and from the ability to provide quantitation of tracer uptake due to accurate attenuation correction. With the detection of gamma-ray pairs by detectors outside the human body, tomographic images of the distribution of positron-labeled compounds can be generated. The medical importance of positron imaging lies in the existence of isotopes (^{11}C, ^{13}N, ^{15}O, ^{18}F) which are essential elements of all living organisms, and their physiological processes. Hence, tissue-specific and chemistry-specific tracers can be synthesized and injected into humans/animals to study the physiological functions of normal or pathological tissues in vivo. With proper tracer-dynamic modeling, the distribution of these positron-labeled compounds, as depicted by the tomographic images, may be converted into images of functional parameters such as metabolic rates, blood perfusion rates, and receptor densities.

Nuclear Properties

A positron (β+) is an antiparticle of an electron (β-). It is an electron with a positive electrical charge and can be created from the radionuclear decay of a nucleus that is deficient in neutrons. The atomic nucleus is made up of protons and neutrons. The neutrons provide an attractive, strong force that binds nuclear particles together and compensates for the repulsive electrostatic force caused by the repulsion of like-charges of the protons that would otherwise break up the nucleus. When the nucleus has too few neutrons to prevent protons from breaking away, radio decay transmutates the nucleus into a more stable

Table 5.1. Properties of commonly used isotopes for positron imaging

Positron isotopes	^{11}C	^{13}N	^{15}O	^{18}F	^{68}Ga[a]
Half-life (min)	20.4	9.96	2.07	109.7	68.3
Average β+ energy (MeV)	0.3	0.4	0.6	0.2	0.7
Average positioning error (mm)	0.28			0.22	1.35

[a] ^{68}Ga is generated from a ^{68}Ga/^{68}Ge generator (the parent ^{68}Ge has a half-life of 275 days)

state. One of the allowed pathways to stabilize the neutron-deficient, i.e., proton-excess, nucleus is through the transmutation of a proton into a neutron and a positron, which is then expelled from the nucleus due to its positive charge.

Because of nuclear instability and the physics of β decay, positron-emitting nuclei have very short lives. Hence, positrons do not occur in nature but can be generated in nuclear reactors or particle accelerators. Because the most useful positron isotopes for biological studies are ^{11}C, ^{15}O, and ^{18}F, which have only six to nine protons in the nucleus, the electrostatic repulsive force, which is encountered by the accelerated particles (protons/deuterons) on their way to penetrate the nucleus to initiate a reaction, is small. Hence, a small cyclotron that can accelerate protons to the 10–17 MeV range is sufficient to overcome electrostatic repulsion and to thereby produce the nuclear reactions required for biomedical positron imaging [1]. Small linear accelerators can also be used. The half-lives of the positron isotopes used most frequently in medical imaging are listed in Table 5.1 [2–4].

The positrons are emitted from the nucleus with some kinetic energy (Table 5.1). The emitted positron has to be slowed down to nearly zero energy through scattering in the tissue before it can annihilate with an electron to generate the two gamma-rays used for tomographic imaging. Hence, the emitted positron travels a short distance (0.2–2 mm) before generating the gamma-ray pair. This implies that the site of positron emission, i.e., the site of the positron-labeled molecule, and the site detected by the positron emission tomography (PET) as the source of gamma generation are slightly different. A higher positron energy will produce a larger imaging error because of the positron-range. This positron-range error contributes to the fundamental resolution limit of PET imaging (Table 5.1). However, the practical resolution limitation to PET imaging is the gamma-ray detection system of a PET camera, which will be discussed later.

Tomographic Properties

After a positron slows to near-zero velocity, it spends a long enough time in the proximity of a nearby electron to cause an annihilation. The annihilation process of mater-antimatter results in the conversion of the total mass (mass-energy) into a gamma-ray pair with the same energy ($E=mc^2$); the matter-antimatter vanishes in the process. Because an electron and a positron have an individual mass–energy of 511 KeV, two 511-KeV gamma-rays are produced in the annihilation process. From Newton's first law (conservation of momentum), the two 511-KeV gamma rays have to be emitted back to back, because the net momentum of two identical objects moving in opposite directions is zero. The back-to-back 180° emission of the gamma pair provides the special tomographic and quantitative properties of positron imaging.

The tomographic property is derived from the detection of the annihilation gamma-ray pair at the same time (coincidence detection) by detectors placed at opposite sides of the imaged subject. A true coincidental detection implies that a positron-tracer molecule existed along the line joining the two detectors (Fig. 5.1). If a point in space has positron tracers, the emission of coincidence pairs from that point will be uniformly distributed over all angles, because the emissions are random, i.e., they have no preferential direction. If these uniformly distributed detection lines are drawn, a blurred image of the point will emerge. This image-reconstruction process is called back-projection. The back-projection process is performed by a computer with a fast processor. To obtain a sharper image of the point, the spatial distribution of the coincidence data is filtered numerically before the back-projection process. This is the filtered back-projection image-reconstruction process, which is also performed by X-ray computed tomography (CT) and single photon-emission computed tomography (SPECT) cameras [5–8]. Because the subject to be imaged can be considered a collection of point sources with different activity levels, an image of the subject can be obtained with coincidence-detection data and the filtered back-projection-reconstruction algorithm. This property allows positron tracers to be used as an effective tomographic-imaging agent.

The quantitative imaging property is also derived from the 180° emission of the gamma-ray pair. In conventional nuclear or single-photon imaging, the attenuation of gamma-rays by the body cannot be calculated exactly or measured with an external radioactive source, which hinders the use of the image as a tool for in vivo quantitative measurement of the tracer distribution. However, with the 180° emission of two gamma rays, the positron tracer allows the attenuating effect of the body to be measured exactly by an external radioactive source. This attenuation correction process is mathematically exact and allows the PET camera to be used as an in vivo quantitative assay device. This quantitative property is very important for generating accurate tracer biodistribution and quantitative parametric images of physiological function, and for studying tracer dynamics in organs.

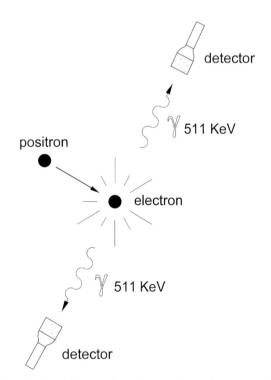

Fig. 5.1. Annihilation of a positron with an electron in tissue to generate the two 180° gamma rays, which are detected in coincidence by two external scintillation detectors

The Positron Cameras

Any camera that can image positron tracers can be called a positron camera, and can range from a simple one-head NaI(Tl) gamma camera, using a lead collimator, to a multi-million-dollar dedicated PET camera. There is wide gradation in the comparison of economics with performance. Designing and buying a camera involve the art of compromise. Generally, there are four classes of positron cameras (Fig. 5.2): (1) a NaI(Tl) gamma or SPECT camera with lead collimators, (2) a dual-head rotating NaI(Tl) camera (SPECT) with modified electronics for coincidence detection and lead collimator removed [9], (3) a dedicated NaI(Tl) PET camera with a ring detection system [10], and (4) a dedicated PET camera with a ring detection system made from the high sensitivity detector material bismuth germanate (BGO) [11, 12]. Class (4) can be further divided into two subclasses: one with a full detection ring and the other with a partial detection ring.

NaI(Tl) Gamma Cameras with Lead Collimators

Using the NaI(Tl) gamma camera with lead collimator is the most inexpensive way to image positron tracer because it uses existing gamma cameras in nuclear medicine operations. This is also the camera with the lowest detection sensitivity for positron imaging. There are two reasons for its low sensitivity. The use of lead collimation to define the direction of the detected gamma ray is very inefficient because the collimator absorbs 95% or more of the incoming gamma ray. In a camera that uses coincidence detection electronics to define the direction of the incoming gamma rays, lead collimation is not needed, and sensitivity is significantly higher (by 1–2 orders of magnitude). The second reason for the lower sensitivity is the thin NaI(Tl) detector, which is optimized for stopping the 140-KeV gamma ray to produce ^{99m}Tc imaging. Many of the higher-energy (511-KeV) gamma rays emitted by positron tracers will penetrate without being detected (70% escape fraction). Hence, a combined total of only 2% of the positron gamma rays that reach the gamma camera are detected. This low detection efficiency implies that only very large lesions (2.5–3 cm) can be detected. This class of camera provides a way to take advantage of the more tumor-specific positron tracers without incurring the expense of buying and operating a dedicated PET camera. Some recent articles [13] have reported the use of this type of camera for breast cancer imaging using the positron tracer, F-18-deoxyglucose (FDG).

Dual-Head Rotating NaI(Tl) Camera with Coincidence Detection Electronics

The dual-head rotating NaI(Tl) camera with coincidence detection electronics is basically a dual-head SPECT camera with coincidence electronics added [9]. With coincidence detection, the direction of the detected gamma rays are defined by

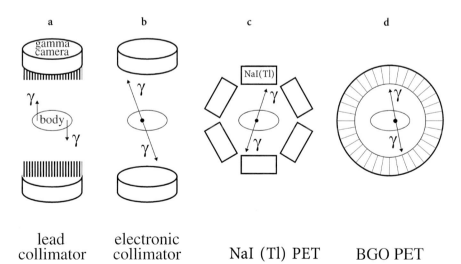

Fig. 5.2a–d. Four classes of positron cameras. **a** Regular single- or dual-head gamma cameras with lead collimators. **b** Regular dual-head single photon-emission computed tomography (SPECT) with coincidence detection circuit added and lead collimators removed. **c** Dedicated positron-emission tomography (PET) camera using large NaI(Tl) detectors. **d** Dedicated PET camera using small bismuth germanate (BGO) detectors

two locations on opposite sides of the subject and the inefficient lead collimator is no longer needed. Elimination of the lead collimator increases the detection sensitivity by 20 times or more relative to the regular gamma camera type. However, the thin NaI(Tl) detector still has low sensitivity for detecting 511-KeV gamma rays. Because the probability of detection is 0.3 for each partner of the gamma-ray pair, the joint probability of detecting both partners of a positron emission to form a coincidence detection is 0.3×0.3=0.09. Hence the detection efficiency is 9% for all the coincidence gamma pairs that reach the two opposing camera heads. When compared with a dedicated PET camera, which uses much thicker detectors made of BGO scintillation material, the sensitivity of this modified SPECT camera type is nine to ten times lower for identical detection areas. Nevertheless, the detection sensitivity of this class of camera is a substantial improvement (5–10×) over the lead collimator type. Recent reports [14] show that this camera type can detect lesions as small as 1.5–2.0 cm. Hence, for a relatively small investment, this camera type may be a better compromise than the lead collimator gamma camera for taking advantage of more tumor-specific positron tracers.

Even though the detection efficiency is improved five to ten times, a new problem arises when the lead collimator is removed. The head of each gamma camera is basically one large detector, and when a gamma ray is detected, the whole camera head is inactive until all the stimulated scintillation light caused by the gamma detection is emitted. If there is a second incoming gamma ray, the signals pile up in the detector and combine, yielding to an erroneous determination of energy and position. With the removal of the lead collimator, gamma-ray flux causes severe signal-pileup problems in the NaI(Tl) detector of this type of camera. As such, the injected dose has to be reduced by 80% compared with that which is used for imaging with a dedicated BGO PET camera; this produces a further reduction in the quality of the image over and above the nine to ten times lower detection efficiency. Another deficiency of this camera design is that the coincidence detection efficiency is geometrically dependent; the region near the center of rotation has the highest efficiency but the coincidence efficiency reduces to zero at the edge of the camera (Fig. 5.2b). Hence, it is important for this camera type to be larger than the field of view to yield usable efficiency at the edge of the patient.

Dedicated PET Camera with a NaI(Tl) Detector Ring

With the advantages reflected in increased purchasing and operating costs, the dedicated PET camera with NaI(Tl) detector ring is yet another improvement over the two previously mentioned camera types. This camera is similar to the dual-head NaI(Tl) gamma camera with coincidence detection electronics, but the dedicated PET has six heads [10]. The six heads are configured to form a fixed ring around the patient. Furthermore, because the camera is designed to be a dedicated PET camera instead of also performing ^{99m}Tc imaging, the thickness of the NaI(Tl) detector is increased from 1 cm to 2.5 cm to increase the camera's detection sensitivity. This increased detector thickness contributes to a four times increase in coincidence detection efficiency compared with a dual-head coincidence camera (with the same active detection area). Furthermore, with the detectors completely surrounding the patient, the detection efficiency is uniform in the transaxial field of view. However, because the detector design is basically that of a gamma camera, signal pileup can still be a problem if the injected dose is not reduced, although such cameras generally use electronic processing to shorten the detector dead time [10]. The injected dose is generally reduced by 60–80% from that of a dedicated PET using BGO scintillation detectors. Although the intrinsic resolution of this camera can rival that of the more expensive BGO camera, the more limited-image counts cause the practical/clinical image resolution to be lower. However, the lower production cost of this dedicated PET makes it a viable option for imaging positron tracers.

Dedicated PET Camera with BGO Detector Rings

The most efficient, fastest-counting camera with the highest image quality is the dedicated PET camera with BGO detector rings; it is also the most expensive. Unlike the cameras discussed above, which are based on the gamma-camera technology, using a single, large NaI(Tl) detector, the BGO camera uses thousands of small, discrete BGO detectors [11, 12]. The discrete BGO detectors are packed into many detector rings surrounding the patient, which eliminates the need to rotate the detection system. The elimination of camera rotation during imaging may be important for imaging tracers that change rapidly with time, such as ^{15}O or ^{13}N. For FDG imaging, camera rotation is generally tolerable.

The multiplicity of detectors in this camera type allows the camera to operate at much higher count rates (3–6×), which translates to a higher injected dose and, consequently, a higher quality image. Furthermore, BGO has higher density (2×) and higher atomic number than NaI(Tl), as well as a significantly higher detection sensitivity for the higher-energy gamma rays emitted by positron tracers. Hence, the detected counts-per-unit injected dose is also higher with the dedicated PET/BGO than with the other three camera types that use NaI(Tl) detectors; this results in a further improvement in image quality. Practical resolution and image quality are highest with this camera type. However, it is also the most expensive positron camera type. Presently, the highest intrinsic spatial resolution of this camera type is 4.2–4.5 mm. The practical image resolution is lower, depending on the number of counts collected. Under optimal conditions, such as brain imaging with FDG, a 6-mm practical image resolution may be achieved. For whole-body imaging, the resolution will be lower because of severe gamma-ray attenuation by the body. For FDG cancer imaging, the smallest detectable lesion size also depends on the ratio of tumor uptake to normal tissue uptake. With this camera type, smaller tumors (6–10 mm) are detectable.

Future Development in Positron Cameras

Recent trends in the development of positron cameras have been largely concentrated on lowering the production costs. For a dedicated PET camera with BGO detectors, the production cost of the detection system is often 50% of the total. Hence, most of the developmental effort is targeted at lowering the detection system cost. The

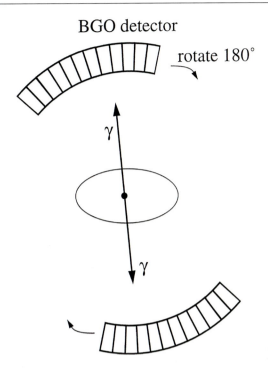

Fig. 5.3. Rotational dedicated positron-emission tomography (PET) camera with a partial ring of bismuth germanate (BGO) detectors

recently introduced rotating BGO camera is one example [15] (Fig. 5.3). This rotating camera is basically the BGO ring camera described above, but with two-thirds of the detectors removed from the ring such that only two opposing sectors of the detection system remain. This reduces the camera cost by 50% and reduces sensitivity by 66% for small objects and 80% for large objects.

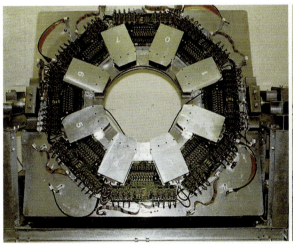
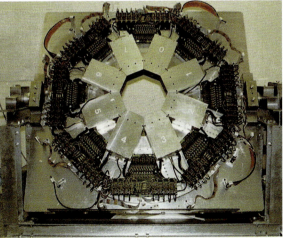

Fig. 5.4. A variable field-of-view-dedicated positron-emission tomography (PET) camera using bismuth germanate (BGO) detectors. *Left* whole-body mode; *right* brain, breast and animal mode

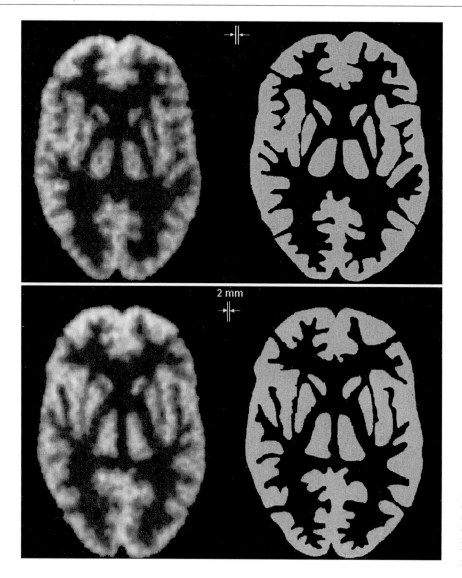

Fig. 5.5. Two image slices of a brain [17] phantom acquired by a prototype variable field-of-view PET operating in the brain/breast mode [37]. The true phantom maps are shown on the right side

A second development that reduces the production cost utilizes a new detector design, photomultiplier-quadrant sharing [16], and a convertible geometry [17]. In this convertible design, there are gaps in the BGO detection rings of the system which reduce cost when the camera is imaging the whole body (Fig. 5.4), but with some sacrifice of detection sensitivity. However, in imaging small objects, such as the brain, breast, and animals, the convertible geometry allows shrinking to a smaller field of view with a full ring of detectors. This mode can increase the detection sensitivity for imaging smaller objects above that of a conventional whole-body camera, because the detection ring is fully populated and the detectors are closer to the object; this increases the probability of capturing the gamma-rays emitted from the subject. Hence, the convertible design has higher sensitivity for smaller objects and lower sensitivity for whole-body images, with a lower overall camera cost. A high-resolution prototype camera has been constructed with this design [17, 37]. This low-cost prototype BGO camera achieves 3.0 mm image resolution (Fig. 5.5).

Another recent effort is the development of a combination SPECT/PET camera using a new detection material made from lutetium orthosilicate (LSO) and NaI(Tl) [18]. This dual-purpose camera is basically a conventional SPECT with two modifications: (1) a new detection material LSO, which has higher sensitivity than NaI(Tl) for detecting the higher-energy positron gamma rays; and (2) the adoption of the lower-cost, discrete-detector design of the photomultiplier-quadrant-sharing detector that is used in the convertible camera mentioned above. The NaI(Tl) detectors are positioned in front of the LSO detector layer and are for conventional single-photon or SPECT imaging; the LSO detector is for positron coincidence imaging. Another advantage of the LSO detector is that it is capable of counting six times faster than NaI(Tl). Hence, LSO allows the camera to detect positron gamma rays at a much higher rate than a regular dual-head SPECT, in addition to being much more sensitive. A prototype camera is being developed with this design [18].

Another recent development in positron imaging is the dedicated breast cameras. These are generally small lower-cost cameras that have two opposing camera heads with very high resolution [19, 20]. These cameras are generally designed to image the compressed breast in the projection mode (similar to X-ray mammography) instead of the tomography mode. This camera type takes advantage of the much higher diagnostic accuracy of positron imaging than X-ray mammography, and the compressed-breast imaging mode allows for easy comparison with X-ray mammography. The disadvantage is that very small lesions or lesions with low contrast may not be detected due to overlap of cancer and normal breast signals in this projection or non-tomographic imaging mode. Although the intrinsic camera resolution is generally 2 mm or less, the smallest breast tumor detected may be larger than that.

With improved instrumentation in the future, positron cameras will be more cost-effective, and the image quality will also be improved. The intrinsic image resolution can be improved from the current industrial standard of 4.2–4.5 mm to 3 mm. An experimental, multi-slice, whole-body PET camera using BGO detectors has demonstrated an intrinsic image resolution of 3 mm in the transaxial and axial planes [17] (Fig. 5.5). Some small experimental cameras designed for rat/mice animal models have already demonstrated 1.5- to 2-mm resolution [21] for imaging F-18, which has the lowest positron-range blurring effect.

Quantitation and Parametric Imaging

One important advantage of PET imaging is that accurate attenuation correction allows tracer uptake and dynamics to be accurately quantified from the image data. However, note that there should be an accurate calibration to correlate the image-pixel value to the tissue activity density (μCi/gm tissue) and that the image-pixel value is not an arbitrary relative number scaled to fit the dynamic range of our vision or the display device. With tracer-transport modeling and multiple scans over a time period (dynamic imaging), functional parameters can be quantified. Some common physiological parameters generated by PET are blood flow [22–24], metabolic rate [25], blood volume [26, 27] and receptor density. These quantified parameters may be more useful than a simple tracer-uptake image. For example, a region that has a high relative uptake of FDG may be either an area of high blood volume/perfusion, especially if the images are taken right after injection, or an area of high glucose metabolism; quantified parametric images of glucose metabolic rate and blood space would eliminate such ambiguity.

The quantitation can be carried out in two different ways, depending on the complexity of the tracer transport model and the quality of the raw image data: (1) if the model is complex, involving many parameters coupled with noisy image data, it would be better to draw a region of interest in the image data, e.g., on a suspected tumor site, and compute the average functional parameters within the region or (2) if the model is simple (1–2 parameters) and the image quality is high, it may be more useful to generate a parametric image set to present the parameters on a pixel-by-pixel basis. A set of parametric images that display separately the metabolic-rate and blood-volume distributions can be useful, clinically, for cancer detection and treatment monitoring. Quantitation is especially important for accurately monitoring the efficacy of therapy if a similar quantitation is performed before treatment.

Tracer modeling and parametric quantitation techniques for FDG, the most clinically useful cancer imaging tracer today, have been studied extensively with different degrees of refinement, simplification, and compromise between practicality and accuracy [25, 28]. Most FDG methods are based on the three compartment models, (Fig. 5.6). The physiological parameters to be deduced are the rate constants k_1^*, k_2^*, k_3^*, and k_4^*, shown in Fig. 5.6. One way to find the rate constants for a lesion is by drawing a ROI in the image set and extracting the time-activity data. The ROI time-activity data are then combined with the time-activity data of the blood-plasma tracer concentration input to a curve-fitting computer program that analyzes the three-compartment model. The curve-fitting program outputs the rate constants [29]. This procedure generates the average rate constants for the ROI instead of a set of parametric images of the rate constants. Conceptually, the same method can be applied pixel by pixel to generate a set of parametric images of the

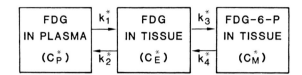

Fig. 5.6. F-18-deoxyglucose (FDG) three-compartment model

rate constants. However, such an image-processing procedure requires the image quality of the original uptake data to be very high so that statistical error for all the pixels is small. Furthermore, the curve-fitting time for all the image pixels may be impractically lengthy compared with the present computing technology.

A more practical method of generating an FDG metabolic image is based on the unidirectional flow model [26, 27], sometimes called the Patlak-plot method, which is basically a three-compartment model as in Fig. 5.6, except that k_4^* is assumed to be insignificantly small. A negligible k_4^* implies that there is no leakage of the tracer from the trapped cell space. This simplifies the model from four parameters (k_1^*, k_2^*, k_3^*, and k_4^*) to two parameters (Ki, Vd), where Ki is the macro metabolic rate constant and Vd is the blood distribution volume and vascular space. Mathematically, the macro metabolic rate constant Ki of the tissue-bound compartment is equivalent to $k_1^* \times k_3^* / [k_2^* + k_3^*]$ in the three-compartment model. This method is computationally fast and less demanding of the raw image data quality. However, even this simplified method requires the measurement of the tracer input function, the blood time-activity curve. Generally, all parametric imaging methods require the measurement of the tracer input function. The extraction of 30 blood samples over the imaging time and the effort required to measure the blood activity information contained in these samples make this procedure rather demanding – especially for clinical studies. As PET imaging moves into the clinics, many different ways of reducing the amount of blood sampling have been proposed, but the most accurate and simplest way is with the use of an automated blood detector [30, 31].

For clinical FDG cancer studies, the most widely used semi-quantitative parameters are the standard uptake value (SUV) or differential uptake ratio (DUR) [32, 33] defined as,

SUV (DUR) = [tissue activity in µCi/g]/
 [injected dose in mCi
 per kg body weight].

For FDG, the tissue activity used is generally the tracer uptake between 30 min and 60 min [32, 33]. There is much variability in this measurement, depending on the exact implementation in each clinical site. To minimize variability for comparison purposes, all studies in the same site should use the same quality-control parameters, such as waiting time after injection, duration of imaging and fasting protocols. To further minimize variability, plasma glucose level correction [34, 35] should also be applied:

SUV (corrected) = SUV × [plasma glucose/100]

In addition, there should be a body-fat correction term [33, 36] to account for the reduced uptake of FDG in body fat. The SUV can be extracted either as the peak value in an ROI or by displaying the SUV pixel by pixel as a pseudo-color-quantitation SUV image. The SUV quantitation is not as accurate as the three-compartment model or the unidirectional model, but it is very simple to implement and requires no blood sampling, which may make it more practical for a clinical environment.

References

1. Fowler JS, Wolf AP (1986) Positron emitter-labeled compounds: priorities and problems. In: Phelps M, Mazziotta J, Schelbert H (eds) Positron emission tomography and autoradiography: principles and applications for the brain and heart. Raven Press, New York, pp 391–450
2. Derenzo SE (1979) Precision measurement of annihilation point spread distributions for medically important positron emitters. Proceedings of the 5th International Conference on Positron Annihilation, Sendai, Japan, pp. 819–824
3. Phelps ME, Mazziotta JC, Schelbert HR (eds) (1986) Positron emission tomography and autoradiography principles and applications for the brain and heart. Raven Press, New York
4. Phelps ME, Sorenson JA (eds) (1987) Physics in nuclear medicine, 2nd edn. Saunders, Philadelphia
5. Bracewell RN, Riddle AC (1967) Inversion of fan-beam scans in radioastronomy. Astrophys J 150:427–434
6. Brooks RA, DiChiro G (1975) Theory of image reconstruction in computed tomography. Radiology 117: 561–572
7. Brownell GL, Burnham CA, Chesler CA, et al. (1977) Transverse section imaging of radionuclide distribution in heart, lung and brain. In: Ter-Pogossian MM, Phelps ME, and Brownell GL (eds) Reconstruction tomography in diagnostic radiology and nuclear medicine. University Park Press, Baltimore, pp 293–307
8. Shepp LA, Logan BF (1974) The fourier reconstruction of a head section. IEEE Trans Nucl Sci NS-21:21–43
9. Muehllehner M, Geagan P, Countryman P, Nellemann P (1995) SPECT scanner with PET coincidence capability (abstract). J Nucl Med 36:70p
10. Karp JS, Muehllehner G, Mankoff D, et al. (1990) Continous-Slice PENN-PET: A Positron Tomography with Volume Imaging Capability. J Nucl Med 31:617–627
11. Adam LE, Zaers J, Ostertag H, et al. (1997) Performance evaluation of the whole-body PET scanner ECAT EXACT HR+ following the IEC standard. IEEE Trans Nucl Sci 44:1172–1179

12. DeGrado T, Turkington T, Williams J, Stearns C, Hoffman J (1994) Performance characteristics of a whole-body PET scanner. J Nucl Med 35:1398-1406
13. Holle LH, Trampert L, Lung-Kurt S, et al. (1996) Investigations of breast tumors with fluorine-18-fluorodeoxyglucose and SPECT. J Nucl Med 36:615-622
14. Ziegler SI, Enterottacher G, Boning P, et al. (1997) Performance characteristics of a dual head coincidence camera for the detection of small lesions. Proceedings of the 44th Annual Meeting, J Nucl Med 38:206
15. Townsend D, Wensveen M, Byars L, et al. (1991) A rotating PET camera using BGO block detectors. Conference Record of the 1991 IEEE Nuclear Science Symposium and Medical Imaging Conference 3:1658-1662
16. Wong WH, Uribe J, Hicks K, Zambelli M, Hu G (1994) A 2-dimensional detector decoding study on BGO arrays with quadrant sharing photomultipliers. IEEE Trans Nucl Sci 41:1453-1457
17. Wong WH, Uribe J, Lu W, et al. (1996) Design of a variable field prototype PET camera. IEEE Trans Nucl Sci 43:1915-1925
18. Dahlbom M, MacDonald LR, Eriksson L, et al. (1997) Performance of a YSO/LSO phoswich detector for use in a PET/SPECT system. IEEE Trans Nucl Sci 44:1114-1119
19. Freifelder R, Karp JS (1997) Dedicated PET scanners for breast imaging. Phys Med Biol 42:2463-2480
20. Thompson CJ, Murthy K, Picard Y, et al. (1995) Positron emission mammography (PEM): a promising technique for detecting breast cancer. IEEE Trans Nucl Sci 42:1012-1017
21. Cherry SR, Shao Y, Silverman RW, et al. (1997) MicroPET: a high resolution PET scanner for imaging small animals. IEEE Trans Nucl Sci 44:1161-1166
22. Frackowiak RSJ, Lenzi G-L, Jones T, Heather JD (1980) Quantitative measurement of emission tomography: theory, procedure and normal values. J Comput Assist Tomogr 4:727-736
23. Huang S-C, Carson RE, Hoffman EJ, et al. (1983) Quantitative measurement of local cerebral blood flow in humans by positron computed tomography and ^{15}O-water. J Cereb Blood Flow Metab 3:141-153
24. Ruotsalainen U, Raitakari M, Nuutila P, et al. (1997) Quantitative blood flow measurement of skeletal muscle using oxygen-15-water and PET. J Nucl Med 38:314-319
25. Phelps ME, Huang SC, Hoffman EJ, et al. (1979) Tomographic measurements of local cerebral glucose metabolic rate in humans with [^{18}F]2-fluoro-2-deoxy-D-glucose: validation of method. Ann Neuro 6:371-388
26. Patlak C, Blasberg R, Fenstermacher J (1983) Graphical evaluation of blood-to-brain transfer constants from multiple-time uptake data. J Cereb Blood Flow Metab 3:1-7
27. Gjedde A (1982) Calculation of cerebral glucose phosphorylation from brain uptake of glucose analogs in vivo: a re-examination. Brain Res Rev 4:237-274
28. Sokoloff L, Reivich M, Kennedy C, et al. (1977) The (^{14}C)-deoxyglucose method for the measurement of local cerebral glucose utilization: theory, procedure and normal values in the conscious and anesthetized albino rat. J Neurochem 28:897-916
29. Carson RE (1986) Parameter estimation in positron emission tomography. In: Phelps M, Mazziotta J, and Schelbert H (eds) Positron emission tomography and autoradiography: principles and applications for the brain and heart. Raven Press, New York, pp. 347-390
30. Hutchins GD, Hichwa RD, Koeppe RA (1986) A continuous flow input function detector for $H_2{}^{15}O$ blood flow studies in positron emission tomography. IEEE Trans Nucl Sci NS 33:546-549
31. Eriksson L, Holte S, Bohm C, et al. (1988) Automated blood sampling systems for positron emission tomography. IEEE Trans Nucl Sci NS 35:703-707
32. Hanburg LM, Hunter GT, Alpert NM, et al. (1994) The dose uptake ratio as an index of glucose metabolism: useful parameter or over simplification? J Nucl Med 35:1308-1312
33. Zasadny KR, Wahl RL (1993) Standardized uptake values of normal tissues at PET with 2-[fluorine-18-]-fluoro-2-deoxy-D-glucose: variations with body weight and a method for correction. Radiology 189:847-850
34. Lindholm P, Minn H, Leskinen-Kallio S, et al. (1993) Influence of the blood glucose concentration on FDG uptake in cancer – a PET study. J Nucl Med 34:1-6
35. Langen K-J, Braun U, Kops ER, et al. (1993) The influence of plasma glucose levels on fluorine-18-fluorodeoxyglucose uptake in bronchial carcinomas. J Nucl Med 34:355-359
36. Kim CK, Gupta NC, Chandramouli B, Alavi A (1994) Standardized uptake values of FDG: body surface area correction is preferable to body weight correction. J Nucl Med 35:164-167
37. Uribe J, Baghaei H, Li H, et al. (1998) Basic Imaging Performance characteristics of a Variable Field of View PET Camera Using Quadrant Sharing Detector Design. IEEE 1998 Nuclear Science Symposium and Medical Imaging Conference Record. Submitted to IEEE Transactions on Nuclear Science

Radiopharmaceuticals for Tumor Imaging and Magnetic Resonance Imaging Contrast Agents

D. J. Yang, S. Ilgan, E. E. Kim

Radiopharmaceuticals

Basic Considerations

The major role of radiopharmaceuticals in clinical oncology is in tumor imaging, which includes evaluating specific organs or the entire body for the presence of tumors. Oncologists use these agents in the initial evaluation of the tumor extent (staging) and in the subsequent management of the patient with cancer – to assess therapeutic response, detect early relapse, and assist in making treatment decisions. Other roles for radiopharmaceuticals include their use in combined-modality treatment programs, as labels for antibodies or as drugs administered in diagnosis and treatment, and in the prediction of therapeutic response.

Localization of a radiopharmaceutical agent in a tumor is best conceptualized in terms of altered regional physiology due to the presence of the tumor. Tumors, certain areas of inflammation, and certain phases of infarct development are characterized by increased permeability of their capillary beds to macromolecules. This permeability is largely due to neovascularization and the large intercapillary pores associated with new growth of capillary beds. Total perfusion of such lesions is increased in comparison with surrounding normal tissue. There may be also a delay in new lymphatic vessel growth, thereby adding to the residence time of the macromolecules in the interstitial fluid space. The increased macrophage activity associated with tissue necrosis may result in ingestion of the labeled macromolecules. There may be specific receptor sites on the cell membrane for the macromolecule. Another mechanism may be the altered cell permeability.

To improve the diagnosis and the planning and monitoring of cancer treatment, various radiolabeled metabolic imaging ligands were developed. These analogues are functional ligands, which should provide information useful for the prediction or monitoring of tumor responses to treatment.

Markers of Estrogen Receptor Tissue

Each year in the United States, 175,000 women are affected by, and approximately 44,000 die of, breast cancer. These numbers are increasing over time and the disease is becoming one of the leading causes of death in women. The presence of sex hormone receptors in both primary and secondary breast tumors is an important indicator for prognosis and for the choice of therapy [1]. Currently, receptors are determined by in vitro analysis of biopsy specimens and the use of anti-estrogens. Tamoxifen is the therapy of choice for estrogen receptor-positive (ER+) tumors. Detecting and measuring ER+ tumors using a radiolabeled ligand should serve as a useful tool for detecting primary and secondary tumors, selecting and following the results of therapy, and for predicting treatment outcome. To this end, a number of variations of substituted estradiols have been prepared that contain radioisotopes in positions 16 or 17 [2-4]. Detecting ER-rich tissue in vivo has been relatively successful using these compounds; however, their ability to provide quantitative information about receptor concentration in either animal models or in humans has been less clearly demonstrated.

Tamoxifen therapy results are positive in 30% of unselected patients with breast cancer. A response rate of 50–60% was obtained in patients with ER+ tumors [5]. Patients with metastatic cancer who respond to the treatment have a response duration of 10–18 months and prolonged survival [6]. Obviously, a radiolabeled tamoxifen ligand would be useful in diagnosing diseases that produce high levels of ERs, such as ovarian cancer, endometriosis, endometrial carcinoma, and meningioma. Our rationale is that if binding of the ligands with tumors can be detected with positron emission tomography (PET) or single photon-emission computed tomography (SPECT), then such ligands may predict responses to anti-cancer agents. Radiolabeled tamoxifen would also be useful for investigating tamoxifen's mechanisms of action, since it would provide accurate information about the effectiveness of antiestrogen (tamoxifen) therapy. In addition, such ligands might help to determine the causes of occasional failure of tamoxifen therapy when biopsy indicators are ER+.

Several halogenated tamoxifen analogues were developed [7, 8]. These analogues had higher ER affinity than tamoxifen [9, 10]. For instance, using pig uterine cytosol, bromotamoxifen was 150 times better than tamoxifen, and fluorotamoxifen had a binding power 30 times that of tamoxifen. In vivo imaging studies demonstrated the specificity of fluorotamoxifen [11], which can be prepared as an analog of tamoxifen (which has a high specificity) [12, 13]. In this report, [^{18}F]fluorotamoxifen in ten ER+ breast cancer patients and [^{131}I]iodotamoxifen and [^{111}In]DTPA-TX in animal models are reported.

Markers of Tumor Hypoxia

Misonidazole (MISO) is a hypoxic cell sensitizer, and labeling it with different halogenated radioisotopes, e.g., fluorine-18 or iodine-123, could be useful for differentiating a hypoxic, but metabolically active, tumor from a well-oxygenated active tumor, using PET or planar scintigraphy [14–19]. [^{18}F]Fluoromisonidazole (FMISO) has been used to assess the hypoxic component in brain ischemia, myocardial infarction and various tumors [20–25]. Moreover, the assessment of tumor hypoxia with labeled MISO prior to radiation therapy would provide a rational means for selecting patients for treatment with radiosensitizing or bioreductive drugs, e.g. mitomycin C. Such selection would permit more accurate evaluation because their use of these modalities could be limited to patients with hypoxic tumors. It is also possible to select proper modalities of radiotherapy (neutron versus photon) by correlating labeled MISO results with tumor response.

It has been reported that MISO produced peripheral sensory neuropathy at the dose level required for radiosensitization [26, 27]. Thus, more hydrophilic MISO analogues are suggested. In this report, autoradiograms and radionuclide imaging of 2-nitroimidazole analogues were evaluated for their usefulness in diagnosing tumor hypoxia and for monitoring the therapeutic effects of anticancer drugs.

Markers of Tumor Cell Proliferation

Noninvasive imaging assessment of tumor cell proliferation could be helpful in the evaluation of tumor growth potential, the degree of malignancy, and could provide an early assessment of treatment response prior to changes in tumor size. Radiolabeled nucleoside/nucleotide analogues should provide proliferative imaging information about primary and secondary tumors [28–33]. It may also assist in selecting and following the most favorable nucleoside/nucleotide therapy and in following-up its outcome. Our rationale is that if the binding of nucleoside/nucleotide to tumor cell DNA/RNA can be detected with PET, then an analogue may be useful for evaluating tumor response to nucleoside/nucleotide (5-fluorouracil, 5-fluorodeoxyuridine, 5-bromodeoxyuridine, cytidine, cytarabine) therapy. To assess tumor proliferative activity, autoradiograms and radionuclide imaging of [^{18}F]-adenosine, [^{131}I]adenosine and 5-[^{131}I]iodo-2′-methyluridine were reported.

Marker of Lipid Peroxidase Inhibitors

Numerous studies have shown that antioxidant/antiangiogenesis agents, such as vitamin A (retinoic acid, retinal and retinol), provide a promising new approach in the prevention and treatment of cancer. For instance, retinoic acid (RA) has been used as a clinically effective treatment for promyelocytic leukemia and juvenile myelogenous leukemia in a majority of patients [34]. RA is also active against papillomas, squamous cell carcinoma and other skin diseases, e.g., acne, psoriasis [35–38]. It was hypothesized that these disorders may be due to high levels of superoxides and/or abnormal gene expression of RA receptors. At least two subtypes of RA receptors, RARs and RXRs, are important in biological actions [39, 40]. RA receptors may act to upregulate gap junction communication, stabilize normal cells by increasing the secretion of TGF-β (transforming growth factor) against subsequent transformation and, thus, decrease cell proliferation [41].

Free radicals, i.e., superoxides, are involved in various degenerative diseases. Reactive superoxides are involved in cancer initiation and promotion. In healthy postmenopausal women, estrogen and antioxidant levels are both low. Higher levels of serum lipid peroxides and estrogen have been reported in patients with untreated benign and malignant breast tumors than in healthy controls [42, 43]. The results could be due to an increase in the rate of lipid peroxidation in the cancerous state and to subsequent increases in the production of estrogen, which leaks into the bloodstream.

It has been shown that the concentrations of serum selenium and vitamins A, C, and E were increased significantly in patients treated with tamoxifen for 3–6 months [44–46]. The results suggest that tamoxifen therapy exerts significant positive effects on the rate of lipid peroxidation and on protective systems in postmenopausal women with breast cancer. In a cancerous stress condition, the requirement for vitamins and antioxidants increases progressively; hence, the decrease in vitamin levels in women with untreated breast cancer relative to normal control subjects. Thus, a combination of vitamin A and tamoxifen could improve tamoxifen efficacy in breast cancer therapy, as both are antioxidants and serve to prevent lipid peroxidation. Moreover, vitamin A reduces the rate of lipid peroxidation; this, in turn, decreases endogenous estrogen levels and subsequently increases tamoxifen's ability to target ER sites. Others have reported that tamoxifen efficacy increases when 13-cis-retinoic acid and tamoxifen are combined [47]. Therefore, a radiolabeled antioxidant may monitor combined 13-cis-retinoic acid and tamoxifen therapy in breast cancer. In this report, [^{111}In] DTPA-retinal was prepared and its radionuclide imaging studies were conducted.

Markers of ER Tissue

PET Imaging of ER+ Breast Tumors Using [^{18}F]Fluorotamoxifen (FTX)

The patient was supine in the scanner so that the detector rings spanned the entire breast. A 20-min attenuation scan was performed with a 4-mCi [^{68}Ge]-ring source prior to administering [^{18}F]FTX. After each patient received [^{18}F]FTX (2–12 mCi, i.v.), six consecutive 20-min scans were taken. Serial transaxial images were performed using a scanner (POSICAM 6.5, Positron Corporation, Houston, Tex.), for which the field-of-view was 42 cm on the transverse and 12 cm on the coronal plane. The axial resolution in the reconstructed plane was 1.2 cm. Twenty-one transaxial slices, separated by 5.2 mm, were reconstructed. Visual inspection, as well as semiquantitative evaluation using standard uptake value (SUV; activity in tumor/injected dose × body weight) were used. Before PET scanning, the position of breast tumors was also determined by contrast-enhanced computed tomography (CT) (High Speed Advantages, General Electric Company, Milwaukee, Wis.) or magnetic resonance imaging using a 1.5-T scanner (GE Medical System, Milwaukee, Wis.). Of ten patients, eight were on tamoxifen therapy after the PET study. Responses to tamoxifen therapy were evaluated after 6 months.

Autoradiogram of [^{131}I]Iodotamoxifen in Ovarian-Tumor-Bearing Rats

[^{131}I]Iodotamoxifen was synthesized using previously described procedures [8, 12]. Ovarian-tumor-bearing mice ($n=3$) were killed 24 h after receiving [^{131}I]iodotamoxifen (50 μCi, i.v.). Each rat body was fixed in carboxymethyl cellulose (4%). The frozen body was mounted onto a cryostat (LKB 2250 cryomicrotome) and cut into 40-μm coronal sections. Each section was thawed and mounted on a slide. The slide was then placed in contact with X-ray film (X-Omat AR, Kodak, Rochester, N.Y.) and exposed for 48 h.

Radiosynthesis of [^{111}In]-DTPA-Tamoxifen (TX) Conjugate

A stirred solution of aminoethylanilide-DTPA (100 mg, 0.195 mmol) [48] and aldotamoxifen (83.3 mg, 1 equivalent, 0.195 mmol) [49, 50] in CH_3CN-H_2O (1:1) (8 ml) was treated with a solution of $NaCNBH_3$ (1 M in THF) (0.13 ml, 0.67 equivalent, 0.13 mmol). The mixture was stirred for 2 h in a nitrogen atmosphere at room temperature. The solvent was then evaporated. The unreacted aldotamoxifen was removed by excessive washing with CH_2Cl_2 (3×5 ml). The final product was used without further purification. DTPA-TX conjugate (5 mg) was dissolved in 1 ml of ethanol/water (2:1) mixture. An aliquot containing 0.1 mg DTPA-TX was added with ^{111}InCl$_3$ (0.7 mCi, in 20 μl, 0.04 N HCl; NEN Dupont, Boston, Mass.). Then, sodium acetate (0.6 N, 20 μl) and sodium citrate (0.06 N, 20 μl) were added. The mixture stood for 30 min. The final solution was then formulated in 5% ethanol/saline solution. Radiochemical purity was determined to be greater than 99% (using $CHCl_3/MeOH$; 1:1, $R_f = 0.2$, Bioscan, Wash.).

Gamma Scintigraphic Imaging of Studies

Gamma scintigraphic images were obtained with a GE Starport System (GE Company) equipped with high-resolution, medium-energy, and a parallel-hole collimator. Five breast-tumor-bearing rats were administered [^{111}In]-DTPA-TX (300 μCi, i.v.). Three rabbits simulated with endometriosis were administered [^{131}I]iodotamoxifen (300 μCi, i.v.). Whole-body planar images were obtained at 30 min, and at 2, 4, 24 and 48 h; 300,000 counts were acquired in 128×128 matrix.

Markers of Tumor Hypoxia

Robotic Synthesis of [^{18}F]FMISO and [^{18}F]FETNIM

[^{18}F]fluoride was produced by the M. D. Anderson cyclotron (42 MeV, Cyclotron Corporation) by means of proton irradiation of enriched [^{18}O]-water in a small-volume silver target. The target was filled with 0.8 ml [^{18}O] water. Aliquots containing 500–800 mCi [^{18}F] activity after a 1-h beam time (18 µA current) were collected. The irradiated water was combined with kryptofix-2, 2, 2 (26 mg) and anhydrous potassium carbonate (4.6 mg), heated under reduced pressure to remove [^{18}O] water, and dried by azeotropic distillation with acetonitrile (3×1.5 ml). The tosyl analogue of 2-nitroimidazole [16, 26] (20 mg) was dissolved in acetonitrile (1.5 ml), added to the kryptofix-fluoride complex, and then warmed at 95 °C for 7 min. After cooling, the reaction mixture was passed through a silica gel Sep-Pak column (Whatman Incorporated, Clifton, N.J.) and eluted with ether (2×2.5 ml). The solvent was evaporated and the resulting mixture hydrolyzed with 2 N HCl (1 ml) at 105 °C for 7 min. The mixture was cooled under N_2 and neutralized with 2 N NaOH (0.8 ml) and 1 N $NaHCO_3$ (1 ml). The mixture was passed through a short alumina column, a C-18 Sep-Pak column, and a 0.22-µm millipore filter. This was followed by eluting 6 ml of 10% ethanol/saline. A yield of 80–100 mCi of pure product was isolated (25–40% yield, decay corrected) with the end of bombardment (EOB) at 60 min. High-performance liquid chromatography (HPLC) was performed on a C-18 ODS-120-T column, 4.6×25 mm, with water/acetonitrile, (80/20), using a flow rate of 1 ml/min. The no-carrier-added product corresponded to the retention time (6. 12 min) of the unlabeled FMISO under similar conditions. The radiochemical purity was greater than 99%. Under the UV detector (310 nm), there were no other impurities. A radio-thin-layer chromatography (TLC) scanner (Bioscan) showed a retardation factor of 0.6 for FMISO, using a 5×20 cm silica gel plate (Whatman, Incorporated), eluted with chloroform:methanol (7:3), which corresponds to the unlabeled FMISO. In addition, kryptofix-2, 2, 2 was not visualized (developed in the iodine chamber) on the silica gel-coated plate using 0.1% (by vol.) triethylamine in methanol as an eluant. Using a similar procedure described for FMISO, fluoroerythronitroimidazole (FETNIM) was prepared. The specific activity of [^{18}F]FMISO and [^{18}F]FETNIM determined was 1 Ci/µmol, based on UV and radioactivity detection of a sample of known mass and radioactivity.

PET Imaging of Head and Neck Tumor Hypoxia Using [^{18}F]FMISO

In a typical study, a patient is positioned supine in the scanner so that the detector rings span the entire head and neck. A 20-min attenuation scan is performed with a 4 mCi [^{68}Ge]-ring source prior to administering [^{18}F]FMISO. After each patient receives 10 mCi of [^{18}F]FMISO, six consecutive 20-min scans were taken. Serial transaxial images were taken using the scanner described above. Before PET scanning, the position of head and neck tumors was also determined by contrast-enhanced CT (High Speed Advantages, GE Medical System).

Radiosynthesis of [^{111}I]IMISO and [^{111}I]IETNIM

[^{131}I]IMISO and [^{131}I]IETNIM were prepared using the same tosyl analogue of 2-nitroimidazole [16–26] (20 mg) precursor. Briefly, 5 mg of tosyl precursor was dissolved in acetonitrile (1 ml), and Na^{131}I (1 mCi in 0.1 ml 1 N NaOH; specific activity 5.32 Ci/mg) (Dupont New England Nuclear) was added. The reaction mixture was heated for 1 h at 80 °C. The solvent was evaporated under nitrogen, and the mixture reconstituted in chloroform (2 ml). The free iodine was removed by adding 2 ml sodium thiosulfate (5%). The chloroform layer was evaporated to dryness over magnesium sulfate. Radio-TLC indicated an Rf value of 0.72 for this unhydrolyzed product, using chloroform:methanol (7:3) as an eluant. Hydrolysis was performed using HCl (2 N, 1 ml) at 100 °C for 5 min. The pH value of the final product was adjusted by adding NaOH (2 N, 0.8 ml) and NaHCO$_3$ (1 N, 1 ml). The final product was filtered through a 0.22-µm millipore filter and 0.6–0.7 mCi (60–70% yield) was obtained. Radio-TLC indicated Rf values of 0.01 for [^{131}I]IMISO and [^{131}I]IETNIM, using chloroform methanol (7:3) as an eluant.

Application of [^{131}I]Iodomisonidazole (IMISO) to Monitor Therapy Response of Breast Tumors with Cisplatin (CDDP)

To ascertain whether [^{131}I]IMISO could follow-up treatment response of CDDP and poly(D, L-lactide) microspheres (PLA CDDP MS) [51], a group of tumor-bearing rats were administered [^{131}I]IMISO (50 µCi, i.v.) on day 5 after therapy with CDDP and PLA CDDP MS. Planar scintigraphic images were obtained with a GE Starport System (GE Company). The image was displayed at 1, 2, and 3 h on the terminal monitor. The graphic processor displayed 256×256 pixels; each pixel was 14 bits. The percentage of tumor uptake (region of interest) was quantified by computer-image analyzer and expressed as percentage of injected dose (%ID) per pixel.

Autoradiographic Studies of Misonidazole Analogues in Tumor-Bearing Rats

One hour after receiving [^{18}F]FMISO, [^{18}F]FETNIM (i.v. 1.5 mCi) or [^{131}I]IMISO, [^{131}I]IETNIM (i.v. 40–50 µCi,), Fischer 344 female breast-tumor-bearing rats (3/ligand) were euthanized. The rat body was fixed in a carboxymethyl cellulose (4%) block. The frozen body in the block was mounted on a cryostat (LKB 2250 cryo-microtome, Ijamsville, Md.), and 50-µm coronal sections were made. The section was freeze-dried and then placed on X-ray film (X-Omat AR, Kodak) for 24 h.

Synthesis and Evaluation of Acetylacetone-2-Nitroimidazole

2-Nitroimidazole, dissolved in N, N-dimethylformamide was reacted with chloro-ACAC in the presence of cesium carbonate. After column purification, 70–80% of acetylacetone-2-nitroimidazole (ACACNIM) was obtained. [^{111}In]-ACACNIM was prepared using a procedure similar to that described for [^{111}In]-DTPA-TX. The biodistribution and planar scintigraphy of [^{111}In]-ACACNIM (100 µg of ACACNIM/mouse) were conducted at 0.5, 4, 24 and 48 h in mammary-tumor-bearing rats (n=3/time interval).

Polar Graphic Oxygen Needle Probe Measurements

To confirm hypoxic tumors detected by imaging, intratumoral pO$_2$ measurements were performed using the Eppendorf computerized histographic system. Twenty to twenty-five pO$_2$ measurements along each of two to three linear tracks were performed at 0.4-mm intervals on each tumor (40–75 measurements in total). Tumor pO$_2$ measurements were made on three tumor-bearing rats and three rabbits. Using an on-line computer system, the pO$_2$ measurements of each track were expressed as absolute values relative to the location of the measuring point along the track, and as relative frequencies within a pO$_2$ histogram between 0 mmHg and 100 mmHg, with a class width of 2.5 mm.

Markers of Tumor Cell Proliferation

Synthesis of [^{18}F]Fluoro- and [^{131}I]Iodo-2′-deoxyadenosine [9-(2′-deoxy-2′-Fluoro (or Iodo-)-β-D-Arabinofuranosyl)Adenine] (FAD and IAD)

2′-O-p-Toluenesulfonyladenosine (100 mg, 0.238 mmol) [52, 53] was derivatized along with N^6, O-3′, and O-5′ acetylated analogues by dissolving in tetrahydrofuran (5 ml), acetic anhydride (2 ml) along with pyridine (2 ml). The reaction was stirred overnight. The solvent, excess pyridine, and unreacted acetic anhydride were removed by evaporation, and the residue was chromatographed on silica gel (with ethyl acetate as eluant). Aliquots containing 20–40 mCi of [^{18}F]fluoride were combined with kryptofix-2, 2, 2 and anhydrous potassium carbonate and heated to remove [^{18}O]H$_2$O. The triacetylated tosyl analogue of adenosine was dissolved in acetonitrile, added to the kryptofix-fluoride (fluorine-18) complex, and then heated at 95 °C for 10 min. After cooling, the mixture was passed through a silica-gel-packed column (SPE-500 mg) and eluted with ACN (2 ml). After solvent evaporation, the acetyl groups were deprotected with 2 N HCl (1 ml) at 105 °C for 10 min. The product was neutralized with 2 N NaOH (0.8 ml) and 1 N NaHCO$_3$ (1 ml). The product was then eluted through a reverse phase C-18 column (Sep-Pak Cartridge, Waters) and a 0.22-mm filter, followed by saline (3 ml). The radioactivity of the final product was 7–15 mCi (50–60%, decay corrected) with the end of bombardment at 70 min.

Using a procedure similar to that described for the radiosynthesis of [^{131}I]IMISO, [^{131}I]iodo-2′-deoxyadenosine was prepared (scheme 1). Briefly, 5 mg of N^6, O-3′, and O-5′ acetylated analogue was dissolved in acetonitrile (1 ml), and Na^{131}I (1 mCi in 0.1 ml 1 N NaOH; specific activity 5.32 Ci/mg) (Dupont New England Nuclear) was added. The mixture was heated for 1 h at 80 °C. The solvent was evaporated under nitrogen, and the mixtures reconstituted in chloroform (2 ml). The free iodine was removed by adding 2 ml sodium thiosulfate (5%). The chloroform layer was dried (evaporated) over magnesium sulfate. Hydrolysis was performed using HCl (2 N, 1 ml) at 100 °C for 5 min. The pH value of the final product was adjusted by adding NaOH (2 N, 0.8 ml) and NaHCO$_3$ (1 N, 1 ml). The product was filtered through a 0.22-µm Millipore filter and 0.45–0.50 mCi (45–50% yield) was obtained. Radio-TLC (chloroform: methanol 7:3) was used to monitor the reactions.

Synthesis of 5-[^{131}I]Iodo-2'-O-Methyluridine

5-[^{131}I]Iodo-2'-O-methyluridine (IMU) was prepared from 2'-O-methyluridine (10 mg) and Na^{131}I (2.1 mCi, specific activity 10 Ci/mg) in 100 ml water. The mixture was warmed at 40 °C for 1 h in an iodogen-coated vial. After cooling, the solution was diluted with 300 µl water. The reaction mixture was passed through a 0.45-µm PTFE filter into a C-18 silica column (500 mg). The column was eluted with water (10 ml) to remove excess Na^{131}I. The product was eluted with ethanol (1.5 ml, 95%), yielding 1.3 mCi (70%). The ethanol was evaporated and reconstituted in saline prior to experiments.

Autoradiograms of [^{131}I]IAD and [^{131}I]IMU

Similar to the procedures described for the preparation of [^{18}F]FAD autoradiographs [52, 53], female Fischer 344 rats ($n=3$/ligand) were inoculated with breast-tumor cells (13762 NF, 100,000 cells per rat, i.m., right leg). When the tumor reached 2 cm in diameter, each rat was given [^{131}I]IAD and [^{131}I]IMU (50 mCi/rat, i.v.), respectively. The rats were sacrificed at 2 h and 24 h following injection of [^{131}I]IAD and [^{131}I]IMU. Each rat body was fixed in a block of 4% carboxymethylcellulose. This block was then mounted on a Cryostat microtome (LKB 2250, Cambridge Instruments Company) and 50- to 60-µm coronal sections were made. These sections were then freeze-dried and placed over X-ray film (X-OMAT AR, Eastman Kodak) for 1 h.

Marker of Lipid Peroxidase Inhibitors

Radiosynthesis of [^{111}In]-DTPA-Retinal

A stirred solution of aminoethylanilide-DTPA (100 mg, 0.195 mmol) [47–53] and retinal (83.3 mg, 1 equivalent, 0.195 mmol) in CH$_3$CN-H$_2$O (1:1) (8 ml) was treated with a solution of NaCNBH$_3$ (1 M in THF) (0.13 ml, 0.67 equivalent, 0.13 mmol). The mixture was stirred under nitrogen atmosphere at room temperature for 2 h. The solvent was then evaporated. The unreacted aldotamoxifen was removed by excessive washing with CH$_2$Cl$_2$ (3×5 ml). The final product was used without further purification. DTPA-retinal conjugate (5 mg) was dissolved in 1 ml ethanol/water (2:1) mixture. An aliquot containing 0.1 mg DTPA-TX was added with [^{111}In]InCl$_3$ (0.7 mCi, in 20 µl, 0.04 N HCl; NEN Dupont). Then, sodium acetate (0.6 N, 20 µl) and sodium citrate (0.06 N, 20 µl) were added. The mixture stood for 30 min. The final solution was formulated in 5% ethanol/saline solution. Radiochemical purity was determined to be greater than 99% (using CHCl$_3$/MeOH; 1:1, Rf=0.2, Bioscan).

Gamma Scintigraphic Imaging of Studies

Gamma scintigraphic images were obtained with a GE Starport System (GE Company) equipped with high-resolution, medium-energy, and parallel-hole collimator. Breast-tumor-bearing rats were administered [^{111}In]-DTPA-retinal (300 µCi/rat, i.v.). Whole-body planar images were obtained at 30 min and at 2, 4, 24 and 48 h; 300,000 counts were acquired in 128×128 matrix.

Results

Markers of ER Tissues

[^{18}F]-labeled tamoxifen ligand (2–12 mCi, i.v.) was used to image ten patients with ER+ breast tumors by PET. It was possible to visualize both primary and metastatic breast tumors by their uptake of the radiolabeled tamoxifen ligand (Fig. 6.1). Of the ten patients, three had tumors that showed good uptake of the radiolabeled ligand and positive responses to tamoxifen therapy (Table 6.1). However, high uptake in the liver and lung was observed; this affected the imaging and created difficulties in interpreting tumors near these organs. Others have also reported that liver and lung tamoxifen-uptake levels can remain high after tamoxifen administration. Autoradiogram and SPECT of [^{131}I]iodotamoxifen (ITX) for noninvasive detection of ovarian tumors (Fig. 6.2) and endometriosis (Fig. 6.3) are demonstrated in

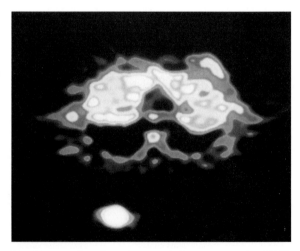

Fig. 6.1. A selected positron-emission tomography (PET) using ^{18}F-fluorotamoxifen demonstrates that it is possible to visualize both primary left breast tumor and metastasis in the right axillary node

Table 6.1. Evaluation of [^{18}F]fluorotamoxifen positron-emission tomography (PET) in ten patients

Patient	Age (years)	Follow-up duration (months)	Lesion location	Number of lesions	Lesion size (cm)	Visual interpretation	SUV	Receptor assay ER (fmol/mg of cytosol protein)	Response to therapy for patient	Response to therapy for lesion	Comment
1 ⟨?6⟩	55 ⟨?6⟩	7 ⟨?6⟩	Left breast	1	3.0×3.0	−	1.6	125 ⟨?6⟩	Progression ⟨?6⟩	Poor	Died 7 months later ⟨?6⟩
			Spines ⟨?3⟩	4 ⟨?3⟩	2.0×3.0	±	6.2			Poor	
					2.5×3.0	±	3.0			Poor	
					2.0×3.0	±	4.3			Poor	
					2.5×2.5	±	4.3			Poor	
			Sternum	1	2.5×6.0	±	4.2			Poor	
			Left axilla	1	ND	−	0.7			Poor	
2	58	5	Mediastinum	1	4×4	−	1.8	95[a]	Progression	Poor	Died 5 months later
3 ⟨?7⟩	52 ⟨?7⟩	24 ⟨?7⟩	Left breast	1	4.5×4.0	+	2.6	173 ⟨?7⟩	PR ⟨?7⟩	Good	Improvement of spine and liver lesions on CT scan ⟨?2⟩
			Right axilla	1	1.5×1.5	+	2.2			Good	
			Right breast	1	7.5×6.0	+	1.6			Good	
			Left axilla	1	2.0×1.0	+	2.6			Good	Improvement of spine lesions on bone scan ⟨?5⟩
			Spines ⟨?3⟩	4 ⟨?3⟩	3.5×2.5	+	3.0			Good	
					2.0×3.0	+	3.0			Good	
					2.5×2.5	+	3.0			Good	
					2.5×3.0	+	3.0			Good	
4	56	13	Right axilla	1	1.5×2.0	− (TN)	1.3	30[a]	NE	−	
5	66	14	Lung	1	1.5×1.5	±	3.3	185[a]	CR	Good	Lung lesion improved
6	65	26	Left axilla	1	3.0×3.0	+	2.9	19[b]	Not done	−	Surgical resection after PET study ⟨?1⟩
7	54	8	Skull	1	3.0×4.0	−	0.9	54[a]	NC	Poor	
8	62	24	Neck	1	3.0×2.5	− (TN)	2.4	39[a]	Not done	−	Chemotherapy with 5-fluorouracil, doxorubicin and cyclophosphamide
9	63	24	Scapula	1	2.5×2.5	− (TN)	1.3	1132[a]	NE	−	No evidence of metastases in biopsy specimen
10	68	13	Spine	1	2.0×2.5	+	6.3	54[a]	PR	Good	Carcinoembryonic antigen down; Improved pain and lesion on bone scan

True positive ratio: patients: 5/7 (71.4%); lesion: 16/20 (80.0%). *SUV* standardized uptake value; *ND* not defined; *TN* true negative; *PR* partial response; *CR* complete response; *NC* no change; *NE* nonevaluable; *ER* estrogen receptor
[a] ER concentration in the primary lesion removed before PET scan
[b] ER concentration in the left axillar lesion

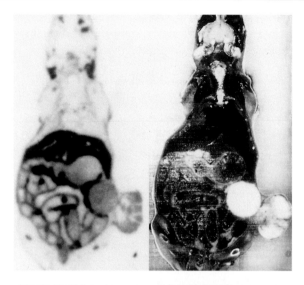

Fig. 6.2. Autoradiogram of [^{131}I]ITX (45 µCi, 24 h, i.v.) (*left*) in ovarian-tumor-bearing mouse; corresponding anatomy photograph shown at *right*

animals. The tumor-to-blood count ratio of [^{131}I]-labeled tamoxifen is optimal at 24 h post-injection. Gamma scintigraphy of [^{111}In]-DTPA-tamoxifen indicates that hydrophilic tamoxifen analogue has greater tumor-to-tissue ratios than the halogenated tamoxifen analogue (Fig. 6.4). The data suggest that either a delay in imaging or imaging with a hydrophilic tamoxifen ligand would decrease the amounts of drug taken up by liver and lung. [^{111}In]-DTPA-TX provides better images of ER+ tumors, due to higher tumor-to-tissue ratios. These ligands have potential application in the detection of ER+ lesions, e.g., uterine cancer, ovar-

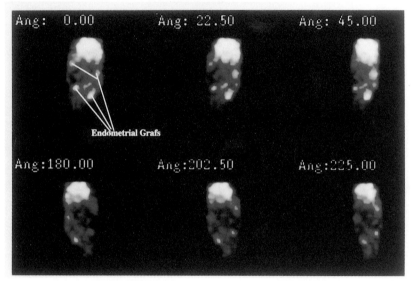

Fig. 6.3. Single photon-emission computed tomography (SPECT) images, 24 h post-injection (i.v.), of [^{131}I]iodotamoxifen in a rabbit simulated with endometriosis

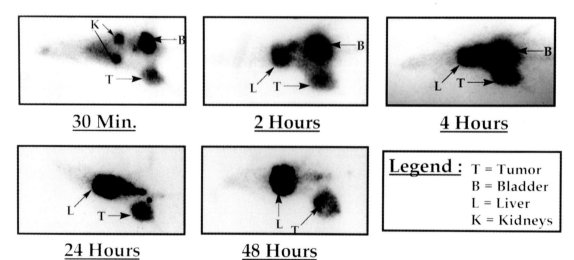

Fig. 6.4. Anterior view of breast-tumor-bearing rats receiving [^{111}In]-DTPA-tamoxifen (300 µCi, i.v.) showing increased uptake in tumor as a function of time

Fig. 6.5. a Computerized tomography (CT) image showed a large neoplasm in the left tonsil extended to the soft palate, the base of the tongue, and into the posterior wall of the oropharynx. There was also cervical adenopathy, with an increase in size and number of the left upper and middle jugular lymphatic chains. **b** Positron-emission tomography (PET) using [^{18}F]FMISO demonstrated a significant uptake in the tumors

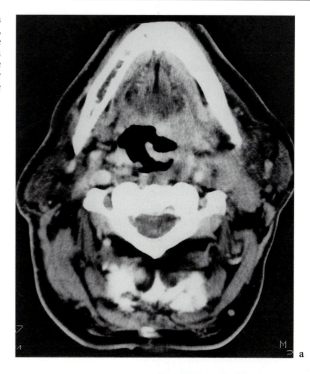

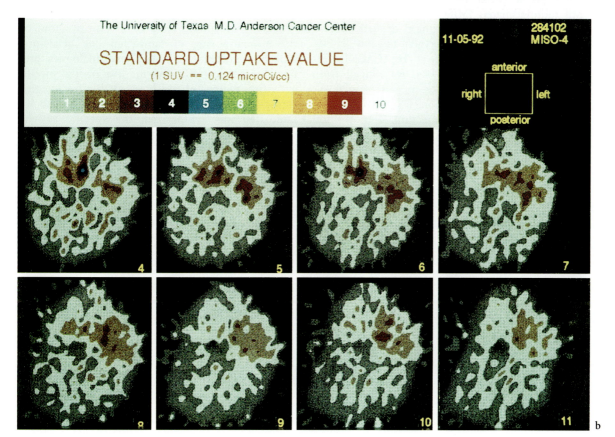

ian cancer, endometriosis, meningioma and breast cancer.

Markers of Tumor Hypoxia

PET-[^{18}F]FMISO imaging studies revealed that the hypoxic tumors could be visualized well at 1 h post-injection (Fig. 6.5A, B). On day 5, rats treated with CDDP or PLA-CDDP M and examined using planar scintigraphy at 1 h post-injection of [^{131}I]IMISO (50 µCi/rat, i.v.) showed decreased uptake relative to control subjects (Fig. 6.6). In rats treated with CDDP and PLA-CDDP MS, followed by [^{131}I]IMISO, tumor %ID/pixel decreased 40% from 0.036+0.001 (control) to 0.029+0.002 (CDDP) and 0.023+0.002 (PLA-CDDP MS) (Table 6.2). There was also a 40% decrease in tumor volume. The results indicate the treatment response of CDDP and PLA-CDDP MS could be monitored by [^{131}I]IMISO.

The tumors could be visualized well on all four misonidazole analogues tested. Autoradiographs of [^{18}F]FMISO and [^{18}F]FETNIM showed that tumor hypoxia could be differentiated (Fig. 6.7). Both radioiodinated IMISO and IETNIM showed high tumor uptake. The tumor oxygen tension was 3–6 mmHg; normal oxygen tension is 30–40 mmHg. Biodistribution of [^{111}In]ACACNIM indicates that tumor uptake (%ID/g) ranged from 0.03–0.25 and kidney uptake ranged from 0.28–1.14 at 0.5–24 h post-injection. The optimum tumor uptake was 2 h post-injection. Tumor/blood and tumor/muscle count density ratios ranged from 0.8–4.1 and 4.7–15.3, respectively (Table 6.3). These ratios were higher than those using [^{18}F]FMISO and [^{131}I]IMISO in the same animal model. Planar scintigraphy on mammary-tumor-bearing rats showed that the tumor could be visualized at 0.5–48 h (Fig. 6.8). The findings indicate that these analogues can selectively detect the hypoxic region of the tumor and, thus, have potential to aid in evaluating responses to radiation and chemotherapy.

Markers of Tumor Cell Proliferation

Tumor-to-blood and tumor-to-muscle count density ratios of [^{18}F]FAD, [^{131}I]IAD and [^{131}I]IMU increased as a function of time (Table 6.4). [^{18}F]FAD shows a better image than [^{131}I]IAD and [^{131}I]IMU, due to higher tumor-to-blood count density ratios. Autoradiograms of [^{131}I]IAD and [^{131}I]IMU showed that the tumors could be well visualized at 2 h and 24 h post-injection (Figs. 6.9 and 6.10).

Marker of Lipid Peroxidase Inhibitors

Planar scintigraphy of [^{111}In]-DTPA-retinal on mammary-tumor-bearing rats showed that tumors could be visualized at 0.5–48 h (Fig. 6.11). Liver and kidneys of both ligands had high uptake.

Placing an iodine atom or a fluorine atom on the aromatic ring of tamoxifen has been previously reported [54, 55]. These analogues produced either low affinities for ERs or low specific activities, neither of which is suitable for imaging estrogen-responsive tissues. When [^{11}C]-labeled tamoxifen was synthesized, the specific activity was also low [56]. Placing a chlorine atom on the aliphatic side chain of tamoxifen produced a higher affinity than for tamoxifen [57, 58]. However, this compound is not suitable for imaging

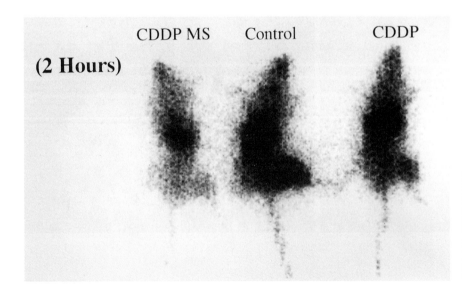

Fig. 6.6. Planar scintigraphy of breast tumor bearing rats treated with cisplatin and microencapsulated cisplatin 5 days prior to receiving [^{131}I]-IMISO (50 µCi, i.v.) demonstrated that [^{131}I]-IMISO could monitor treatment of breast cancer with CDDP

Table 6.2. Evaluation of breast cancer treatment response using [^{131}I] Iodomisonidazole (IMISO)[a]

	Control	Cisplatin (CDDP)	PLA-CDDP MS
1 h			
ID (%)	16.82±0.03	9.62±0.03	8.28±0.03
ID/Pixel (%)	0.036±0.001	0.029±0.002[b]	0.023±0.002[b]
T/M	1.83±0.01	1.54±0.01	1.38±0.02
2 h			
ID (%)	18.06±0.02	7.71±0.03	8.55±0.03
ID/Pixel (%)	0.039±0.001	0.023±0.002[b]	0.024±0.002[b]
T/M	2.06±0.01	1.15±0.01[b]	1.36±0.02[b]

ID percentage of injected dose; T/M tumor-to-muscle ratio
[a] Each tumor-bearing rat (n=3/group) was treated with CDDP or PLA-CDDP MS 5 days prior to receiving [^{131}I]IMISO (50 µCi, i.v.)
[b] Significant difference ($P<0.05$, student t-test) between control and treated groups

Table 6.3. Tumor-to-tissue ratios of 2-nitroimidazole analogues. 13762 cell line (dimethylbenzaanthracene-induced tumors) was inoculated into rats (s.c. 10^5 cells/rat). When tumor size reached 1–2 cm, each rat was administered 10 µCi tracer (n=3/time interval, i.v.)

[^{131}I]IMISO	1 h	2 h	4 h
Tumor	1.083±0.2417	0.795±0.0313	0.679±0.1110
Tumor/blood	0.836±0.0678	0.877±0.0871	0.989±0.1459
Tumor/muscle	5.823±0.6170	6.149±0.8883	8.071±1.5914
[^{18}F]FMISO	1 h	2 h	4 h
Tumor	0.899±0.1132	1.047±0.1107	0.691±0.0967
Tumor/blood	1.566±0.1879	2.239±0.2042	3.780±0.6762
Tumor/muscle	1.516±0.1754	2.201±0.1576	3.246±0.2994
[^{111}In]ACACNIM	0.5 h	4 h	24 h
Tumor	0.244±0.0210	0.032±0.0027	0.030±0.0021
Tumor/blood	0.820±0.0501	2.800±0.1903	4.100±0.7409
Tumor/muscle	4.700±0.4607	13.000±0.9105	15.300±0.6602

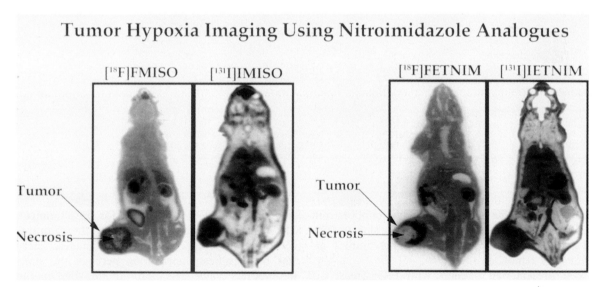

Fig. 6.7. Autoradiographs of [^{18}F]- and [^{131}I]-labeled misonidazole analogues demonstrated that breast tumor hypoxia could be diagnosed at 1 h post-injection (i.v.)

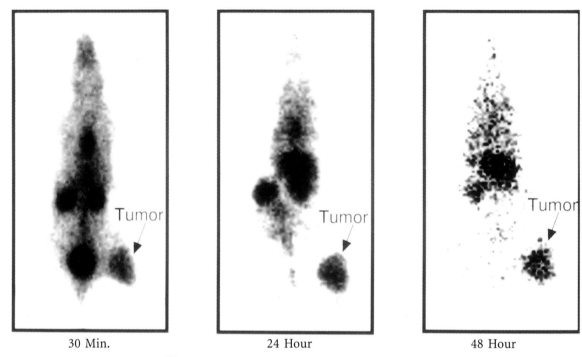

Fig. 6.8. Gamma scintigraphy of [^{111}In]acetylacetone-2-nitroimidazole (50 µCi, i.v.) in a breast-tumor-bearing rat. The tumor is located on the right leg

Table 6.4. Tumor-to-tissue ratios of radiohalogenated nucleoside analogues. 13762 cell line (dimethylbenzaanthracene-induced tumors) was inoculated into rats (s.c. 10^5 cells/rat). When tumor size reached 1–2cm, each rat was administered 10 µCi tracer ($n=3$/time interval, i.v.)

	1 h	2 h	4 h
[^{131}I]Iodoadenosine			
Tumor	0.732±0.0453	0.547±0.0198	0.382±0.0692
Tumor/blood	0.692±0.0468	0.628±0.0630	0.669±0.0330
Tumor/muscle	5.114±0.2212	4.941±0.1609	4.941±0.4145
[^{18}F]Fluoroadenosine			
Tumor	0.886±0.2783	0.759±0.1225	0.661±0.1666
Tumor/blood	1.830±0.8249	2.770±0.1989	5.250±1.9000
Tumor/muscle	3.050±1.0800	5.280±0.8713	14.340±6.2200
[^{131}I]Iodomethyluridine			
Tumor	0.359±0.0438	0.268±0.0858	0.171±0.0267
Tumor/blood	0.693±0.0479	0.938±0.2822	0.719±0.0474
Tumor/muscle	2.234±0.1215	5.897±1.6990	4.455±0.7902

purposes, since there is no existing cyclotron-produced isotope for chlorine. Previous studies from our group indicate that replacing a chlorine with a halomethyl group develops a higher binding affinity for tamoxifen [8].

At present, ten patients with ER+ breast tumors (IND 40,589) were imaged by PET, using [^{18}F]-labeled tamoxifen ligand (2–12 mCi, i.v.). Both primary and metastatic breast tumors could be diagnosed by [^{18}F]-labeled tamoxifen ligands. Three lesions in three patients were considered to be negative for breast cancer on the basis of biopsy specimens and/or clinical course. Five of seven patients (71.4%) and 16 of 20 lesions (80%) were interpreted to be positive for breast cancer. The mean standard uptake value of the radiotracer in tumor was 2.8 on delayed images. There was no significant correlation between the standard uptake value of [^{18}F]fluorotamoxifen in the lesion and the ER concentration in primary or metastatic lesions. Eight of ten patients received tamoxifen therapy after the PET study. Three patients who had a good response to tamoxifen therapy showed a standard [^{18}F]fluorotamoxifen uptake of more than 2.4 in the tumor, whereas four of five patients who had a poor response to

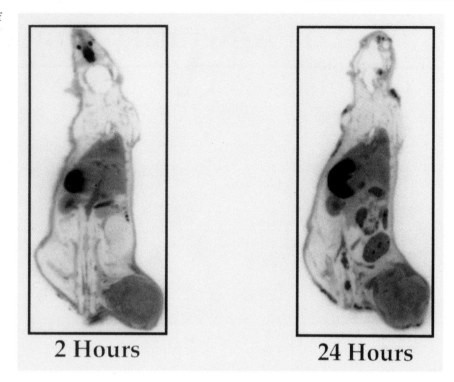

Fig. 6.9. Autoradiographs of the post-injection of breast-tumor-bearing rats injected with 2'-[^{131}I]iododeoxyadenosine (30–40 µCi, i.v.) demonstrated that the tumor could be visualized at 2 h and 24 h

2 Hours

24 Hours

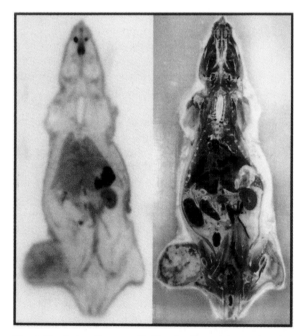

Fig. 6.10. Autoradiogram (*left*) of a breast-tumor-bearing rat administered with [^{131}I]iodomethyluridine (50 µCi, i.v., 2 h, post-injection). The tumor (on the right leg) can be well visualized. Matching photograph on the *right*

tamoxifen therapy showed a standard uptake of less than 2.0. PET imaging using [^{18}F]fluorotamoxifen as the radiotracer provides useful information for predicting the effect of tamoxifen therapy in patients with recurrent or metastatic ER+ breast cancer. Results from the present study also indicate that radioiodinated and In-labeled tamoxifen analogues are useful in the diagnosis of ER+ lesions.

The key to developing [^{18}F]FMISO or [^{131}I]IMISO is to prepare (2'-nitro-1'-imidazolyl)-2-O-acetyl-3-O-tosylpropanol precursor. This intermediate could be prepared easily by treatment of 2-acetyl-1, 3-ditosyl glycerol and 2-nitroimidazole, as described previously [16]. Both labeled compounds produced sufficient radioactivity and high radiochemical purity. Others have used [^{18}F]epifluorohydrin with 2-nitroimidazole or 1, 3-ditosyl-O-tetrahydropyran to react with 2-nitroimidazole, followed by [^{18}F]-displacement [17–19, 59, 60]. These reactions either take more synthetic steps, have longer reaction times or provide lower radiochemical yield. Additionally, [^{131}I]iodomisonidazole has not been synthesized using the same precursor. Numerous in vitro and in vivo experiments have shown that cells irradiated under low oxygen tensions are more resistant to the lethal effects of low linear energy transfer (LET) ionized radiation compared with cells irradiated under normal oxygen tensions [61, 62]. Clinical trials with PET de-

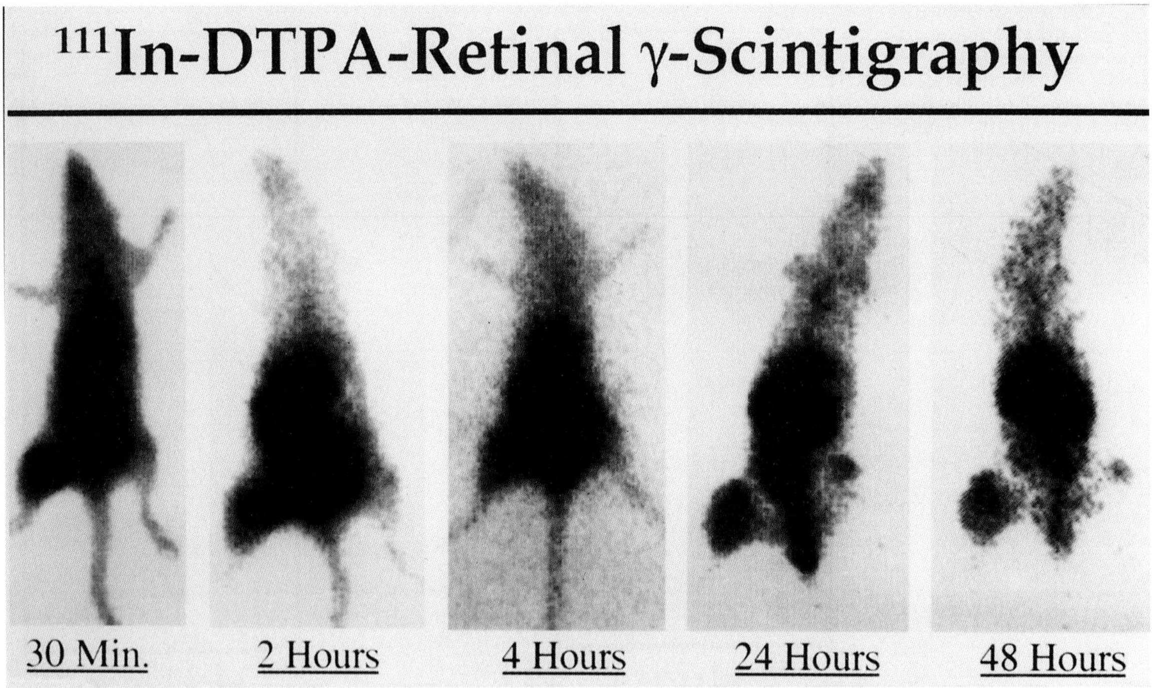

^{111}In-DTPA-Retinal γ-Scintigraphy

Fig. 6.11. Anterior view of breast-tumor-bearing rats receiving [^{111}In]-DTPA-retinal (200 µCi, i.v.) showed increased uptake in the tumor as a function of time

monstrated that [^{18}F]FMISO is capable of providing functional images of tumor hypoxia. Autoradiographs of all four analogues showed that tumor hypoxia could be easily demonstrated in rodents. Tumor oxygen tension was determined to be 3.2–6.0 mmHg, whereas normal muscle tissue had 30–40 mmHg. Attachment of an acetyl acetone moiety to nitroimidazole was achieved; the [^{111}In]-labeled analogue demonstrates the feasibility of using this analogue as a diagnostic tool for defining tumor hypoxia. To evaluate microscopic tumor uptake of these analogues, microautoradiographs should be employed in the future investigation of both compounds. Additionally, [^{131}I]IMISO could be used for chemotherapeutic follow-up treatment and for quantification of tumor hypoxia uptake at 1 h post-injection.

To enhance biological activity and increase chemical or metabolic stability, fluorine substitution at the C2′ position of the sugar moiety (arabino configuration) has been investigated widely in drug research [63–66]. Due to the Van-der-Waals radii between the C-H bond and C-halogen bond, [^{18}F]FAD, [^{131}I]IAD and [^{131}I]IMU are structurally similar to 2′-deoxyadenosine and IUDR. Deep-seated tumors in blood-rich organs may require significantly higher ratios for the assessment of proliferation. Tumor-to-muscle ratios of [^{18}F]FAD at 2 h and 4 h post-injection were 5.2 and 14.3, respectively. Tumor-to-blood ratios at the same time intervals were 2.8 and 5.3, respectively. These data were considered to be acceptable for a tumor-imaging agent. [^{18}F]FAD appears to be a better imaging agent than [^{131}I]IAD, due to higher tumor-to-nontumor tissue count density ratios. Tumors, or portions of actively growing tumors, were well-visualized on autoradiography using [^{131}I]IAD and [^{131}I]IMU. Although many other radiopharmaceuticals could be used for assessing tumor proliferation and/or metabolic activity [67–71], the choice should be determined not only by the biological behavior of radiopharmaceuticals, but also by the ease of preparation and the logistics of imaging. The results indicated that [^{18}F]FAD, [^{131}I]IAD and [^{131}I]IMU could be easily prepared and might be helpful in assessing tumor cell proliferation.

Using a similar synthetic approach, DTPA-retinal (vitamin A) was prepared by treating retinal with aminoethylanilide-DTPA and following with a reduction reaction. Planar scintigraphy of both conjugates of this ligand showed that tumor uptake remained steady throughout the time periods. Our data suggests that DTPA-retinal may have potential use in monitoring the treatment of breast cancer with tamoxifen and vitamin A.

In summary, for markers of ER+ tissues, we prepared [^{18}F]fluorotamoxifen, [^{131}I]iodotamoxifen and [^{111}In]-DTPA-tamoxifen; for markers of tumor hypoxia, we prepared [^{18}F]fluoromisonidazole, [^{131}I]iodomisonidazole, [^{18}F]fluoroerythronitroimidazole, [^{131}I]iodoerythronitroimidazole and [^{111}In]acetylacetonenitroimidazole; for markers of tumor proliferation, we prepared [^{18}F]fluoroadenosine, [^{131}I]iodoadenosine and 5-[^{131}I]iodo-2'-O-methyluridine; for markers of antiangiogenesis, we prepared [^{111}In]-DTPA-retinal and [^{111}In]-DTPA-taxol. All these ligands provide functional imaging of oncology.

MR Contrast Agents

Basic Principles

The primary purpose of magnetic resonance (MR) imaging is to visualize the contrast between tissues that arises from differences in perceived signals from inherent compartments. The detected signal arises from the relaxation of protons in the water molecules that are associated with the tissue. Image contrast occurs in MRI when the signal intensities of two tissues differ.

The process by which a difference in signal intensity is maximized is called contrast enhancement. The difference between signal intensities can be accentuated by introducing a material that selectively changes one of the intrinsic MR properties in one tissue more than in another. Positive contrast enhancement brightens the target tissue, and negative contrast enhancement darkens the target tissue. The contrast may be increased by administering a pharmaceutical that alters the physical characteristics of the tissue. The contrast-enhanced agents must change the signal intensity and be distributed differentially to normal or abnormal tissues. They must not produce a significant adverse reaction.

Electric charges in motion induce a magnetic field, and the magnetic moment (μ) of the electron is about 700 times stronger than the μ of the nuclear proton. All magnetic fields interact, and this interaction tends to align the magnetic moment of the proton. There are two quasi-stable states for this alignment, and the net magnetic field is the sum of all the fields. The magnetic moments are small, but there are about 10^{22} dipoles in 1 ml of matter. More than 95% of the dipoles are protons in water, lipids, or macromolecules. The precessional frequency of hydrogen is a basic property of its magnetic composition and is 42.57 MHz/T of magnetic field; this value is known as the Larmor frequency.

The MR signal is generated by a net magnetization precessing in the transverse plane which, in turn, induces a voltage in a receiving coil. When the new magnetic field is turned off, the proton magnetic vectors return instantly to the former precessional frequency and more slowly back to their initial net orientation. The process of realignment is called relaxation. Within an external magnetic field, the proton vectors are partially aligned along the main magnetic field, B_0. The direction of B_0 is along the z axis and usually corresponds to the long direction of the human body. At thermal equilibrium, there are more protons in the low-energy state along the direction of B_0. To reach equilibrium, the excess high-energy spins must jump from the high-energy cone surface and release a quantum of energy to the thermal environment, or lattice. This process is called longitudinal, spin-lattice, or T_1 relaxation.

An absolute requirement of an MR pulse sequence is to produce a net magnetic vector in the transverse plane. The measured signal, called free-induction decay (FID), reflects only the behavior of transverse magnetization of the tissues and is degraded by local magnetic field inhomogeneities at a rate referred to as T_2^*. The rate of amplitude decay between refocused echoes represents the T_2 relaxation due to tissue interactions. T_2 relaxation is also know as spin-spin relaxation.

Each proton contains a single spin, so the spin-spin exchange must occur with another proton. The protons may not only exchange their spins, but may also physically change positions (chemical exchange). An exchange between bulk water protons (free protons) and protons on macromolecules (protons of restricted mobility) has consequences for relaxation processes [72, 73]. The oriented magnetic vectors from proton spins are called dipoles. Relaxation stimulated by proton interactions with other biomolecules during routine MRI is indistinguishable from that caused by contrast agents.

Effective contrast-enhancing agents include:
1. Materials with no hydrogen nuclei – carbon dioxide gas, perfluorocarbon and deuterated water. These reduce the total proton spin density within volume elements.
2. Paramagnetic materials – molecular oxygen, free radical and metal ions Gd^{+++}, Fe^{+++} and Mn^{++}. These decrease T_1 and T_2 proton relaxation times.
3. Superparamagnetic and ferromagnetic particles and [^{17}O] cause a reduction in T_2 that is many times greater than the reduction in T_1, resulting in a dramatic drop in signal intensity. Signal intensity increases when proton spin density increases, T_1 relaxation time decreases, or T_2 relaxation time increases.

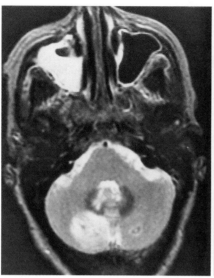 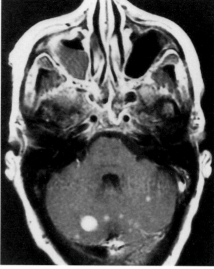

Fig. 6.12. T_2-weighted axial image (*left*) of the cerebellum shows metastatic lesions of breast cancer in bilateral cerebellar hemispheres. T_1-weighted axial image (*right*) after injection of gadolinium (Gd)-DTPA shows additional small metastases. Note a retention cyst in the right maxillary sinus

Paramagnetic Contrast Agents

Paramagnetic materials have unpaired electrons that generate large fluctuating magnetic fields. The relaxation effect is proportional to the square of the magnetic moment of the paramagnetic material; this value varies with the number of unpaired electrons, e.g., gadolinium has 7, iron and manganese have 5, and nitroxides have 1. Although the relaxation effect decreases rapidly with the sixth power of the separation distance between proton and paramagnetic, the paramagnetic center field is sufficiently large that the ion can be caged or encapsulated within a chemical structure. With the possible exception of manganese chloride given orally, paramagnetic materials are highly toxic [74]. Small molecular chelates behave as centers with favorable T_1 and T_2 relaxivities and possess the pharmacokinetics of diethylenetriamine pentaacetic acid (DTPA) complexes (Fig. 6.12). These agents have been clinically available (Gd-DTPA, gadopentetate, Magnevist; Gd-DTPA-BMA, gadodiamide, Omniscan; Gd-DOTA, Dotarem; Gd-HP-D03 A, gadoteridol, Prohance) (Fig. 6.13). By adding side chains that target receptors responsible for clearing into bile via hepatocytes, small hepatobiliary agents can be created. Mangafodipir (Mn-DPDP) is also a mixed hepatobiliary contrast agent (Fig. 6.14) [75]. Some hepatomas retain the ability to enhance with Mn-DPDP [76], and this may also be true for Gd-BOPTA and Gd-EOB-DTPA, which utilize the hepatocyte transport system [77].

Extracellular agents usually distribute into only 25% of the tissue space and blood-pool agents distribute into 3–15% of tissue volume. Pharmaceutical design has created paramagnetic chelates that are bound strongly to macromolecules, which tumble more slowly than small chelates.

Superparamagnetic Contrast Agents

Iron oxides can form magnetically ordered nanoparticles [78] and have a much larger magnetic moment than paramagnetic chelates. Ferumoxide (AMI-25, Feridex) is a crystal aggregate with dextran coating and a very large T_2 relaxivity. Ferumoxtram (AMI-227, Sinerem) is composed of smaller particles with less T_2 relaxivity and more T_1 relaxivity. Particles comprised of iron oxides with a diameter less than approximately 15 nm can act as single magnetic domains. They create large magnetic gradients which act as local field inhomogeneities. Water protons diffusing through these gradients experience constantly changing magnetic moments, leading to rapid dephasing of the spins and to the shortening of T_2 relaxation times. The amplitude and intensity of the spin-echo signal decreases; this can be seen as a darkening of tissue on images. Increasing the nanoparticle size from 6 nm to 50 nm increases potency, but even bigger particles reach a plateau of effectiveness. Superparamagnetic particles are very effective even at low doses. They can be made tissue specific, and accumulation in target organs makes the biodistribution more favorable.

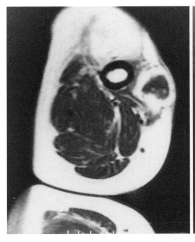 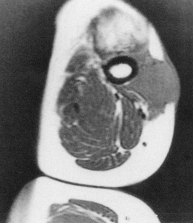 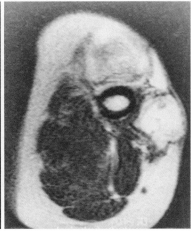

Fig. 6.13. T$_2$-weighted axial image of the right upper thigh (*left*) shows recurrent malignant fibrous histiocytomas masses in the anterior and lateral aspects of anterior soft tissue compartment. T$_1$-weighted axial images before (*middle*) and after (*right*) injection of Gd-DTPA-BMA show necrotic mass in the anterior aspect and hemorrhagic mass in the lateral aspect

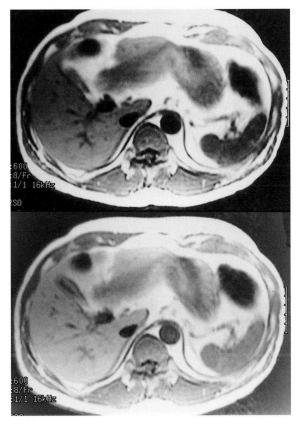

Fig. 6.14. T$_1$-weighted axial image of the upper abdomen at 5 min after injection of Mn-DPDP shows a diffuse enhancement of liver and spleen (*bottom*). Note also enhanced walls of stomach and gallbladder. Pre-contrast image (*top*)

A surface that is easily opsonized will lead to a rapid clearance by the reticuloendothelial system and a short blood-life. The blood half-life of ferumoxide is less than 15 min, whereas that for ferumoxtran is more than 12 h. A long blood-life allows targeting to lymph nodes and is also key for receptor localization [79].

Targeted Contrast Agents

Altering tissue signal intensities with contrast agents can be used to improve lesion detection (higher sensitivity), improve lesion characterization (higher specificity), or assess treatment efficacy. Target-specific agents hold promise for imaging specific cellular and subcellular components, for example, receptors and antigens. Ideal agents should be stable in vivo, have a high affinity for the target, be circulating and not readily removed from circulation, result in tissue concentration, and be metabolized to nontoxic products. It is desirable that target tissues possess a large number of specific binding sites, have adequate regional blood flow, and allow the carrier to efficiently traverse the capillary wall.

A variety of vector and carrier molecules have been developed to deliver magnetic labels to specific target sites. Antibodies demonstrate high specificity and have been labeled with superparamagnetic iron oxides or paramagnetic polylanthanides [80]. Unfortunately, there are problems, such as low concentration of antibody, scarcity of target antigen, low specificity in vivo, rapid clearance of certain antibody-magnetic label constructs, and decreased affinity of antibody.

An alternative approach to antibody imaging has been to direct immuno-conjugates toward normal components of tissue. Cholecystokinin (CCK) has been attached to monocrystalline iron oxide, and the complex (CCK-MION) has been tested to improve detection of pancreatic cancer [81]. Asialoglycoproteins (ASG) have been used as targeting agents for MR imaging. Hepatocyte-directed iron oxides have several advantages over Kupffer-cell-directed iron oxides, including lower dose requirements, the ability to assess hepatic function, and differentiation of receptor-positive versus receptor-negative hepatomas [82]. ASG receptor activity has been demonstrated in normal liver, focal nodular hyperplasia and adenoma. Neither primary nor metastatic tumors show significant levels of accumulation of receptor agents [83]. A variety of polysaccharides, such as dextran, have been used to coat magnetic particles or to synthesize paramagnetic macromolecular agents such as dextran-polylysine.

Because of a long blood half-life, small iron oxides (USPIO, MION, AMI-227) accumulate in considerable amounts in lymph nodes. Lymph node uptake is believed to occur either by direct extravasation of the agent within the capillaries of the nodes or by the clearance of lymphatic fluid once the particles reach tissue interstitium. Most studies have found accumulation in normal and hyperplastic – but not in tumorous – lymph nodes [84].

Magnetically labeled macromolecular polymers have been investigated for blood-pool imaging, tissue perfusion, vascular anatomy, and capillary permeability. MPEG-Pl-Gd-DTPA has also been used to assess tumor neovascularity, which has been shown to correlate with the malignant potential of a tumor [85]. Liposomes are artificial lipid vesicles of nano-to-micrometer scale that are composed either of single or multiple concentric spherical lipid bilayers, and can be prepared to encapsulate or surface-bind magnetic labels [86]. During the vascular distribution phase, magnetic liposomes act as blood-pool agents, similar to the other paramagnetic micellar agents. Because they become trapped by phagocytic cells, magnetic liposomes have been exploited as contrast agents for the liver and spleen [87]. T cells can be labeled with superparamagnetic iron oxide by endocytosis without interfering with cell function or viability [88]. The availability of such labeled cells offers an opportunity to use MRI to track the migration of different cell types.

References

1. Fernandez MD, Burn JI, Sauven PD, Parmar G, White JO, Myatt L (1984) Activated estrogen receptors in breast cancer and response to endocrine therapy. Eur J Cancer Clin Oncol 20:41–46
2. McGuire AH, Dehdashti F, Siegel BA, Lyss AP, Brodack JW, Mathias CJ, Mintun MA, Katzenellenbogen JA, Welch MJ (1991) Positron tomographic assessment of 16-alpha-[^{18}F] fluoro-17-beta-estradiol uptake in metastatic breast carcinoma. J Nucl Med 32:1526–1531
3. McManaway ME, Jagoda EM, Kasid A, Echelman WC, Francis BE, Larson SM, Gibson RE, Reba RC, Lippman ME (1987) [^{125}I]17-beta-iodovinyl-11-beta-methoxyestradiol interaction in vivo with estrogen receptors in hormone-independent MCF-7 human breast cancer transfected with the v-rasH oncogene. Cancer Res 47:2945–2949
4. Jagoda EM, Gibson RE, Goodgold H, Ferreira N, Francis BE, Reba RC, Rzeszotarski WJ, Eckelman WC (1984) [^{125}I]17 alpha-iodovinyl-11-beta-methoxyestradiol: in vivo and in vitro properties of a high affinity estrogen-receptor radiopharmaceutical. J Nucl Med 25:472–477
5. Hamm JT, Allegra JC (1991) Hormonal therapy for cancer. In: Witts RE (ed.) Manual of oncologic therapeutics. Lippincott, New York, pp 122–126
6. Wittliff JL (1984) Steroid-hormone receptor in breast cancer. Cancer Res 53:630–643
7. Yang DJ, Cherif A, Tansey W, Kuang LR, Wright KC, Li C, Kim EE, Wallace S (1992) N,N-diethylfluoromethyltamoxifen: synthesis assignment of ^{1}H and ^{13}C spectra and receptor assay. Eur J Med Chem 27:919–924
8. Yang DJ, Tewson T, Tansey W, Kuang L-R, Reger G, Cherif A, Wright K, Moult R, Tilbury RS, Kim EE, Wallace S (1992) Halogenated analogs of tamoxifen: synthesis, receptor assay and inhibition of MCF7 cells. J Pharm Sci 81:622–625
9. Yang D, Wallace S (1993) High affinity tamoxifen derivatives and uses thereof. United States Patent Number 5, 192, 525; March 1992
10. Yang D, Wallace S, Wright KC, Price JE, Kuang L-R, Kim EE (1992) Imaging of estrogen receptors with PET using ^{18}F-fluoro analogue of tamoxifen. Radiology 182:185–186
11. Yang DJ, Kuang LR, Cherif A, Tansey W, Li C, Lin WJ, Liu C-W, Kim EE, Wallace S (1993) Synthesis of ^{18}F-alanine and ^{18}F-tamoxifen for breast tumor imaging. J Drug Targeting 1:259–267
12. Yang DJ, Li C, Kuang LR, Tansey W, Cherif A, Price J, Buzdar A, Gretzer M, Kim EE, Wallace S (1994) Imaging, biodistribution and therapy potential of halogenated tamoxifen analogues. Life Sci 55:53–67
13. Yang DJ, Wallace S (1993) High affinity halogenated tamoxifen derivatives and uses thereof. US Patent June 15; Number 5:219:548
14. Koh WJ, Rasey JS, Evans ML, Grierson JR, Lewellen TK, Graham MM, Krohn KA, Griffin TW (1992) Imaging of hypoxia in human tumors with ^{18}F fluoromisonidazole. Int J Radiat Oncol Biol Phys 22:199–212
15. Rasey JS, Nelson NJ, Chin L, Evans ML, Grunbaum Z (1990) Characterization of the binding of labeled fluoromisonidazole in cells in vitro. Radiat Res 122:301–308
16. Cherif A, Yang DJ, Tansey W, Kim EE, Wallace S (1994) Synthesis of [^{18}F]fluoro-misonidazole. Pharm Res 11:466–469
17. Hwang DR, Dence CS, Bonasera TA, Welch MJ (1989) No-carrier-added synthesis of 3-[^{18}F]fluoro-1-(2-nitro-1-imidazolyl)-2-propanol: a potential PET agent for detecting hypoxic but viable tissues. Int J Radiat Appl Instrum A 40:117–126

18. Jerabeck PA, Patrick TB, Kilbourn D, Dischino D, Welch MJ (1986) Synthesis and biodistribution of [18F]-labeled fluoronitroimidazoles: potential in vivo markers of hypoxic tissue. Appl Radiat Isot 37:599–605
19. Parliament MB, Chapman JD, Urtasun RC, McEwan AJ, Golberg L, Mercer JR, Mannan RH, Wiebe LI (1992) Noninvasive assessment of human tumor hypoxia with [123I]-iodoazomycin arabinoside: preliminary report of a clinical study. Br J Cancer 65:90–95
20. Valk PET, Mathis CA, Prados MD, Gilbert JC, Budinger TF (1992) Hypoxia in human gliomas: demonstration by PET with [18F]fluoromisonidazole. J Nucl Med 33:2133–2137
21. Martin GV, Caldwell JH, Rasey JS, Grunbaum Z, Cerqueia M, Krohn KA (1989) Enhanced binding of the hypoxic cell marker [18F]fluoromisonidazole in ischemic myocardium. J Nucl Med 30:194–201
22. Martin GV, Cardwell JH, Graham MM, Grierson JR, Kroll K, Cowan MJ, Lewellen TK, Rasey JS, Casciari JJ, Krohn KA (1992) Noninvasive detection of hypoxic myocardium using [18F]fluoromisonidazole and PET. J Nucl Med 33:2202–2208
23. Yeh SH, Liu RS, Hu HH, Chang CP, Chu LS, Chou KL, Wu LC (1994) Ischemic penumbra in acute stroke: demonstration by PET with fluorine-18 fluoromisonidazole (abstract). J Nucl Med 35:5:205
24. Yeh SH, Wu LC, Liu RS, Yang DJ, Yen SH, Yu TW (1994) Fluorine-18 fluoromisonidazole tumor: muscle retention ratio in detecting hypoxia in nasopharyngeal carcinoma (abstract). J Nucl Med 35:5:142
25. Liu RS, Chu LS, Yen SH, Chang CP, Chon KL, Wu LC, Chang CW, Lui MT, Chen KY, Yeh SHOURS (1996) Detection of odontogenic infections by [18F] fluoromisonidazole. Eur J Nucl Med 23:1384–1387
26. Yang DJ, Wallace S, Cherif A, Li C, Gretzer MB, Kim EE, Podoloff DA (1995) Development of F-18-labeled fluoroerythronitroimidazole as a PET agent for imaging tumor hypoxia. Radiology 194:795–800
27. Cherif A, Wallace S, Yang DJ, Newman R, Wilson V, Nornoo A, Inoue T, Kim C, Kuang LR, Kim EE, Podoloff DA (1996) Development of new markers for hypoxic cells: [131I]iodomisonidazole and [131I]iodoerythronitroimidazole. J Drug Targeting 4:31–39
28. Tjuvajev J, Muraki A, Ginos J, Berk J, Koutcher J, Ballon D, Beattie B, Finn R, Dahighian F, Blasberg R (1993) Iododeoxyuridine uptake and retention as a measure of tumor growth. J Nucl Med 34:1152–1162
29. Abe Y, Fukuda H, Ishiwata K, Yoshioka S, Yamada K, Endo S, Kubota K, Sato T, Matsuzawa T, Takahashi T, Ido T (1983) Studies on [18F]-labeled pyrimidines tumor uptakes of [18F]-5-fluorouracil, [18F]-5-fluorouridine, and [18F]-5-fluorodeoxyuridine in animals. Eur J Nucl Med 8:258–261
30. Wright JA, Taylor NF, Fox JJ (1969) Nucleosides LX, fluorocarbohydrates XXII, synthesis of 2-deoxy-2-fluoro-D-arabinose and 9-(2-deoxy-2-fluoro-alpha- and beta-D-arabinofuranosyl) adenines. J Org Chem 34:2632–2636
31. Chu CK, Matulic-Adamic J, Huang JT, Chou TC, Burchenal JH, Fox JJ, Watanabe KA (1989) Nucleosides CXXXV. Synthesis of some 9-(2-deoxy-2-fluoro-beta-D-arabinofuranosyl)-9H-purines and their biological activities. Chem Pharm Bull 37:336–339
32. Zhuang Z-P, Kung M-P, Liang B, Kung HF (1997) Synthesis and characterization of iodinated adenosine derivatives as selective A_1 and A_2 receptor imaging agents. XIIth International Symposium on Radiopharmaceutical Chemistry. 12:85–87
33. Griengle H, Wanek E, Schwarz W, Streicher W, Rosenwirth B, Clercq ED (1987) 2'-Fluorinated arabinonucleosides of 5-(2-haloalkyl)uracil: synthesis and antiviral activity. J Med Chem 30:1199–1204
34. Folkman J (1975) Tumor angiogenesis. In: Becker FF (ed) Cancer biology: biology of tumors. (vol 3) Plenum, New York, pp 355–388
35. Warrell RP Jr, Frankel SR, Miller WH Jr, Scheinberg DA, Itri LM, Hittelman WN, Vyas R, Andreeff M, Tafuri A, Jakubowski A (1991) Differentiation therapy of acute promyelocytic leukemia with tretinoin (all-trans-retinoic acid). N Engl J Med 324:1385–1393
36. Davies RE (1967) Effects of vitamin A on 7, 12-dimethylbenz(a)-anathracene-induced papillomas in rhino mouse skin. Cancer Res 27:237–241
37. Bollag W (1979) Retinoids and cancer. Cancer Chemother Pharmacol 3:207–215
38. Smith EL, Tegeler JJ (1989) Advances in dermatology. Annu Rep Med Chem 24:177–186
39. Lippman SM, Meyskens FL (1987) Treatment of advanced squamous cell carcinoma of the skin with isotretinoin. Ann Intern Med 107:499–501
40. Hu L, Crowe DL, Rheinwald JG, Chambon P, Gudas LJ (1991) Abnormal expression of retinoic acid receptors and keratin 19 by human oral and epidermal squamous cell carcinoma cell lines. Cancer Res 51:3972–3981
41. Blomhoff R, Green MH, Berg T, Norum KR (1990) Transport and storage of Vitamin A. Science 250:399–404
42. Bertram JS (1991) Cancer chemoprevention by retinoids and carotenoids: proposed role of gap junctional communication. In: Jacobs MM (ed) Vitamins and minerals in the prevention and treatment of cancer. CRC, Boca Raton, pp 32–50
43. Sugioka K, Shimosegawa Y, Nakano M (1991) Estrogens as natural antioxidants of membrane phospholipid formation. FEBS Lett 210:37–39
44. Kumar K, Thangaraju M, Sachdanadam P (1991) Changes observed in antioxidant systems in the blood of postmenopausal women with breast cancer. Biochem Int 25:371–380
45. Thangaraju M, Vijayalakshmi T, Phil M, Sachdanandam P (1994) Effect of tamoxifen on lipid peroxide and antioxidative system in postmenopausal women with breast cancer. Cancer 74:78–82
46. Wiseman H, Laughton MJ, Armsteinn HRV (1990) The antioxidant action of tamoxifen and its metabolites. FEBS Lett 263:192–194
47. Eisemann JL, Sentz D, Rosen DM, Ramsland TS (1995) Combination trial of 13-cis retinoic acid and tamoxifen and fenretinide and tamoxifen in MCF-7 tumor xenograft model (abstract). Proc Am Assoc Cancer Res 36:408
48. Paik CH, Quadri SM, Reba RC (1989) Interposition of different chemical linkages between antibody and In-111 DTPA to accelerate clearance from non-target organs and blood. Nucl Med Biol 16:475–481
49. Yang DJ, Delpassand ES, Cherif A, Kuang LR, Wallace S, Podoloff DA (1995) Development of DTPA-tamoxifen conjugate as a new imaging kit for estrogen receptor tissues. Pharm Res 12:132
50. Yang DJ, Wallace S, Delpassand E, Cherif A, Kim EE, Podoloff DA (1995) DTPA-tamoxifen and DTPA-retinal: a new combined radiotracer to target breast tumors (abstract). Radiology 197(P):320
51. Yang DJ, Kuang LR, Li C, Wallace S (1994) CT liver enhancement imaging studies using poly(d-l-lactide) microcapsules. Invest Radiol 29:267–270
52. Kim CG, Yang DJ, Kim EE, Cherif A, Kuang LR, Li C, Tansey W, Liu CW, Li SC, Wallace S, Podoloff DA (1996) Assessment of tumor cell proliferation using [18F] fluorodeoxyadenosine and [18F]fluoroethyluracil. J Pharm Sciences 85:339–344
53. Cherif A, Yang DJ, Tansey W, Lee KW, Kim EE, Wallace S (1995) Radiosynthesis and biodistribution studies of [18F]fluoroadenosine and [I-131]-5-iodo-2'-O-methyl-uridine for the assessment of tumor proliferation rate. Pharm Res 12:128

54. Shani J, Gazit A, Livshitz T, Brian S (1995) Synthesis and receptor binding of fluorotamoxifen, a possible receptor imaging agent. J Med Chem 28:1504–1511
55. Hanson RN, Seitz DE (1982) Tissue distribution of the radiolabeled antiestrogen [^{125}I] iodotamoxifen. Int J Nucl Med Biol 9:105–107
56. Ram S, Spicer LD (1989) Synthesis of ^{11}C-labeled tamoxifen. J Labeled Compounds Radiopharm 27:661–668
57. Kangas L, Nieminen AL, Blanco G, Gronroos M, Kallio S, Karjalainen A, Perila M, Sodervall M, Toivola R (1986) A new triphenylethylene, Fc-1157a.II: Antitumor effects. Cancer Chemother Pharmacol 17:109–113
58. Kallio S, Kangas L, Blanco G, Johansson R, Karjalainen A, Perila M, Pippo I, Sundquist H, Sodervall M, Toivola R (1986) A new triphenylethylene, Fc-1157a.I. Hormonal effects. Cancer Chemother Pharmacol 17:103–108
59. Grierson JR, Link JM, Mathis CA, Rasey JS (1989) A radiosynthesis of fluorine-18-fluoromisonidazole. J Nucl Med 30:343–350
60. Lim JL, Berridge M (1993) Efficient radiosynthesis of [^{18}F]fluoromisonidazole suitable for routine PET. J Labeled Compounds Radiopharm 22:541–543
61. Hall EJ (1988) The oxygen effect and reoxygenation. In: Hall EJ (ed) Radiobiology for the radiobiologist, 3rd edn. Lippincott, Philadelphia, pp 137–160
62. Bush RS, Jenkin RD, Allt WE, Beale FA, Bean H, Dembo AJ, Pringle JF (1978) Definitive evidence for hypoxic cells influencing cure in cancer therapy. Br J Cancer 37:302–306
64. Kawai G, Yamamoto Y, Kamimura T, Masegi T, Sekine M, Hata T, Iimori T, Watanabe T, Miyazawa T, Yokohama S (1992) Coformational rigidity of specific pyrimidine residues in tRNA arises from posttranscriptional modifications that enhance steric interaction between the base and the 2′-hydroxyl group. Biochem 31:1040–1046
64. Uesugi S, Kaneyasu T, Ikehara M (1982) Synthesis and properties of ApU Analogues containing 2′-halo-2′-deoxyadenosine. Effect of 2′ substituents on oligonucleotide conformation. Biochem 21:5870–5877
65. Ikehara M, Miki H. (1978) Studies of nucleosides and nucleotides. Cyclonucleosides. Synthesis and properties of 2′-halogeno-2′-deoxyadenosines. Chem Pharm Bull 26:2449–2453
66. Malspeis L, Grever MR, Staubus AE, Young D (1982) Pharmacokinetics of 2-F-are-A (9-B-D-arabinofuranosyl-2-fluoroadenine) in cancer patients during the phase I clinical investigation of fludarabine phosphate. Semin Oncol 17:18–32
67. Goethals P, Eijkeren MV, Lodewyck W, Dams R (1995) Measurement of [methyl-carbon-11]thymidine and its metabolites in head and neck tumors. J Nucl Med 36:880–882
68. Martiat PH, Ferrant A, Labar D, Cogneau M, Bol A, Michel C, Michaux JL, Sokal G (1988) In vivo measurement of carbon-11 thymidine uptake in non-hodgkin's lymphoma using positron emission tomography. J Nucl Med 29:1633–1637
69. Shields AF, Lim K, Grierson J, Lin J, Krohn KA (1990) Utilization of labeled thymidine in DNA synthesis: studies for PET. J Nucl Med 31:337–342
70. Tjuvajev J, Macapinlac HA, Daghighian F, Scott AM, Ginos JZ, Finn RD, Kothari P, Desai R, Zhang J, Beattie B (1994) Imaging of brain tumor proliferative activity with iodine-131-iododeoxyuridine. J Nucl Med 35:1407–1417
71. Willemsen AT, van Waarde A, Paans AM, Pruim J, Luurtsema G, Go KG, Vaalburg W (1995) In vivo protein synthesis rate determination in primary or recurrent brain tumor using L-[1-^{11}C]-tyrosine and PET. J Nucl Med 36:411–419
72. Brooks D, Kuwata K, Schleich T (1994) Determination of proton magnetization transfer rate constants in heterogeneous biological systems. Magn Reson Med 31:331–336
73. Yang H, Schleich T (1994) T_2 discrimination contributions to proton magnetization transfer in heterogeneous biological systems. Magn Reson Med 32:16–20
74. Burnett DR, Goldstein EJ, Wolf GL (1984) The oral administration of $MnCl_2$: a potential alternative to IV injection for tissue contrast enhancement in magnetic resonance imaging. Magn Reson Imaging 2:307–312
75. Gehl HB, Vorwerk D, Klose KC (1991) Pancreatic enhancement after low-dose infusion of Mn-DPDP. Radiology 180:337–341
76. Rofsky NM, Weinreb JC (1992) Manganese (II) N,N′-diphyridoxylethylenediamine-N,N′-diacetate 5, 5′-bis (phosphate): clinical experience with a new contrast agent. Magn Reson Imaging 8:156–162
77. deHaen C, Gozzini L (1993) Soluble-type hepatobiliary contrast agents for MRI imaging. J Magn Reson Imaging 3:170–184
78. Hardy PA, Henkelman RM (1989) Transverse relaxation rate enhancement caused by magnetic particulates. Magn Reson Imaging 7:265–271
79. Weissleder R, Elizondo G, Josephson L (1989) Experimental lymph node metastases: enhanced detection with MR lymphography. Radiology 171:835–840
80. Gupta H, Weissleder R (1996) Targeted contrast agents in MR imaging. MRI Clin North Am 4:171–183
81. Reimer P, Weissleder R, Shen T (1994) Pancreatic receptors: initial feasibility studies with a targeted contrast agent for MR imaging. Radiology 193:527–531
82. Schaffer BK, Linker C, Papisov M (1993) MION-ASF: biokinetics of an MR receptor agent. Magn Reson Imaging 11:411–417
83. Reimer P, Weissleder R, Wittenberg J (1992) Receptor-directed contrast agents for MR imaging. Preclinical evaluation with affinity assays. Radiology 182:565–569
84. Vassallo P, Matei C, Hston WD (1994) AMI-227-enhanced MR lymphography: usefulness for differentiating reactive from tumor-bearing lymph nodes. Radiology 193:501–506
85. Weidner N, Folkman J, Pozza F (1992) Tumor angiogenesis: a new significant and independent prognostic indicator in early-stage breast carcinoma. J Natl Cancer Inst 84:1875–1887
86. Barsky D, Pütz B, Schulten K (1992) Theory of paramagnetic contrast agents in liposome system. Magn Reson Med 24:1–13
87. Niesman MR, Bacic GG, Wright SM (1990) Liposome encapsulated $MnCl_2$ as a liver specific contrast agent for MRI. Invest Radiol 25:545–551
88. Bulte JWM, Ma LD, Magin RL (1993) Selective MRI of labeled human peripheral blood mononuclear cells by liposome mediated incorporation of dextran-magnetite particles. Magn Reson Med 29:32–37

Receptor Imaging

F.C.L. Wong, E.E. Kim

Basic Considerations

Although the idea of a receptor as a molecular entity has been around since the turn of the century, it remained elusive until 1976, when Snyder proved its existence [1]. Before that time, the best evidence of receptors and subtypes of receptors was derived from bioassays. These earlier studies were technically tedious and involved a wide range of variances. Since 1976, the understanding of receptors, subtypes of receptors and development of receptor methodologies has made great advances. The development of receptor technology in pharmacology, indeed, has benefited from earlier studies of antibody-antigen interactions, as pioneered by Yalow [2]. Despite differences in molecular weights of the entities involved, both antibody-antigen interactions and drug-receptor interactions are governed by the same mass-action laws that underlie all ligand-protein reactions.

When different molecules in aqueous solution encounter each other in close proximity, they either attract, repel, pass by without any significant effect or collide with each other. The underlying forces behind the attraction or repulsion of the moieties are governed by the hydrophobic or hydrophilic interactions, electrostatic forces, bulkiness of the entities and hydration of the various moieties. After two molecules collide, they may remain bound either for a short duration or indefinitely. The status of a ligand bound to a protein is referred to as the ligand-protein binding. Such binding is governed by the affinity of the ligand for the protein (or vice versa). In the initial phase, binding is a reversible phenomenon, i.e., the ligand may leave the protein at various rates. However, with time, it may become an irreversible event as conventional chemical reactions form covalent bonds between the ligand and the protein. Such events may occur naturally or may be triggered by other factors, such as other chemicals in the vicinity or radiation-induced free-radical formation and reaction between the ligand and the protein. Therefore, the ligand-protein interactions can be either reversible or irreversible. Furthermore, depending on the manner in which the ligand is bound to the protein, the interaction can also be classified as noncompetitive or competitive, when other ligands with similar chemical structures may interfere with the binding itself.

In molecular pharmacology, reversible saturable competitive ligand-protein binding is the main concern, because it allows the ability to study the structure-activity relationship of various analogs of the ligands and provides a good rationale and explanation of the ligand-protein interactions at the molecular level. High affinity and specificity are the two key requirements for study of a ligand-binding system. Competitive irreversible binding, such as photo-affinity labeling, i.e., covalent crosslinking between the ligand and protein using ultraviolet light, has also been a good biochemical tool. In fact, competitive irreversible binding using tissue-presentation X-ray provides an opportunity to effect in vivo receptor labeling [3]. Noncompetitive binding, whether reversible or irreversible, is typical of lower affinity, but needs to be suppressed or discounted in order to evaluate the more biologically significant saturable competitive reversible interactions between the ligand and the protein.

The above discussion only applies to in vitro homogeneous aqueous environments, such as test tubes in the laboratory. For in vivo imaging, multiple additional factors may affect the resultant ligand binding tremendously. The venous dilution, hepatic metabolism and intravascular metabolism of the ligand may markedly decrease the available ligand in the tissue of interest. The vasculature and the vascular reaction to pathology or to the ligand itself may further alter the access of the ligand to the tissue. The ability of the ligand to cross the barrier between the capillary and the tissue may prevent the ligand from reaching the tissue. The internalization process of the bound ligand on the surface of the cells and subsequent metabolism in the cells may decrease the amount of the ligand detected from the extracorporal imaging device. Other protein binding, whether noncompetitive or irreversible, in the intravascular compartment may decrease the availability of the ligand to the tissue of interest. The metabolism of the ligand itself in the body, whether in the serum or in the liver, may result in release of ligand metabolites into the intravascular compartment and a decrease in signal-to-noise ratio because of rising background tracer activities. Lastly, endogenous or exogenous ligands may compete with the tracer. Therefore, the translation of in vitro ligand-protein binding studies into in vivo imaging requires careful consideration of each of the above pharmacokinetic and pharmacodynamic factors. These factors may operate both in this certainly heterogeneous environment of body-fluid and tissue, as well as across the multiple biological membrane barriers.

Receptors and Human Disease

Receptors mediate many vital communications between extrinsic chemicals and nervous and muscular systems, as demonstrated by the various types of neurotransmitter-receptor pathways. Aberrations in these types of receptors may lead to different forms of myasthenia gravis. Receptors also mediate the communication between different organs in the human body via the endocrine system. Aberrations in the receptors may lead to endocrinopathy such as Graves' disease. Additionally, receptors mediate the communication between cells and also with the cell itself through the environment via the autocrine system. Aberrations in the receptors along this system may result in uncontrolled growth of the cell lines to become tumors.

Abnormalities at the receptor level, either because of altered affinity or density, may be the primary cause of an ailment; alternatively, these could also be results of the up- or downregulation of or interaction with other molecular entities or receptor systems within the cells. Therefore, evaluation of receptors alone does not provide the specific etiology of the disease. Changes in receptor affinity and density may be nonspecifically correlated with disease processes, but not necessarily causally related.

Multiple in vitro and in vivo techniques have been devised to study specific receptor systems related to human disease. In the clinical practice of oncology, elevated levels of somatostatin receptors have been found in tumors such as small cell lung cancer, different forms of pancreatic cancer, carcinoid tumor, meningioma and, to a lesser degree, lymphoma.

Early detailed receptor imaging studies were mostly in the study of human brain diseases. For instance, the first human receptor imaging was reported on the dopamine (D) receptors using positron emission tomography (PET) [4]. By using ^{11}C-labeled 3-N-methylspiperone (NMSP), it was found that D2 receptors are elevated in patients with schizophrenia [5] and depression [6]. Subsequent developments in single-photon-emission computed tomography (SPECT) tracer led to the use of ^{123}I-labeled iodobenzamide for the SPECT imaging of human D2 receptors [7].

Prerequisites of Receptor Imaging

Eckelman outlined 16 categories of study in the development of a receptor-binding system for in vivo imaging [8]. These categories include the determination of the dissociation constant (K_d) for the parent compound, in vitro displacement of the labeled compound by a nonradioactive derivative, the determination of the K_d for the radioactive derivative, the use of active and inactive stereoisomers of the radioactive derivative as well as the confirmation of animal distribution pattern of the tracer compound in humans.

The choice of a receptor system should originally be based on the in vitro binding affinity and specificity data. In general, because of the high specific activity available with radioactive ligands (up to 30 Ci/mmol/molecule) and the concern of excessive dosimetry to humans, K_d as a measure of the affinity of the ligand to the receptor should be in the range 0.1–50 nM. When the affinity is too high, i.e., with very small K_d or a very high association rate constant, the radioactivity determined in the target organ is independent of the receptor concentration. The rate-limiting step becomes a measure of flow rate or membrane transport rather than the ligand-receptor binding processes. With a low affinity constant, i.e., when K_d is greater than 50 nM, a large amount of unbound free tracer will be in the circulation and the signal-to-noise ratio may be significantly decreased. The resultant images may become a measure of other factors, such as vasculature or blood volume in the tissue of interest instead of a reflection of the receptors.

Since the optimum condition for detection of changes in binding occurs when the ligand-receptor ratio is between 0.2 and 0.8, too much or too little tracer ligand in the vasculature will decrease the ability to detect significant alterations. The quantification of receptor-ligand interactions is beyond the scope of this chapter, but may be referred to in the study by Vera et al. [9].

Other requirements of ligand-receptor systems for human imaging studies include the relatively nontoxic nature of the tracer ligand at the dose prescribed. It also should have relatively good stability in the intravascular compartment during the imaging session.

In other words, considerations for in vivo human receptor imaging start with an existing in vitro ligand-receptor binding system, with additional attention to details of the pharmacokinetic characteristics, such as intravascular dilution, permeability, biodistribution, metabolism and endogenous ligand competitions.

A less-preferred approach to receptor imaging is to conduct empirical studies using putative ligands. Such an approach suffers from the criticism that the interaction between the receptor and the ligand have not been characterized and therefore any findings or images may reflect the various physiologic and pathologic processes other than those at the receptor levels. Therefore, even though impressive images may be obtained, validation studies still have to be carried out to verify the receptor-ligand interaction.

Imaging of Receptors in Tumors

Most of the earlier receptor imaging studies were performed with regard to the central nervous system because of the abundant basic research data on the different neurotransmitter pathways. Imaging of receptors in tumors started as a transition from the brain to brain tumors. Dopamine receptors were found to be markedly elevated in human pituitary adenomas by a PET study using ^{11}C-NMSP [10] and visualization of brain lesions, as well as tumors using compounds such as ^{11}C-PK 11195 [11]. These earlier studies benefited from the abundant basic research, including animal work and in vitro studies. A good example of the transition between in vitro and in vivo receptor studies is illustrated by Raderer [12], who compared in vitro receptor density and affinity to the imaging characteristics of ^{123}I-labeled vasoactive intestinal peptide (VIP) in human tissue and cancer cells. He also compared the ^{123}I VIP system to ^{111}In-CYT-103 monoclonal antibody in vitro and in vivo imaging characteristics. This is the preferred mode of development of receptor-binding studies from in vitro to in vivo clinical studies.

In the case of PK-11195 binding to gliomas, in vitro studies found at least a 20-fold-elevated receptor density on the tumor cells [13]. Ex vivo autoradiography confirmed only about a sixfold-elevated receptor density when the tissue was sectioned into thin layers and exposed to the ligand [14]. Subsequent PET images only found a twofold increase in the signal detected in the tumor compared with that of the surrounding brain tissues. This same experience of decreased signal-to-noise ratio from the in vitro study to the in vivo imaging is, again, confirmed in the above-mentioned ^{123}I VIP study [12], with the initial tumor receptor density of 1000-fold higher by the in vitro study decreasing probably to give a less than tenfold difference in the signal detected in the tumor by an in vivo method. The explanation for this loss of signal-to-noise ratio may be explained by the multiple factors involved in the delivery of the ligand to the receptor site and the subsequent detection of the signal in the living organism. This reduction in signal-to-noise ratio will direct the search for a suitable receptor-ligand system for oncologic imaging to those receptors that are markedly elevated in tumors. Using PK 11195 as an example, a minimum of 20-fold receptor-density difference will be required for visualization of the receptors in the tumor using PET. When less-sensitive instrumentation such as SPECT is used, as in the case of the ^{123}I VIP, the requirement of the receptor-density elevation in tumors will be even higher, for instance, greater than 100-fold in order for the tumor to be visualized.

The requirement of a high in vitro signal-to-noise receptor-density ratio is not unique to receptors found on the surface of tumor cells. Since cytosolic estrogen receptors are elevated with breast cancer, PET studies have been reported with ^{18}F-labeled estrogen analogs. For 16α-^{18}F-fluoro-17β-estradiol, which has a target background ratio of 80:1 from in vitro studies, a signal-to-noise ratio of 2:2 is noted in breast cancer with human PET [15].

Obviously, multiple other factors, such as perfusion, size of tumor, intravascular and hepatic metabolism, affinity, internalization rate of the ligand and competition from endogenous ligands are all factors that potentially affect the threshold of the receptor-density difference for the tumor to be visualized. Since in vivo quantitative evaluation of receptors requires meticulous attention to technical details, arterial blood sampling, and stringent and multiple time sequences of imaging sessions, they are not routinely performed in the clinical setting. Instead, optimum imaging conditions derived from the above quantitative studies are typically chosen, and routine clinical imaging of receptors in oncology is performed without blood sampling.

^{111}In-Labeled-Somatostatin-Receptor Imaging in Oncology

Early successful imaging of human tumors involved somatostatin analogs using ^{123}I labels [16, 17]. The K_d of the radioiodinated compound, ^{123}I Tyr-octreotide ranges between 0.5 nM and 1.5 nM, well within the suitable range of affinity constant for imaging [18]. The somatostatin receptor density is barely detectable in neuroendocrine tissues, but markedly elevated in malignant tissues, from 80 fmole/mg to 2000 fmole/mg protein [19]. ^{111}In-[diethylenetriaminepentaacetic acid (DTPA) D-phenylalanine (Phe)] octreotide has been used in subsequent development of somatostatin-receptor scintigraphy because of the more favorable stability and imaging characteristics in the delayed images.

Somatostatin is a peptide that exists in either a 14-amino acid or a 28-amino acid form. It is present in the hypothalamus, brain stem and gastrointestinal tract as well as the pancreas. Somatostatin receptors are found on activated lymphocytes and cells of neuroendocrine origin, such as the anterior pituitary, pancreatic islet cells and thyroid C cells. Five subtypes of somatostatin receptors have been identified and cloned. All of these subtypes exert their effects by inhibiting adenylyl cyclase activity. Subtype 2 has high affinity, or low K_d, in the range of 0.1 nM to 1 nM, while subtypes 3 and 5 are in the 10–100 nM range; subtypes 1 and 4 exhibit affinity >1000 nM [20]. Therefore, only subtype 2 is suitable for imaging. In fact, subtype 2 is the one most frequently expressed in tumors, and antiproliferative effects have been observed with activation of subtypes 1 and 2 [21].

Typically, 5 mCi of ^{111}In [DTPA D-Phe] octreotide is injected intravenously and whole-body images obtained after clearance of intravascular activities, typically at 4 h. More delayed images are obtained typically after 24 h. The images may further be studied by SPECT, either at 4 h or 24 h. It has been argued that SPECT at 4 h is adequate. Images obtained after 48 h are seldom performed, and may hardly provide any additional useful information. Comparison with anatomic imaging is important to further ascertain the location of the radioactivity. Typically, a strong signal-to-background ratio is identified in the tumor sites. For instance, in a patient with neuroblastoma, suspected sites of adenopathy in the neck are confirmed to be metastatic tumors by histology (Fig. 7.1).

In vivo imaging studies using ^{111}In [DTPA D-Phe] octreotide have demonstrated high sensitiv-

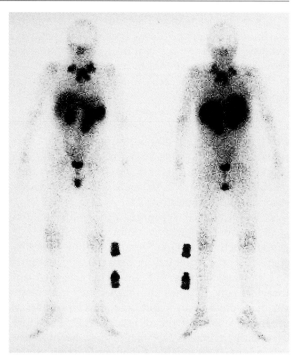

Fig. 7.1. Whole-body anterior (*left*) and posterior (*right*) images at 4 h following the injection of ^{111}In octreotide show markedly increased activities in proven metastatic neuroblastoma masses in the superior mediastinum and bilateral supraclavicular lymphatic chains. A small mass in the left adrenal gland is obscured by the intensely increased activities in the adjacent kidney and spleen

ity of tumor detection in most tumors of neuroectodermal origin (Figs. 7.1 and 7.2). These findings are also confirmed by in vitro analysis in pituitary tumors, gastrinomas, insulinomas, paragangliomas, small cell lung cancers, meningiomas, astrocytomas, thyroid cancers, lymphoma and amine-precursor-uptake-and-decarboxylation tumors [19]. However, sarcoidosis, rheumatoid arthritis, tuberculosis and post-radiation effects have all been reported to have elevated the frequency of octreotide-avid lesions, as confirmed by in vivo imaging as well as in vitro tissue analyses. Part of the explanation of the uptake of octreotide in the non-malignant lesions may be the accumulation of activated lymphocytes in the vicinity.

^{111}In-labeled octreotide has the disadvantage that it emits beta-electrons, therefore limiting the dose of the tracer. Other somatostatin-receptor imaging agents have been developed. More specific fragments of somatostatin, technetium-labeled P829, have been found to achieve a dosimetry with better photon flux in phase-II studies (Fig. 7.3) [22]. ^{67}Ga and ^{68}Ga deferoxamine-labeled octreotide achieve better dosimetry and quantitation, respectively [23].

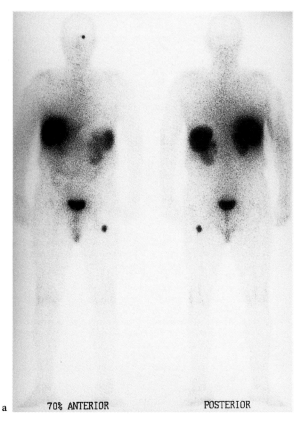
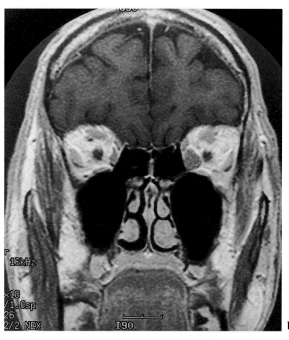
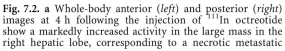

Fig. 7.2. a Whole-body anterior (*left*) and posterior (*right*) images at 4 h following the injection of ^{111}In octreotide show a markedly increased activity in the large mass in the right hepatic lobe, corresponding to a necrotic metastatic pancreatic islet cell tumor on computed tomography. Unexpected small focal areas of markedly increased activities in the left orbit and left thigh also correspond to the mass involving the medial rectus muscle of the left eye and also the left proximal femur seen on the subsequent magnetic resonance imaging examinations. **b** Coronal T_1-weighted image of the head shows a mass in the medial rectus muscle of the left eye

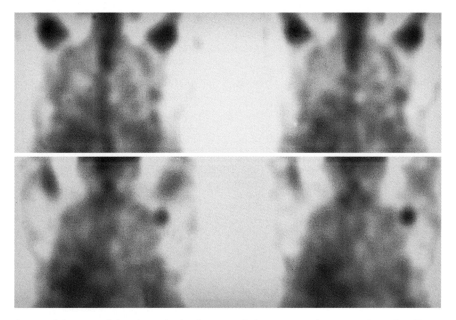

Fig. 7.3. Selected coronal images of the chest single-photon-emission computed tomography using Tc-99m P829 peptide show metastatic melanomas in the left breast (*upper*) and left axilla (*lower*)

The advantage of receptor imaging in oncology is that the receptor is not a biological product, so its production is not subject to animal variation as in antibody production. Furthermore, because of the fact that they are small molecules, biodistribution is more favorable because these small molecules may be able to pass different biological barriers by mere diffusion. Currently, cost and availability are still constraints that limit the wide use of receptor imaging. However, with more support from basic research in receptors and the development of alternative, better and less-expensive tracers, receptor imaging may be the best example of applying basic science directly to patient care.

References

1. Snyder SM, Bennett JD (1976) Neurotransmitter receptors in the brain: biochemical identification. Ann Rev Physiol 38:153–175
2. Yalow RS, Berson SA (1971) Introduction and general considerations. In: Odele WD, Daughaday WH (eds) Principles of competitive protein binding assays. Lippincott, Philadelphia, p 1
3. Wong FCL, Ho B, Lu IG, Fan SH, Myen R, Yang DJ, Kim EE (1993) Affinity labeling of neuroreceptors using gamma rays. J Nucl Med 34[suppl]:26
4. Wagner HN, Barns HD, Dannals RJ, Wong DF, Langstrum B, Duelfer T, Frost JJ, Ravert HT, Links JM, Rosenbloom SB, Lukas SE, Kramer AV, Kuher MJ (1983) Imaging human dopamine receptors in the human brain. Science 221:1264–1266
5. Wong DF, Wagner HN, Tune LE, Dannals RF, Pearlson GD, Links JM, Tamminga CA, Broussolle EP, Ravert HT, Wilson AA, Toung JKT, Malat J, Williams JA, O'Tauma LA, Snyder SH, Kuhar MJ, Gjedde A (1986) Positron emission tomography reveals elevated D2 dopamine receptors in drug-naive schizophrenics. Science 234:1558-1563
6. Wong DF, Pearlson G, Tune LE, et al. (1987) In vivo measurements of D2 dopamine receptor abnormalities in drug-naive and treated manic depressive patients. J Nucl Med 28:611
7. Kung HF, Slavi A, Chang W, King MP, Keyes JW Jr, Velchik MG, Billings J, Pan S, Noto R, et al. (1990) In vivo SPECT imaging of CNS D2 dopamine receeptors: initial studies with Iodine-123 IBZM in humans. J Nucl Med 31:573–578
8. Eckelman WC (1982) The testing of putative receptor binding radiotracers in vivo. In: Diksic M, Reba RC (eds) Radiopharmaceuticals and brain pathology studies with PET and SPECT. CRC Press, Boca Raton, pp 42–62
9. Vera DR, Krohn KA, Scheibe PO, Stadolnil RC (1985) Identifiability analysis of an in vivo receptor-binding radiopharmacokinetic system. IEEE Trans Biomed Eng 32:312–322
10. Yung BCK, Wand GS, Blevins L, Dannals RF, Ravert HT, Chan B, Wong DF (1993) In vivo assessment of dopamine receptor density in pituitary macroadenoma and correlation with in vitro assay. J Nucl Med 34:133
11. Junck L, Olson JM, Ciliax BJ, Koeppe RA, Watkins GL, Jewett DM, McKeever PE, Wieland DM, Kilbourn MR, Starosta-Rubinstein S, et al. (1989) PET imaging of human gliomas with ligands for the peripheral benzodiazepine binding sites. Ann Neurol 26:752–758
12. Raderer M, Becherer A, Kurtaran A, Angelberger P, Li S, Leimer M, Weinlaender G, Kornek G, Kletter K, Scheithauer W, Virgolini I (1996) Comparison of Iodine-123-vasoactive intestinal peptide receptor scintigraphy and Indium-111 CFT-103 immunoscintigraphy. J Nucl Med 37:1480–1487
13. Starosta-Rubinstein S, Ciliax BJ, Penney JB, McKeever P, Young A (1980) Imaging of a glioma using peripheral benzodiazepine receptor ligands. Proc Natl Acad Sci U S A 84:891–895
14. Price GW, Ahier RG, Hume SP, Myers R, Manjil L, Cremer JE, Luthra SK, Pascali C, Pike V, Frackowiak RS (1990) In vivo binding to peripheral benzodiazepine binding sites in lesional rat brain: comparison between [^{3}H]-P/C11194 and [F^{18}] PK 14105 as markers for neuronal damages. J Neurochem 55:175–185
15. McGuire AH, Dehdashti F, Siegel BA, Lyss AP, Brodack JW, Mathias CJ, Mintun MA, Katzenellenbogen JA, Welch MJ (1991) Positron tomographic assessment of 16α-F18-fluoro 17-estradiol uptake in metastatic breast carcinoma. J Nucl Med 32:1526–1531
16. Reubi JC, Krenning E, Lamberts SW, Krols L (1990) Somatostatin receptors in malignant tissues. J Steroid Biochem Mol Biol 37:1073–1077
17. Lambert SW, Bakker WH, Reubi JC, Krenning EP (1990) Somatostatin receptor imaging in vivo localization of tumors with a radiolabeled somatostatin analog. J Steroid Biochem Mol Biol 37:1079–1082
18. Bakker WH, Krenning EP, Breeman WA, Koper JW, Kooij PP, Reubi JC, Klijn JG, Visser TJ, Docter R, Lamberts SW (1990) Receptor scintigraphy with a radioiodinated somatostatin analogue: radiolabeling, purification, biologic activity and in vivo application in animals. J Nucl Med 31:1501–1509
19. Faglia G, Bazzoni N, Spada A, Arosio M, Ambrosi B, Spinelli F, Sara R, Bonino C, Lunghi F (1991) In vivo detection of somatostatin receptors in patients with functionless pituitary xadenomas by means of a radioiodinated analog of somatostatin I-123 SD2204-090. J Clin Endocrinol Metab 73:850–856
20. Krenning EP, Kwekkeboom DJ, Panwels S, Kvols K, Reubi JC (1995) Somatostatin receptor scintigraphy. Ann Nucl Med 1:1–50
21. Buscail L, Delesque N, Estéve JP, Saint-Laurent N, Prats H, Clerc P, Robberecht P, Bell GI, Liebow C, Schally AV, et al. (1994) Stimulation of toposine phosphatase and inhibition of cell proliferation by somatostatin analogues:mediation by human somatostatin receptor subtypes SSTR1 and SSTR2. Proc Natl Acad Sci U S A 91:2315–2319
22. Vallabhajosula S, Moyer BR, Lister-James J, McBride BJ, Lipszyc H, Lee H, Bastidas D, Dean RT (1996) Preclinical evaluation of technetium-99.-labeled somatostatin receptor-binding peptides. J Nucl Med 37:1016–1022
23. Smith-Jones PM, Stolz B, Borms C, et al. (1994) Ga-67/Ga-68 [DFO] octreotide-A potential radiopharmaceutical for PET imaging of somatostatin receptor-positive tumors: synthesis and radiolabeling in vitro as preliminary in vivo studies. J Nucl Med 35:317–325

Practical Magnetic Resonance Imaging and Positron Emission Tomography Techniques and Their Artifacts

E. E. Kim

Magnetic Resonance Imaging Techniques

Spin-Echo Imaging

The basic magnetic resonance (MR) signal occurs as an exponentially diminishing sinusoidal oscillation called the free induction decay (FID). This signal decays as a result of loss of transverse magnetization due to dephasing of the protons precessing in the xy plane. The loss of phase coherence is related to slight differences in precessional frequency due to interaction of the protons with neighboring protons (spin-spin interactions) and inhomogeneity in the applied magnetic field. FID would decay with a time constant of T_2, but it decays with a time constant of T_2^*, which represents the observed transverse relaxation time constant. The application of a selective 90° radiofrequency (RF) pulse followed by one or more selective 180° pulses forms the basis of SE imaging. The 90° pulse tips the magnetization vector into the xy plane. The protons begin to lose phase coherence, partly as a result of spin-spin interactions (T_2 relaxation), and partly as a result of magnetic-field inhomogeneity. The loss of phase coherence results in a fanning-out of the proton's net transverse magnetization vectors. In the process of dephasing, the protons with faster precessional rates get ahead of the slower protons, which fall behind. The application of a 180° pulse causes the protons to flip 180° about the x axis so that the faster protons are now behind the slower ones. The rephasing or refocusing of the protons by the 180° RF pulse produces a signal called the spin echo (SE). If the time interval between the 90° and 180° pulses is designated τ, the protons will be back in phase at a time 2τ. The time interval between the 90° pulse and the resulting echo is called the echo time (TE) and is equal to 2τ. The time interval between successive 90° pulses is called the repetition time (TR). The amplitude of the MR signal decreases with long TE due to dissipation of the FID. T_2 information can be maximized by using a long TE (Figs. 8.1–8.4).

Inversion Recovery SE Imaging

The inversion recovery (IR) SE pulse sequence consists of a 180° pulse followed by a 90° pulse and then another 180° pulse. After the 180° pulse, T_1 relaxation begins to take place. A 90° pulse is then applied to tip the net magnetization vector into the xy plane. After a short interval, a 180° refocusing pulse is applied and the signal is measured during the ensuing SE. The time interval between the initial 180° pulse and the 90° pulse is called the inversion time (TI). For each tissue there is a TI at which the signal from that tissue is zero. This is called a null point of the tissue (also called the inflection or bounce point). The degree of T_1 tissue contrast produced with the IR pulse sequence is dramatically affected by the choice of either the phase or magnitude image reconstruction method.

The TE is kept relatively short to minimize T_2 information. The T_1 and T_2 effects tend to cancel one another, diminishing tissue contrast, if a long TE is used. The TR pulse sequence is capable of achieving greater T_1 weighting than the T_1-weighted SE pulse sequence. One must use a longer TR than with the SE sequence to allow greater recovery of Z magnetization. In the short-T_1 inversion recovery (STIR) pulse sequence, a T_1 in the range 0–250 ms is used. If a T_1 of 100–200 ms at the null point of fat is used, the signal from fat is suppressed. When magnitude reconstruction is used, the effects of prolonged T_1 and T_2 are additive, both increasing signal and thus tissue contrast.

Chemical Shift Imaging

The resonance frequency of a given nucleus is affected in a small but detectable manner by its chemical environment. Nuclei in different binding sites experience slight variations in local magnetic-field strength due to the shielding effects of nearby electron orbitals. The changes in the resonant frequency of the detected MR signal are re-

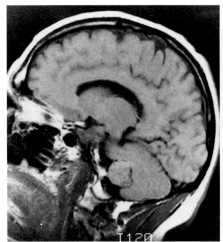 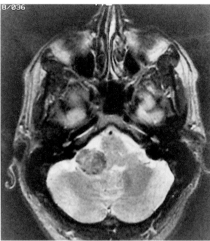

Fig. 8.1. Spin-echo T_1-weighted sagittal (*left*) and T_2-weighted axial (*right*) images of the head show a meningioma in the right cerebellopontine angle with slightly heterogeneous intermediate signal intensity

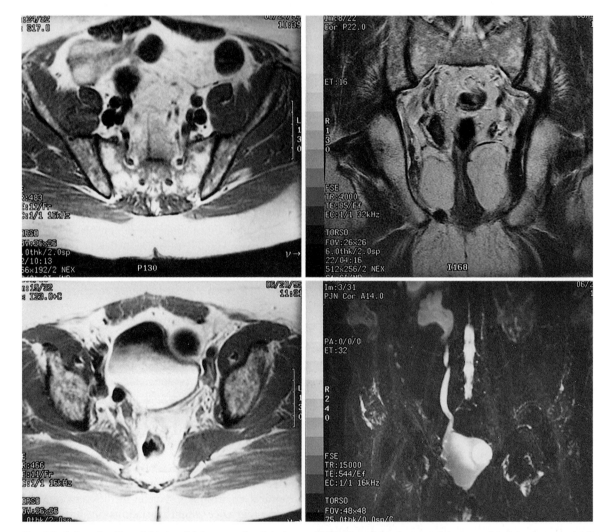

Fig. 8.2. Spin-echo T_1-weighted axial images of pelvis before (*upper left*) and after (*lower left*) injection of gadolinium-diethylenetriaminepentaacetic acid. Fast spin-echo (FSE) T_2-weighted coronal image of pelvis (*upper right*) and magnetic resonance urogram (*lower right*) using heavy T_2-weighted FSE

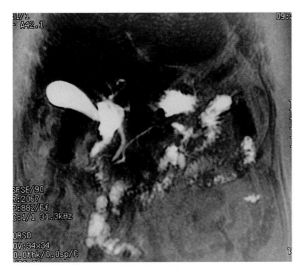

Fig. 8.3. Magnetic resonance pancreatocholangiogram using heavy T_2-weighted fast spin echo shows normal gall bladder, common bile and pancreatic ducts

ferred to as chemical shifts. Water protons precess at a rate of 3–4 ppm faster than fat protons. This difference in resonant frequencies causes a chemical shift artifact in the frequency-encoding direction at water/fat interfaces. In conventional SE imaging, water (w) and fat (f) protons are in-phase. Signal intensity on the resulting in-phase imaging is therefore due to the summation of signals produced by water and fat protons (w+f). In an out-of-phase or opposed image, signal detection occurs when fat and water protons are oriented in opposite directions. The timing of the 180° refocusing pulse and the sampling of the MR signal is altered, and the net transverse magnetization is detected when fat and water protons are aligned in opposite directions. The resulting image expresses the signal which is the difference between water and fat protons (w–f). Adding an in-phase image and its opposed image together results in a pure water image: (w+f)+(w–f)=w. A pure fat image is obtained by subtracting the opposed from the in-phase image: (w+f)–(w–f)=f. Opposed images have been shown to be more sensitive than standard SE techniques for detecting small changes in hepatic fat content. The potential of chemical shift imaging (CSI) to map the distribution of important biological metabolites also holds great interest. Imaging of lactate as a marker of tissue ischemia is an intriguing possibility, and [31]phosphorus CSI can potentially map the relative distributions of adenosine triphosphate, phosphocreatine and inorganic phosphate. Imaging the distribution of sodium is another interesting use, since sodium ion concentration is increased in tumor, ischemia and infarction. CSI

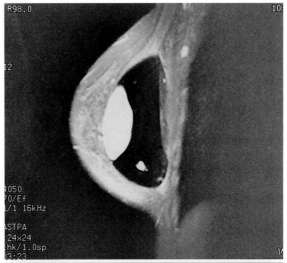

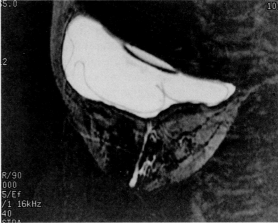

Fig. 8.4. Magnetic resonance mammogram. Sagittal image of the right breast using heavy T_2-weighted fast spin echo shows uniform high signal intensity in a saline implant (*top*). Heavy T_2-weighted axial images using a silicone pulse show a silicone implant and also linear leakage of silicone towards the nipple (*bottom*)

of fluorine can be accomplished with the exogenous administration of various fluoro compounds, such as 2-fluoro-2-deoxyglucose.

Rapid Imaging

Rapid magnetic resonance imaging (MRI) techniques play an important adjunctive role to improve the efficiency of clinical MRI and to decrease artifacts that arise from cardiac, respiratory and other patient motion. Gradient-echo (GE) imaging uses a single RF excitation pulse (usually 10–90°), whereas an SE pulse sequence consists of two separate RF pulses. The 180° pulse in SE imaging rephases spins in the transverse plane, thereby producing a SE. In GE imaging, the echo is produced by reversal of the magnetic-field gradients rather than of a 180° RF pulse. The net effect of the gradient reversal is a rephasing of spins and the production of a GE at time TE. The use of partial-flip angle excitation pulses and elimination of the 180° refocusing pulse typically reduces RF power deposition in GE imaging. The 180° refocusing pulse in SE imaging compensates for spin dephasing due to inhomogeneities in the magnetic field, chemical shift and susceptibility effects. The reversal of imaging gradients in GE imaging does not compensate for these dephasing processes. The appearance of GE images is therefore influenced by T_2^*, which characterizes the sum effect of magnetic field distortions, causing loss of transverse magnetization.

Imaging time (Ti) is a function of TR value, the number of phase-encoding steps (Npe) and the number of data acquisitions (Nda). The TR values used for GE imaging are generally much shorter than those used in SE imaging. The short TR allows too little time for recovery of longitudinal magnetization between excitation pulses. By using an excitation pulse with a flip angle less than 90°, only part of the longitudinal magnetization is converted to transverse magnetization. When TR is less than 100–150 ms, a variable amount of residual transverse magnetization is typically present at the time of the next excitation pulse. Transverse magnetization is either removed by a spoiler gradient or converted into longitudinal magnetization. Both longitudinal and transverse magnetization reach equilibrium and contribute to the steady-state signal. This type of pulse sequence is called GRASS (gradient-recalled acquisition in steady state) or FISP (fast imaging and steady precession). The signal intensity on short-TR GRASS or FISP images is dependent on T_2^*/T_1, producing a bright signal in cerebrospinal fluid (CSF) or urine. However, the conspicuity of pathological lesions such as tumors is diminished compared with SE imaging. The transverse magnetization remaining at the end of the TR interval is destroyed by a spoiler gradient. This sequence is designed to maximize T_1 weighting by minimizing T_2 effects, but signal intensity is still influenced by T_2^*. T_1 weighting is maximized by using short TR, short TE and high (90°) flip angle. T_2 weighting is achieved with longer TR and TE and small-to-intermediate flip angle, and proton-density weighting with long TR, short TE and small flip angle.

GE pulse sequences are often used in conjunction with SE imaging for the examination of joints. Steady-state GE images with short TR and low flip angle provide a myelogram effect for the study of CSF flow dynamics. The combination of rapid scanning and bright intravascular signal has led to the development of dynamic cardiac imaging to visualize regional wall-motion abnormalities and blood-flow disturbances. Modifications of the GE pulse sequence have been applied to MR angiography (Fig. 8.5). Rapid-acquisition spin-echo (RASE) or fast spin-echo (FSE) imaging [1] is an alternative approach to rapid MRI and uses a standard SE pulse sequence with short TR, short TE, and single excitation using half-Fourier sampling. This allows for simultaneous acquisition of multiple imaging sections within a relatively short period of time. Due to the use of a short TR and half-Fourier sampling, RASE technique shows a relatively low signal-to-noise ratio (SNR). With echo-planar imaging (EPI), sampling of the entire raw data space is accomplished following a single RF excitation pulse [2]. The readout gradient is rapidly oscillated following the excitation pulse to generate a train of closely spaced

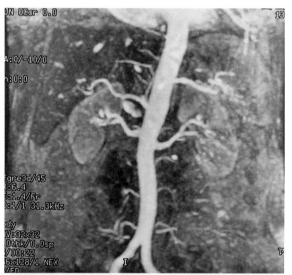

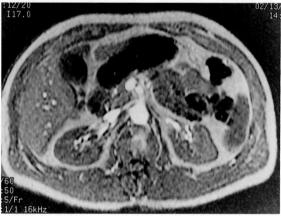

Fig. 8.5. Magnetic resonance angiogram using three-dimensional efficient gradient-echo (GE) image shows bilateral renal arteries (*top*). Axial image of abdomen using 60° GE pulse sequence shows abdominal aorta, renal arteries and inferior vena cava with high signal intensity (*bottom*)

GEs. An increment of phase-encoding gradient is applied between each echo and individual lines are sampled within 10–100 ms. Subsecond scan times have been achieved with a modification of fast low-angle shot (FLASH) GE pulse sequence (Snapshot FLASH or Turbo-FLASH). High bandwidth sampling and reduced RF pulse lengths are used to shorten TR to below 10 ms with this technique. The loss in SNR incurred by the short TR and high bandwidth sampling is partially compensated by the use of very short TE and voxel larger than in conventional GE images. This allows for the acquisition of near-real-time studies of the heart, joint and bowel. In addition, when used in conjunction with various contrast agents, these high-speed dynamic studies may allow determination of organ or tumor perfusion.

Positron-Emission-Tomography Techniques

All patients need to fast (except for water) for at least 4–6 h before imaging and normal blood glucose levels are confirmed. Before the positron trace is administered, transmission scans are obtained with 5 mCi (185 Mbq) gallium-68 (approximately 300 million counts in 30 min) for attenuation correction. Patients are usually given an intravenous bolus injection of radiopharmaceuticals, such as 10 mCi (370 mBq) ^{18}F fluoro-2-deoxy-D-glucose (FDG). The labeling of 2-deoxyglucose as previously described provides the positron-emitting form of the glucose analog [3]. Quality control, sterility and pyrogen tests are performed. Beginning simultaneously with the initiation of the FDG injection, rapid sequential scans are obtained in order to measure the FDG kinetic rate constants and to monitor the uptake and fixation of the isotope in the tissues [4]. Blood samples for determination of ^{18}F plasma activity and glucose concentration are taken from the opposite arm, using direct arterial sampling. Diagnostic static imaging is initiated after a 30-min uptake period, and 2–5 million true coincidences are obtained per slice in the static scans. Patients may be imaged with an indwelling urinary catheter to evaluate pelvic tumors or nodal metastases.

A whole-body eight-ring system usually produces 15 simultaneous transaxial image slices per bed position, and eight-bed interlaced positions are acquired to cover an 81-cm total axial field of view over the patient's upper body, from the top of the head to the upper pelvis. A second eight-bed interlaced acquisition is performed on the lower portion of the body, covering the upper pelvis to the distal tibial level after the patient has voided (Fig. 8.6).

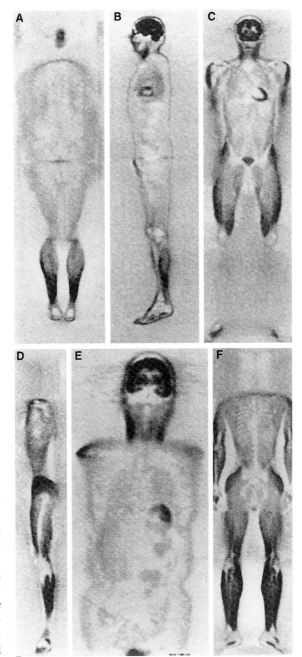

Fig. 8.6 A–F. Whole-body positron-emission-tomography (PET) images using ^{18}F-fluoro-2-deoxy-D-glucose. Note variable activities in skeletal muscles (reprinted with permission from [21])

For studies of blood flow and volume, as well as oxygen extraction and metabolism, ^{15}O-labeled gases, O_2, CO_2 and CO, are administered sequentially in one session to provide maps [4]. The ^{15}O O_2 and CO_2 gases are delivered continuously during the study period at flows of 10 mCi/min at 80 ml/min and 5 mCi/min at 60 ml/min, respectively. Labeled gases are mixed with 200 ml/min medical air, and supplied to the patient through a plastic face mask. Once inhalation of the labeled gas is initiated, equilibrium is established over a 12-min period, followed by medium-resolution scans at the positions described for the FDG study. Typically, 1.5–2.5 million true events are recorded for each ^{15}O O_2 image, and 2–4 million for each ^{15}O CO_2 image. The ^{15}O CO is administered at a rate of 80 mCi/min at 100 ml/min for 4 min, at which time it is discontinued and, after a 1-min equilibrium period, low resolution images are obtained.

For the evaluation of cerebral blood flow in addition to glucose metabolism, 20–30 mCi ^{15}O water can be used together with 10 mCi ^{18}F FDG. Collected counts are reconstructed into (192×192) transaxial images using a standard 0.30 Shepp-Logan filter, which gives a final image resolution of 10.1 mm [5]. The transaxial images are then re-sliced into 32 coronal and 32 sagittal tomographic images. In addition, a set of two-dimensional projection images are formed by re-sorting the raw sinogram data into 32 nontomographic whole-body images for a rotating body on the computer. All images are visually inspected on a high-resolution display. An abnormal focus of tracer uptake is defined as focal activity higher or lower relative to that of surrounding tissue with no similar activity seen in the contralateral side of the body (Fig. 8.7). Images are generally scored as positive, indeterminate or negative for abnormal activity on a patient and anatomical-site basis. Each positive site of disease is scored as a unit increment in that anatomical site to eliminate the need to count every discrete lesion within an involved anatomical site. Lesion and normal sites are also examined by investigating general count-density ratios of circular regions of interest and comparing these with computed tomography (CT) and/or MRI findings. Averaged standardized uptake values (SUVs) are calculated by normalization to injected dose and body weight or surface, and normalization to blood glucose for the FDG study as performed by multiplying SUVs with blood-glucose level. FDG influx constant (ml/min/100 g tissue) is determined from the slope of the linear part of the arterial-input function curve. The tumor size is obtained by analysis of the axial activity profile of the lesions at 70% of the maximum activity values within a lesion [6].

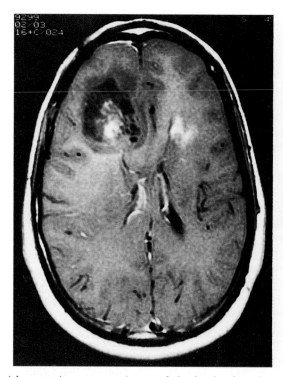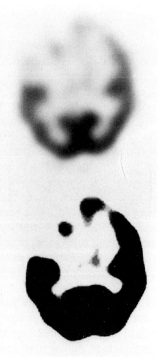

Fig. 8.7. T_1-axial magnetic resonance image of the head after injection of gadolinium-diethylenetriaminepentaacetic acid shows focal areas of contrast enhancement in bilateral frontal deep-subcortical areas and post-surgical cavity in right frontal lobe (*left*). Axial positron-emission-tomography image at the comparable level shows a focal area of increased ^{18}F-fluoro-2-deoxy-D-glucose uptake in the right frontal subcortical area, corresponding to the enhanced lesion on the MR image, indicating recurrent glioblastoma multiforme. Note decreased activity in the cortex of right frontal lobe due to previous irradiation. Note also the variable appearance depending on the setting of the intensity (*right*)

MRI Artifacts

MR image artifacts should be identified to avoid misinterpretations, and appropriate steps can be taken to eliminate them on subsequent examinations. The more commonly encountered MRI artifacts are grouped into four categories: motion-related artifacts, magnetic-field-gradient-related artifacts, RF-field artifacts, and static-magnetic-field artifacts.

Motion-Related Artifacts

Because of the relatively long imaging time of most conventional MRI, any type of macroscopic motion results in image degradation with loss of spatial resolution [7]. Random motion causes image blurring, whereas cyclic or periodic physiologic motion (in addition to causing blurring) results in multiple ghost images (harmonic images) displaced at regular intervals along the phase-encoding axis. The cyclic physiologic motions include respiration, cardiovascular pulsation, and cerebrospinal fluid pulsation (Figs. 8.8 and 8.9) [8]. The separation of ghost images increases with prolonged repetition time and with increasing frequency of the cyclic motion. The phase-encoding gradient is much more sensitive to motion, because phase encoding takes place over numerous repetitions and the phase-encoding gradient is temporally removed from the time of signal sampling [9]. In contrast, the frequency encoding and signal acquisition occur simultaneously over the course of several milliseconds. Various motion-suppression techniques have been developed and range from simple methods, such as physical restraint of the patient or restriction of the field of view, to more complex methods, such as reordered phase encoding or gradient moment nulling [10]. Some motion-reduction techniques require monitoring of the patient, e.g., pseudogating, and increased imaging time, e.g., respiratory gating [11].

Magnetic-Field-Gradient-Related Artifacts

Three orthogonal magnetic field gradients (slice selection, phase and frequency encoding) provide the information necessary for spatial encoding in MRI. Drop off in power of either the phase- or frequency-encoding gradient results in compression of the image along the affected gradient. Instability of the gradient power supply during imaging results in alternating bands of high and low signal intensity projected over the image, producing the zebra-stripe artifact. Truncation or boundary artifacts occur at abrupt transitions between tissues of markedly dissimilar signal intensities [12]. It appears as a series of regularly spaced alternating bands of high and low signal intensity that parallel the boundary of an abrupt signal intensity transition. This periodic-ring artifact is frequently seen at the interface between the inner table of the skull and the adjacent brain, as well as any air-fat, air-water, or bone-fat interfaces. Truncation artifacts occur because the two-dimensional Fourier-transform technique cannot

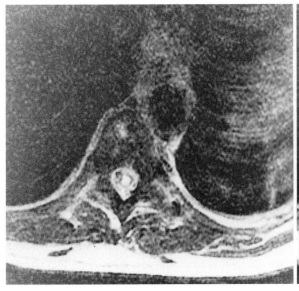
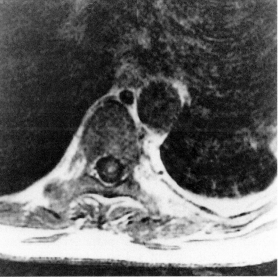

Fig. 8.8. T_2-(*left*) and T_1-(*right*) weighted axial image of the posterior chest shows a metastatic breast cancer involving T7 vertebral body and respiratory-motion artifacts in the left lung along the phase-encoding direction

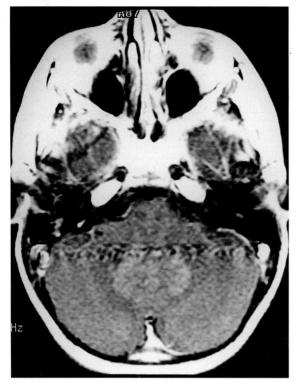

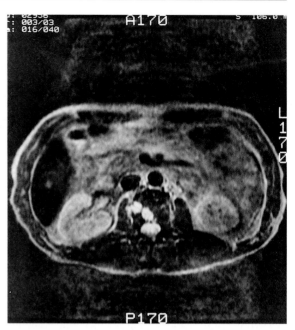

Fig. 8.9. T$_1$-weighted axial image of the head shows a vascular pulsating artifact crossing the anterior portion of the cerebellum

Fig. 8.10. T$_2$-weighted axial image of the abdomen shows a chemical-shift artifact in the periphery of the kidney bilaterally along the frequency-encoding direction. Note also an artifact related to respiratory motion along the phase-encoding direction

accurately represent sudden transitions in signal intensity. The sine and cosine waves that describe abrupt signal-intensity transitions undergo over- and undershoot oscillations about the site of transition, producing curvilinear bands of high and low signal intensity. Truncation artifacts are more prominent in the phase-encoding direction when an asymmetric acquisition matrix is applied. They can be decreased by expanding the matrix size. Addition of a low-pass filter will remove high spatial-frequency information from the signal, thus eliminating much of the truncation effect, but it also decreases image sharpness.

Chemical-Shift Artifacts

Chemical-shift artifacts occur at the interface between fat and water-containing organs. It results from the fact that hydrogen nuclei experience slight variations in local magnetic-field strength depending on their chemical binding sites, causing small differences in the resonant frequencies of the nuclei. The protons in water molecules have a precessional frequency of 3–4 ppm higher than the protons in lipids. Since spatial location along the frequency-encoding axis depends on the rate of proton precession, the difference in resonant frequencies of fat and water protons causes spatial misregistration of their respective signals. The result is an image in which a high-intensity band is present at the fat-water interface on one side of an organ (due to signal overlap) and a low-intensity band at the water-fat interface on the opposite side (due to signal drop out) (Fig. 8.10). Chemical-shift misregistration is more pronounced at higher magnetic field strength and is also more prominent with the use of reduced-bandwidth techniques, due to weaker magnetic-field gradients in the frequency-encoding direction [13].

Aliasing or Wrap-Around Artifacts

Aliasing or wrap-around artifacts occur when the size of the object being imaged exceeds the field of view. The part of the object lying outside the field of view but within the plane of the image is mismapped onto the opposite side of the image. The artifact is seen primarily along the phase-encoding axis, since a band-pass filter can eliminate aliasing in the frequency-encoding direction, which results from the low data-sampling rate for the high-frequency signal being detected (Fig. 8.11). The high-frequency signals from outside the field of view are misinterpreted as lower-

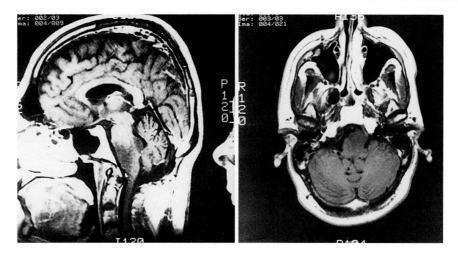

Fig. 8.11. T_1-weighted sagittal image of the head (*left*) shows a wraparound artifact along the phase-encoding direction with the nose behind the occipital head

frequency signals coming from within the imaged volume. In the phase-encoding direction, location is determined by the amount of phase shift occurring during multiple applications of the phase-encoding gradient. Spins outside the field of view accumulate more than one cycle of shift, but are misencoded to a position along the phase-encoding axis. Increasing the number of phase-encoding steps can eliminate aliasing at the expense of time. Increasing the field of view can be applied at the expense of spatial resolution. Surface coils or selective 90° pre-excitation pulses can also be applied to eliminate aliasing artifacts [14].

RF-Field Artifacts

Interference from RF sources can occasionally cause image artifacts, although MR imagers are generally well-shielded from extraneous RF energy. Broad-band RF noise can degrade the entire MR image, and narrow-bandwidth interference results in a linear artifact perpendicular to the frequency-encoding gradient. Objects that can act as inadvertent RF shields include metal-containing surgical dressing and electrode patches. They cause local areas of signal loss or image distortion [8]. Cross-excitation of adjacent slices results in diminished signal in the adjacent slices. If consecutive slices are excited in rapid sequence, partial excitation of tissues in slices adjacent to the selected slice effectively decreases the longitudinal magnetization. Cross-excitation also results in augmented T_1 contrast since the time for recovery for longitudinal magnetization between pulses is reduced. The use of interslice gaps ranging from 20% to 50% of slice thickness is used to minimize cross-excitation.

Zero-Line Artifacts

Zero-line (also called zipper) artifacts appear as a line of alternating high and low signal intensity foci oriented along the frequency-encoding axis. It is due to a direct current (DC) offset from zero of the electronic measurement system. It may also be related to the fact that slice profiles are not perfectly rectangular. When a 180° pulse is applied, extraneous RF energy excites protons outside the selected slice, resulting in residual out-of-slice transverse magnetization that contaminates the slice-selected MR signal. If the DC offset for all phase-encoding steps is constant, a central-point artifact may be produced and appears as a small bright or dark focus in the isocenter of the magnet. Zero-line and central-point artifacts can be eliminated by phase-alternating the pulses and combining the data from two acquisitions. Uneven brightness in an image can occur because of RF tip-angle inhomogeneity related to either coil geometry or RF-transmitter attenuation. If a patient is positioned to one side of the magnet's central bore, an asymmetric signal may result from inhomogeneous power deposition.

Static Magnetic-Field Artifacts

Artifacts due to inhomogeneities in the static magnetic field (B_0) are related to imperfections in the MRI system itself and also extraneous factors. A shimming is required to compensate for inerent B_0 inhomogeneities since no magnet is capable of producing a perfectly homogeneous magnetic field. Inadequate shimming results in image distortion, blurring, or areas of signal loss. Similar artifacts may result from thermal instability of the magnet or from fluctuations in power supply in the case of resistive magnets.

Large ferromagnetic moving objects generate magnetic forces that can cause field inhomogeneity artifacts. Ferromagnetic objects within the patient may include shrapnel, indwelling prostheses, dentures, intracranial shunts, orthopedic fixation devices, heart valves and some surgical clips, as well as external objects such as hairpins, safety pins and zipper-cause artifacts (Fig. 8.12). Cosmetic products, such as mascara and eyeliner, containing iron oxide also produce distortion artifacts [15]. Ferromagnetic objects generally show a focal signal void in addition to local distortion and/or obliteration of the signal from adjacent tissues. Nonferromagnetic-metal objects can cause artifacts due to eddy currents, which are induced by gradient switching and manifested as DC changes in the magnetic field and/or time-dependent magnetic field changes during the pulse sequence and data acquisition, resulting in more rapid dephasing of the transverse magnetization. Artifacts from nonferromagnetic-metal objects appear as focal areas of signal void bordered by a high-signal-intensity rim (Fig. 8.13).

An additional artifact of static magnetic-field inhomogeneity is produced by structures within the image volume that differ in magnetic susceptibility. It occurs frequently at the interface at two adjacent structures whose magnetic susceptibilities differ, and appears as alternating low- and high-signal-intensity lines. Magnetic-susceptibility artifacts are more pronounced on GE images because of the lack of a 180° refocusing pulse compensating for some field inhomogeneity [16].

Pitfalls in PET Scanning

FDG is a tracer of energy substrate metabolism, and increased FDG uptake is not limited to malig-

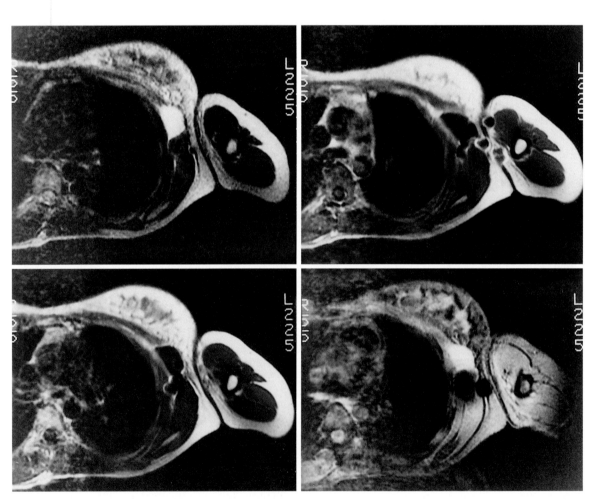

Fig. 8.12. T_2-weighted (*upper left* and *lower right*) and T_1-weighted (*upper right* and *lower left*) images of the upper chest at slightly different levels show postoperative seroma along the left chest wall (high signal intensity on T_2-weighted images) and surgical clip artifacts along the lower-left axilla (*upper right*). Note also the artifacts due to cardiac motion along the phase-encoding direction

CHAPTER 8   Practical Magnetic Resonance Imaging and Positron Emission Tomography Techniques and Their Artifacts   117

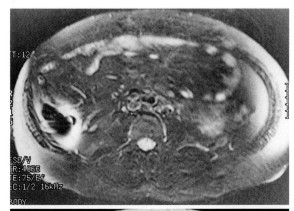

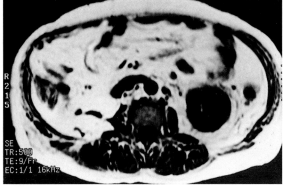

Fig. 8.13. T_2-weighted axial image of the lower abdomen shows a metallic artifact in the posterolateral aspect with focal signal void surrounded by high signal intensity (*top*). Note also nonuniform fat suppression of the subcutaneous fat signals

nant tumors alone. FDG remains trapped in tissue because it does not enter further enzymatic reactions after being converted into FDG-6-phosphate by hexokinase. Glucose-6-phosphatase mediates dephosphorylation, and the accumulation of FDG-6-phosphate is proportional to the glycolytic rate [17]. Tissues with high levels of glucose-6-phosphatase, such as liver, kidney, intestine and resting muscle accumulate smaller amounts of FDG-6-phosphate. It is important to appreciate the physiologic variants of FDG distribution and benign changes that may simulate malignant tumors (Figs. 8.14a and b) [18].

Physiologic Variants

Normal myocardium uses free fatty acids and glucose. Cardiac muscle uptake of ^{18}F-FDG may vary greatly, and maximum uptake is noted by the administration of oral glucose together with insulin to drive FDG into the myocytes. Myocardial activity may interfere with the evaluation of the mediastinum. A fatty meal or drug that increases the circulating fatty acid level is a possible way of en-

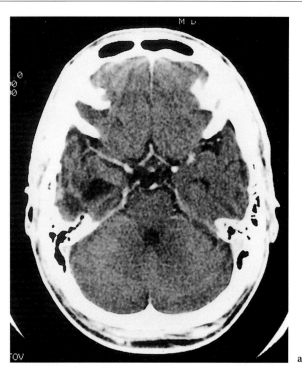

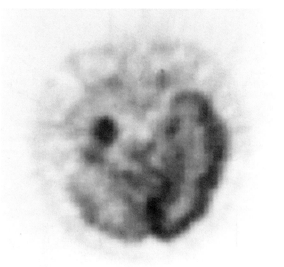

Fig. 8.14. **a** Postcontrast axial computed tomography image of the head shows a postsurgical cavity in the right temporal lobe surrounded by minimal contrast enhancement. **b** Axial positron-emission-tomography image at the comparable level shows a focal increased uptake of ^{18}F-fluoro-2-deoxy-D-glucose in the right temporal lobe, probably due to a seizure developed during the scanning. Biopsy showed only gliosis without the tumor

hancing free fatty acid metabolism rather than glucose. Normal lymphoid tissue in the gastrointestinal tract shows FDG uptake. Tonsillar and adenoidal tissue may be prominent in children [19]. The gastric wall may show moderate uptake,

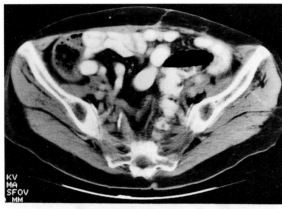

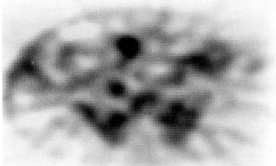

Fig. 8.15. Postcontrast axial computed-tomography image of the pelvis shows contrast-filled bowel loops without a mass lesion (*top*). Axial positron-emission-tomography image at the comparable level shows focal areas of increased uptake of ^{18}F-fluoro-2-deoxy-D-glucose in the bowel loops. Note also some activity in the iliac bone marrow (*bottom*)

producing a ring appearance on coronal images that could be confused with necrotic lymph nodes. Similarly, FDG activity may be seen in the small bowel and more commonly in the large bowel. Cecal or terminal-ileal activity may be marked and caused by uptake into lymphoid tissue. This makes differentiation of malignant tumors from a physiologic variant difficult (Fig. 8.15) [20].

FDG is not totally reabsorbed in the renal tubules, resulting in significant activity that may limit the investigation of renal tumors. Reconstruction artifacts may interfere with visualization of the upper abdomen. Small focal areas of urinary activity may be seen in the ureters, simulating paraaortic lymphadenopathy. Because of high bladder activity, the study of pelvic tumors using FDG is difficult. Diluting urinary activity with hydration and diuretics may be of some help.

Skeletal muscle does not show significant uptake of ^{18}F-FDG at rest, but there is increased uptake after exercise or if contraction takes place (Fig. 8.6) [21]. This is related to increased aerobic glycolysis of active muscle and should be considered carefully in follow-up imaging of sarcoma and melanoma. Chewing gum may cause marked uptake in the mastication muscles. Significant uptake may be also seen in the laryngeal muscles with vocalization; thus, it is essential that patients be prohibited from speaking [21]. It has been

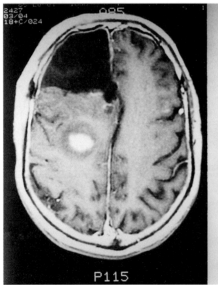

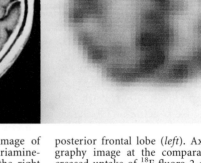

Fig. 8.16. T_1-weighted axial magnetic-resonance image of the head after injection of gadolinium-diethylenetriamine-pentaacetic acid shows a large surgical cavity in the right frontal lobe and also a focal enhanced lesion in the right posterior frontal lobe (*left*). Axial positron-emission-tomography image at the comparable level shows a focal increased uptake of ^{18}F-fluoro-2-deoxy-D-glucose (*right*). Surgery showed an abscess

shown that muscle activity may be abolished by muscle relaxants such as the benzodiazepines [22]. Thymic activity may be seen in children, simulating anterior mediastinal tumors. It can also be noted in patients in their late teens or twenties. Breast uptake of ^{18}F-FDG may be variable, but usually is symmetical, and focal increased uptake may be seen at the nipple. Asymmetric uptake may be seen in a woman who has fed her baby on one side just before scanning.

Pathological Variants

A number of diseases or benign conditions may cause FDG uptake, simulating malignant diseases. Stress-induced muscle tension shows symmetrical FDG uptakes in the paraspinal muscles, in the posterior cervical muscles, and frequently in the trapezius muscles across the shoulders. Focal FDG uptake is often seen at stoma sites, possibly caused by a cutaneous inflammatory reaction. Inflammation in any tissue may cause an increase in FDG accumulation (Figs. 8.16 and 8.17). Active tuberculosis, sarcoidosis and histoplasmosis show increased FDG uptake in the thorax [23]. Increased FDG uptake has been noted in the region of treated brain tumor, possibly related to increased macrophage activity in granulation tissue [24]. High uptake of FDG in the periphery of an active follicular ovarian cyst may simulate a necrotic lymph node. Graves' disease may cause intense diffuse uptake of FDG in the thyroid. Metabolic activity within bones may lead to abnormal FDG uptake. Increased marrow activity in hyperplastic marrow causes increased FDG uptake, which may be difficult to distinguish from diffuse tumor infiltration in patients after chemotherapy. Bone with Paget's disease usually shows absent or low FDG uptake, but some cases demonstrated increased uptake [25].

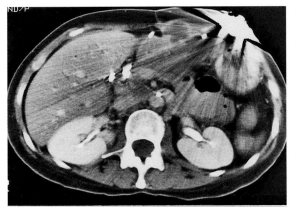

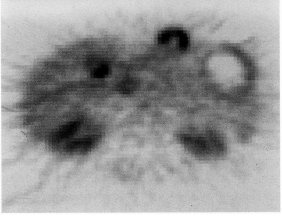

Fig. 8.17. Postcontrast axial computed-tomography (CT) image of the upper abdomen shows a subcutaneous abscess adjacent to the post-operative changes anteriorly (*top*). Axial positron-emission-tomography (PET) image at the comparable level shows an increased uptake of ^{18}F-fluoro-2-deoxy-D-glucose in the anterior periphery of the abscess (*bottom*). Note also activities in the bilateral kidneys and gastric wall. There is a metastatic colon cancer in the medial segment of the left hepatic lobe identified better with PET than with CT

References

1. Henrig J, Nauerth A, Friedburg H (1986) RARE imaging: a fast imaging method for clinical MR. Magn Reson Med 3:823–833
2. Butts K, Riederer SJ, Ehman RL, Thompson RM, Jack CR (1994) Interleaved echo planar imaging on a standard MRI system. Magn Reson Med 31:67–72
3. Wahl RL, Zasadny K, Helvie M, Hutchins GD, Weber B, Cody R (1993) Metabolic monitoring of breast cancer chemohormotherapy using positron emission tomography: initial evaluation. J Clin Oncol 11:2101–2111
4. Tyler JL, Diksic M, Villemure J-G, Evans AC, Meyer E, Yamato YL, Feindel W (1987) Metabolic and hemodynamic evaluation of gliomas using positron emission tomography. J Nucl Med 28:1123–1133
5. Hoh CK, Glaspy J, Rosen P, Dahlborn M, Lee SJ, Kunkel L, Hawkin RA, Maddahi J, Phelps ME (1997) Whole-body FDG-PET imaging for staging of Hodgkin's disease and lymphoma. J Nucl Med 38:343–348
6. Avril N, Bense S, Ziergler SI, Dose J, Weber W, Laubenbacher C, Römer W, Jänicke F, Schwaiger S (1997) Breast imaging with fluorine-18 FDG PET: quantitative image analysis. J Nucl Med 38:1186–1191
7. Ehrman RI, McNamara MT, Brasch RC (1986) Influence of physiologic motion on the appearance of tissue in MR. Radiology 159:777–782
8. Axel L, Summers RM, Kressel HY, Charles C (1986) Respiratory effects in two-dimensional Fourier transformation. Radiology 160:795–801
9. Schultz CL, Alfidi RL, Nelson D (1984) The effect of motion on two-dimensional Fourier transformation magnetic resonance imaging. Radiology 152:117–121
10. Mitchell DG, Vinitski S, Burk DL Jr (1988) Motion artifact reduction in MRI of the abdomen: gradient nulling versus respiratory-sorted phase-encoding. Radiology 169:155–166
11. Wood ML, Runge VM, Henkelman RM (1988) Overcoming motion in abdominal MR imaging. AJR Am J Roentgenol 150:513–522
12. Czervionke LF, Czervionke JM, Daniels DL, Haughton VM (1988) Characteristic features of MR truncation artifacts. AJR Am J Roentgenol 151:1219–1228

13. Dick BW, Mitchell DG, Burk DL, Levy DW, Vinitsky S, Rifkin M (1988) The effect of chemical shift misrepresentation on cortical bone thickness on MR imaging. AJR Am J Roentgenol 151:537–538
14. Porter BA, Hastrup W, Richardson ML (1987) Classification and investigation of artifacts in magnetic resonance imaging. Radiographics 7:271–287
15. Sacco DC, Steiger DA, Bellon EM (1987) Artifacts caused by cosmetics in MR imaging of the head. AJR Am J Roentgenol 148:1001–1004
16. Wendt RE, III, Wilcott MR, III, Nitz W (1988) MR imaging of susceptibility-induced magnetic field inhomogeneities. Radiology 168:837–841
17. Ishizu K, Nishizawa S, Yonekura Y (1994) Effects of hyperglycemia on FDG uptake in human brain glioma. J Nucl Med 35:1104–1109
18. Cook GJR, Fogelman I, Maisey MN (1996) Normal physiological and benign pathological variants of 18-fluoro-2-deoxyglucose positron-emission tomography scanning: potential for error in interpretation. Semin Nucl Med 26:308–314
19. Jabour BA, Choi Y, Hoh CK (1993) Extracranial head and neck: PET imaging with 2-[F-18] fluoro-2-deoxy-D-glucose and MR imaging correlation. Radiology 186:27–35
20. Bischof-Delalove A, Wahl RL (1995) How high a level of FDG abdominal activity is considered normal? (abstract). J Nucl Med 36:106p
21. Engel H, Steinert H, Buck A, Berthold T, Huch Böni RA, von Schulthesis GK (1996) Whole-body PET: physiological and artifactual FDG accumulations. J Nucl Med 37:441–446
22. Barrington SF, Maisey MN (1996) Skeletal muscle uptake of fluorine-18 FDG: effect of oral diazepam. J Nucl Med 37:1127–1129
23. Lewis PJ, Salama A (1994) Uptake of fluorine-18 fluoride-oxyglucose in sarcoidosis. J Nucl Med 35:1–3
24. Kubota R, Kubota K, Yamade S (1995) Methionine uptake by tumour tissue: a microautoradiographic comparison with FDG. J Nucl Med 36:484–492
25. Cook GJR, Maisey MN, Fogelman I (1996) Paget's disease of bone: appearance with F-18 FDG PET (abstract). J Nucl Med 32:27p

Clinical Applications
of MRI, MRS and PET

Lung Cancers

T. INOUE, J. AOKI, E. E. KIM

Basic Considerations

Lung cancer has long been the leading cause of cancer-related mortality in men and, beginning in the late 1980s, lung cancer exceeded breast cancer as the leading cause of cancer-related mortality in women. An estimated 171,500 new cases of lung cancer will be diagnosed in the United States in 1998 [1] Approximately 80% will be non-small-cell lung cancer (NSCLC). Over 70% of patients will present with advanced disease at diagnosis, and fewer than 5% of those with metastatic disease will be alive at 5 years. In the United States, 1 of every 14 deaths from any cause is due to lung cancer. Worldwide, lung cancer is the most common cancer in males, accounting for 17.6% of all cancers in men, and the fifth most common cancer in women. The worldwide mortality rate associated with lung cancer is 86% [2]. Over the last decade, the incidence of lung cancer in men has leveled off to approximately 70 per 1,000,000. However, there has been a sharp rise in the incidence of lung cancer in women [3].

The majority of lung-cancer patients are between 35 years and 75 years old, with a peak incidence between the ages of 55 years and 65 years. Black males have a 40% higher incidence of lung cancer than do white males. Epidemiological studies have demonstrated a clear correlation between tobacco exposure and lung cancer. The *N*-nitrosamines and polycyclic aromatic hydrocarbons are the two major classes of tobacco-related inhaled carcinogens [4]. The association between asbestos exposure and certain lung diseases, such as pulmonary fibrosis, mesothelioma and lung cancer, has been confirmed, and the silicate fiber has been implicated in carcinogenesis [5]. Asbestos most likely acts as a tumor promoter. Radon decays to products that emit heavy ionizing alpha particles, and radon exposure increases the risk of developing lung cancer by as much as ten times [6], and the cancer is usually the small-cell type. Exposure to halogenated ethers has also been associated with an increased risk of small-cell lung cancer (SCLC), which accounts for 20–25% of all lung cancers in the United States. SCLC is the most sensitive to chemotherapy and radiotherapy, yet the overall outcome is poor, with only 5–10% of patients surviving 5 years from diagnosis.

Although the genetic risk factors associated with lung cancer are poorly defined, increasing data suggest the existence of a genetic predisposition to the development of lung cancer. The risk of lung cancer appears to be increased with chronic obstructive pulmonary disease. Cytogenetic studies of lung cancer have revealed a large number of chromosomal abnormalities, and the most commonly identified deletion involves the short arm of chromosome 3. This is even more frequent in SCLC. Mutations in tumor-suppressor genes *p53* and retinoblastoma (*Rb*) have been associated with the development of NSCLC [7]. The *p53* gene is responsible for the production of a nuclear phosphoprotein that is important in DNA repair, growth regulation, cell division and programmed cell death (apoptosis). Mutations in the *p53* tumor-suppressor gene on chromosome 17p are the most commonly identified genetic alterations in human cancers and have been documented in 60–100% of SCLC cell lines and in 77% of tumors [8]. The *Rb* gene codes for a nuclear phosphoprotein that appears to be involved in cell regulation. Frequent cytogenetic alterations at 13q14, the locus for this gene, in SCLC cell lines and tumors were the catalyst for further study. The dominant oncogene *ras* codes for a 21-kDa protein that mediates signal transduction pathways between cell-surface receptors and intracellular molecules. Transfection of a mutated *ras* gene into SCLC cell lines results in a phenotype consistent with NSCLC [9]. The *myc* oncogene family appears to play a role in the pathogenesis of SCLC. In NSCLC, epidermal growth factor binds to the epidermal-growth-factor receptor and stimulates the growth of the tumor [10]. SCLC produces a variety of peptide hormones that act as mitogens and growth factors, e.g., insulin-like growth factor (IGF)-1 and gastrin-releasing peptide. IGF-1 is present in 95% of SCLC tumors and cell lines. Somatostatin analogs inhibit the production of IGF-1 and are active against SCLC xenografts in rats [11]. Activation of opioid receptors on the surface of lung cancer cells results in inhibition of tumor growth. Nicotine has been found to reverse this inhibition [12]. Various cancers lose the cell-surface expression of blood-group determinants. In NSCLC, patients whose tumors do not express AB0 blood-group antigen have shorter survival than patients whose tumors maintain blood-group antigen A and AB expression [13].

The development of drug resistance is one of the most intriguing phenomena in the biology of SCLC. The mechanism for multidrug resistance in cancer cells is overexpression of the multidrug-resistance (*mdr*-1) gene, encoding the multidrug efflux pump termed *p*-glycoprotein. Another transporter gene distantly related to *mdr*-1 and in the same superfamily of ATP-binding cassette transmembrane transporters encodes a protein termed the multidrug-related protein (MRP), whose overexpression has been found in several multidrug-resistant SCLC cell lines [14]. In multidrug-resistant cells that do not overexpress MDR-1 or MRP, changes in activity or in the amount of topoisomerase I or II may be the basis for the resistance to epipodophyllotoxins and anthracyclines or to camptothecin and its analogs, respectively. Topoisomerases modify the topologic structure of DNA without changing the nucleotide sequence. Topoisomerase-targeted drugs stabilize the transient DNA-enzyme complex, the so-called cleavable complex.

Pathology, Diagnosis and Staging

The distinction between NSCLC and SCLC is of major clinical importance, as it significantly alters treatment options. While specific subtypes of NSCLC do not alter overall treatment plans, certain clinical patterns are associated with specific subtypes. Recently, the incidence of adenocarcinoma has increased while the incidence of squamous cell carcinoma (formerly the most frequent subtype) has decreased.

Adenocarcinoma constitutes about 50% of all NSCLC in North America and is associated with smoking. It occurs mostly in peripheral areas and stains positive for keratin as well as carcinoembryonic antigen (CEA). Patients with adenocarcinoma frequently develop symptoms of metastasis and pulmonary osteoarthropathy. The bronchioalveolar subtype may occur as early as the second decade of life, and the characteristic presentation is that of multiple pulmonary nodules. Squamous cell (or epidermoid) carcinoma now accounts for 30%, and arises mostly in the proximal bronchi and causes bronchial obstruction and atelectasis or pneumonia with cavity formation. It has an association with smoking and secretion of a parathyroid-like hormone. Large-cell carcinoma accounts for 20% of NSCLC.

The second World Health Organization (WHO) update in 1977 simplified the SCLC subtyping: oat cell, intermediate small cell, and combined small cell carcinomas. The International Association for the Study of Lung Cancer redefined the subtypes of SCLC in 1984: small cell, variant (small cell/large cell), and combined. SCLC expresses several markers of neuroendocrine differentiation, such as chromogranin and gastrin-releasing peptide.

The signs and symptoms of lung care are related to the location of the cancer and the occurrence of paraneoplastic syndromes. The symptoms of centrally located (SCLC) lesions include cough, hemoptysis, wheezing, stridor, dyspnea, and post-obstructive pneumonia. Peripheral lesions may result in pain from pleural- or chest-wall invasion, cough, or restrictive dyspnea. Pancoast's syndrome is characterized by shoulder pain radiating to the arm in an ulnar distribution and is caused by tumor invasion of the eighth cervical and first thoracic nerves in the superior sulcus. Horner's syndrome consists of enophthalmos, ptosis, meiosis and ipsilateral dyshidrosis, and may be caused by extension of the tumor into the paravertebral sympathetic nerves. Since the left recurrent laryngeal nerve passes through the aortopulmonic window, it is susceptible to injury secondary to mediastinal-node involvement, resulting in hoarseness. Elevation of the hemidiaphragm due to phrenic-nerve paralysis may be caused by tumor invasion into the mediastinum. Superior vena cava syndrome may result from either right-sided tumor or mediastinal nodal involvement. Dysphagia may result from compression of the esophagus, and dyspnea may result from pleural effusion or pericardial invasion. NSCLC frequently metastasizes to hilar and mediastinal lymph nodes, pleura, opposite lung, liver, adrenals, bone, central nervous system (CNS), and other organs in descending order of frequency, and symptoms secondary to the metastatic sites are common. SCLC is particularly notable for producing a variety of paraneoplastic syndromes via the ectopic hormones or hormone-like substances. Classic examples include hyponatremia caused by arginine vasopressin and Cushing's syndrome caused by excessive precursor peptide of adrenocorticotropin (ACTH). One of the most distressing symptoms is weight loss and anorexia, which occurs in nearly one-third of SCLC patients. Hypercalcemia caused by bone metastases or ectopic parathyroid-hormone-related peptide is the most frequent paraneoplastic syndrome in NSCLC, most frequently the squamous cell subtype.

Obtaining a pathological diagnosis is essential to the management of lung cancer since NSCLC is managed differently than SCLC. Sputum cytology is a first study, especially in the case of a central lesion. The next step is usually examination with a flexible fiberoptic bronchoscopy. For lesions that can be visualized endoscopically, diagnoses are made in 97% of tumors with the combination of biopsies, bronchial washings, and bronchial brushings [15]. Percutaneous transthoracic fine-needle aspiration (FNA) of pulmonary nodules is usually performed under fluoroscopic or computed tomography (CT) guidance to evaluate supraclavicular adenopathy, pleural effusion, or metastasis to the liver, bone or adrenal gland. Negative FNA results are frequent and must be considered indeterminate until the diagnosis is established by another method. If a diagnosis still cannot be established, mediastinoscopy with biopsy may be used. If the mediastinal nodes are negative, resection of the nodule will lead to a definite diagnosis. Distinct margins, certain calcification patterns (diffuse central-core bull's eye for granuloma or popcorn ball for hamartoma) or high density on CT scans suggest a benign lesion. Age less than 40 years, nonsmoker, history of tuberculosis exposure, or residence in an endemic area for histoplasmosis are also suggestive of a benign lesion.

Involvement of intra-abdominal organs is noted in 30% of patients undergoing initial staging for SCLC, and CT of the abdomen should be a routine procedure for the staging evaluation. Radionuclide bone scans remain the most valuable test for detecting early bony metastasis, which occurs in nearly 30% of SCLC patients. Bone-marrow involvement is also present in 20–25% of patients with SCLC at diagnosis and, thus, routine unilateral bone-marrow examination is warranted in SCLC. About 10% of SCLC patients have symptoms related to brain metastases and, thus, magnetic resonance imaging (MRI) of the brain is a routine part of comprehensive staging. Serum levels of neuro-nonspecific enolase and CEA may correlate with tumor bulk and response to chemotherapy [16]. Advanced age (older than 60 years), supraclavicular nodal involvement, and many metastatic sites were predictive of a poor prognosis. Other poor signs are: low levels of hemoglobin, platelets, sodium albumin, uric acid, and bicarbonate; elevated levels of leukocytes, lactate dehydrogenase, and CEA; weight loss; slow response to therapy; and being male [17].

To most accurately predict the prognosis of lung cancer, surgical/pathological staging should be considered. Clinical staging often underestimates the true disease extent. The American Joint Committee on Cancer has developed a staging system for lung cancer based on TNM classification (Tables 9.1 and 9.2).

SCLC has also been classified into limited disease (LD) and extensive disease (ED). The original LD included involvement of ipsilateral- and contralateral-hilar, mediastinal, and supraclavicular nodes, as well as ipsilateral pleural effusion. However, as therapy for LD has evolved with the value of chest radiation for a subset of patients, a refined definition of LD, excluding contralateral-hilar and supraclavicular nodal involvement, as well as pleural effusion, is frequently used. ED denotes tumor beyond these limits and usually ac-

Table 9.1. TNM classification of non-small-cell lung cancer

T (primary tumor)	
Tx	Cannot be assessed visually
T0	No evidence
Tis	In situ
T1	<3 cm; no invasion proximal to lobar bronchus
T2	>3 cm; invading visceral pleura; atelectasis or pneumonitis; proximal extent within lobar bronchus or 2 cm distal to carina
T3	Any size, extension to chest wall, diaphragm, pleura or pericardium
T4	Any size, involving mediastinum, heart, great vessel, trachea, carina, esophagus, vertebral body or malignant effusion
N (Node)	
N0	No determination
N1	Peribronchial or ipsilateral hilar nodes, or both
N2	Ipsilateral mediastinal and carinal nodes
N3	Contralateral mediastinal or hilar nodes, or supraclavicular nodes
M (Metastasis)	
M0	No known distant metastasis
M1	Distant metastasis

Table 9.2. Staging of non-small-cell lung cancer based on the TNM system

Occult	Tx, N0, M0
Stage 0	Tis, N0, M0
Stage I	T1 or T2, N0, M0
Stage II	T1 or T2, N1, M0
Stage IIIa	T3, N0 or N1, M0
	T1–3, N2, M0
Stage IIIb	Any T, N3, M0
	T4, any N, M0
Stage IV	Any T, any N, M1

counts for 60–70% of SCLC patients. Survival of more than 3 years occurs almost exclusively in those with LD and long-term survival in patients with ED remains uncommon [18].

Magnetic Resonance Imaging

MRI of the chest has come of age within the last decade because of technical advances, and its sensitivity to flow has made it a preferred modality to assess vascular pathology in the mediastinum (Fig. 9.1). MRI is excellent in the evaluation of thoracic-inlet, apical, perihilar, paracardiac, and peridiaphragmatic regions. MRI can help characterize fibrosis, hemorrhage, or fluid. However, major limitations have hampered the development of MRI as a routine study. Only state-of-the-art MR equipment and artifact reduction can provide adequate information in oncology patients who require repeated follow-up examination.

MRI has a limited role in the T-staging of tumors that are surrounded by lung parenchyma and/or visceral pleura, and these are generally staged with CT. Correct evaluation of tumor extension beyond the visceral pleura is of critical importance for surgical planning (Fig. 9.2). Chest-wall invasion adjacent to a lung tumor may be better seen by MRI than by CT (Fig. 9.3) [19]. A thin extrapleural fat layer seen on T_1-weighted images may be effaced in the presence of early invasion. On T_2-weighted images, chest-wall invasion is characterized by high-signal areas extending into the chest wall from the adjacent tumor. It is notable that high signal on T_2-weighted images is not specific for tumor, but may also represent edema or inflammation. MRI better delineates a small rim of fatty tissue beneath the apical parietal pleura whose integrity excludes the possibility of superior-sulcus (Pancoast) tumor invasions (Fig. 9.4).

Coronal images are valuable in determining the exact extent of the tumor invasion and defining the potential resectability of the carina with reconstructive surgery, and also tumor extension near or into the aortopulmonary (AP) window. Tumor tissue, with its low signal intensity on T_1-weighted images, distinctly contrasts with the bright mediastinal fat (Fig. 9.5).

MRI is helpful in determining pericardial involvement (T3 status) versus cardiac-muscle or intracardiac involvement (T4-unresectable status) (Fig. 9.6). CT better visualizes bronchial relationships of peripheral lung tumors. In patients with cytologically positive malignant pleural effusions, a significant contrast enhancement of the pleural fluid can be seen with the gadolinium-diethylenetriaminepentaacetic acid (Gd-DTPA), possibly through the increased permeability of pleural surfaces involved in metastatic disease [20]. In general, post-treatment fibrosis exhibits a low signal on both T_1- and T_2-weighted images, whereas recurrent tumor shows relatively increased intensity on T_2-weighted images. Contrast enhancement is generally noted in areas of active tumor and not observed in mature fibrosis. However, it is important to know that such differentiation is possible only at a minimum of 6 months after completion of radiation therapy. Inflammatory reactions such as radiation pneumonitis or developing fibrosis with secretions may also lead to high signal intensity on T_2-weighted images. Destruction of the ciliated epithelium secondary to radiation therapy prevents effective clearance of secretions and leads to the development of bronchiectasis. These changes also display a tubular high signal intensity on T_2-weighted images. The postpneumonectomy hemithorax represents a diagnostic challenge because of its complex solid and liquid components. Excellent contrast resolution of MRI facilitates easy identification of solid tissue and fluid, and allows differentiation between recurrent tumor and fibrosis.

In the new staging system, the presence of hilar or paratracheal-ipsilateral or subcarinal lymph nodes does not contraindicate resectability (Figs. 9.7 and 9.8). Previously, the presence of any nodal metastasis in the mediastinum (N2 status) signaled unresectability (Fig. 9.8). CT, with its high spatial resolution, lack of motion artifacts, and low cost, is a usual modality to stage mediastinal nodes. However, in patients with poor vascular opacification or with contraindications to contrast media, MR allows a more confident evaluation. MRI has been found to be more sensitive than CT in detecting small, but pathological, hilar lymph nodes [21]. Although the average T_1 values were different between metastatic nodes and other diseases (640 ms vs 566 ms, respectively), there was too much overlap to allow differentiation [22]. Lung cancers most frequently metastasize to adrenal glands with prevalences up to 38% [21]. Therefore, the adrenal glands are commonly included in the staging of the primary lung cancer. CT appearance of adrenal lesions is not specific, and MRI has the potential to distinguish metastasis from benign adenomas. In general, a small mass measuring less than 1.5 cm in diameter with low signal intensity on T_2-weighted or fat-suppressed (out-of-phase) images is typical for a nonfunctional cortical adenoma. A combination of large size, irregular margins, and high signal on T_2-weighted or fat-suppressed images is characteristic of a metastatic lesion.

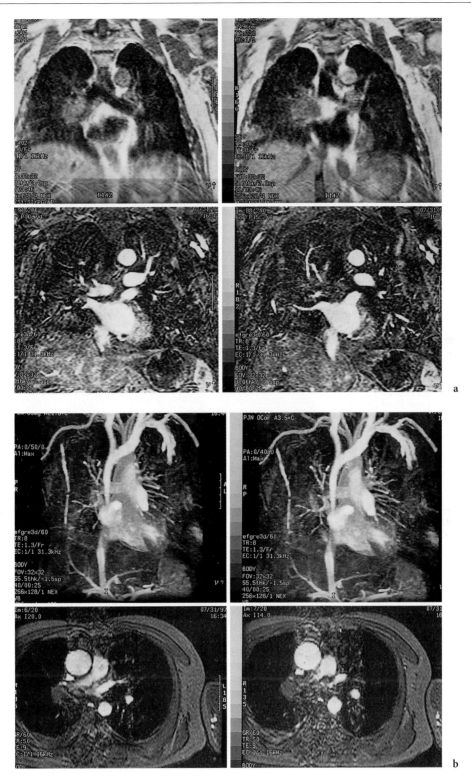

Fig. 9.1. a Coronal spin-echo T_1-weighted images (*upper*) of the chest in slightly different slices show an irregular lung-cancer mass in the right hilum invading the right main pulmonary artery. Coronal 3-D efficient gradient echo images (EFGRE) (*lower*) at 15–20 s following the injection of gadolinium-diethylenetriaminepentaacetic acid (Gd-DTPA) show no contrast agent filling the right pulmonary-arterial segments. **b** The 3-D EFGRE coronal images of the chest obtained at 5–10 s following the injection of Gd-DTPA (*upper*) show a good delineation of superior vena cava and right brachiocephalic vein. Gradient echo axial images of the chest show a thrombosis in the right main pulmonary artery

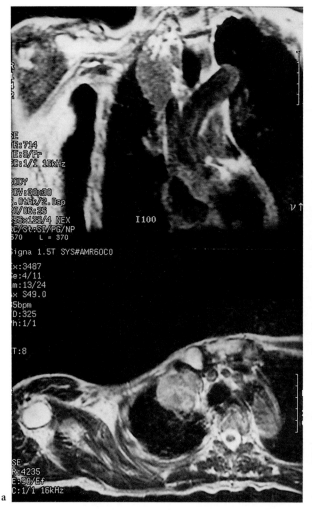 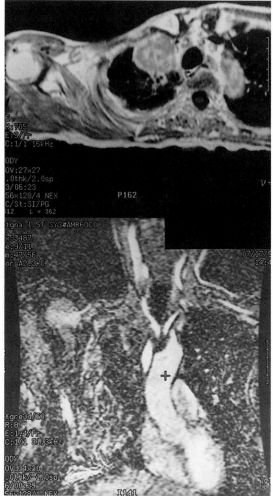

Fig. 9.2. a T$_1$-weighted coronal image of the chest (*upper*) shows a lung cancer mass in the right paratracheal region with slightly heterogeneous signal intensity obstructing the right brachiocephalic vein. Axial T$_2$-weighted image of the right upper chest (*lower*) shows a mass with heterogeneous high signal intensity abutting displaced right brachiocephalic vein. **b** Axial post-gadolinium (Gd) T$_1$-weighted image of the upper chest (*upper*) shows a heterogeneous contrast enhancement of the mass. Coronal 3-D efficient gradient echo image of the chest at 20 s following the injection of Gd-diethylenetriaminepentaacetic acid shows an obstruction of the right brachiocephalic vein by the adjacent mass. Note also the ascending aorta (+)

Magnetic Resonance Spectroscopy

To our knowledge, there have been no published magnetic resonance spectroscopy (MRS) studies in lung cancer. Probable causes for there being no applications of MRS to such a common cancer include the many air-tissue interfaces that give rise to magnetic-field inhomogeneities secondary to the air-tissue susceptibility changes and respiratory motion.

Positron Emission Tomography

Lung cancer is still one of the leading causes of death around the world. Positron emission tomography (PET) applications for lung cancer have been conducted for the past 15 years, mainly by using 2-[^{18}F]-fluoro-2-deoxy-D-glucose (FDG). In this chapter, PET applications for diagnosing and monitoring patients with lung cancer will be discussed by reviewing medical papers published in the 1990s and by presenting our clinical cases.

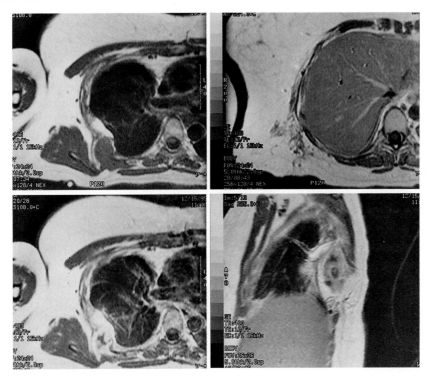

Fig. 9.3. T_1-weighted axial images of the right mid-chest before (*upper left*) and after (*lower left*) injection of gadolinium-diethylenetriaminepentaacetic acid show a contrast-enhanced neurofibrosarcoma involving the posterolateral chest wall. Note heterogeneous contrast enhancement of the mass on the sagittal T_1-weighted image (*lower right*)

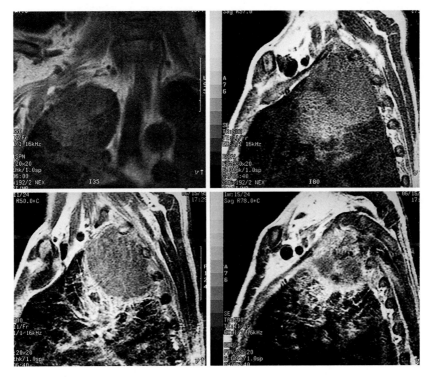

Fig. 9.4. T_1-weighted coronal (*upper left*) and sagittal (*upper right*) images of right upper chest and lower neck show a large superior-sulcus cancer involving chest wall and also first and second ribs. Post-gadolinium sagittal images (*lower*) show a heterogeneous contrast enhancement of the mass. Note intact right brachial plexus branches just above and posterior to subclavian vessels (*upper left* and *lower right*)

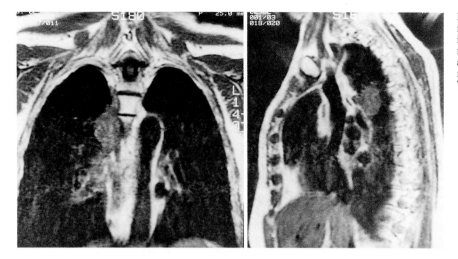

Fig. 9.5. T_1-weighted coronal (*left*) and sagittal (*right*) images of the chest show a mass in the right suprahilar area posteriorly, invading mediastinal fat and abutting T3 and T4 vertebral bodies

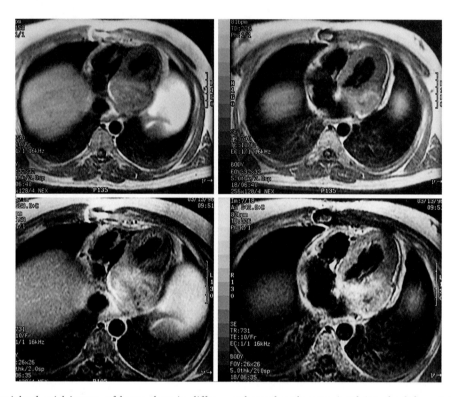

Fig. 9.6. T_1-weighted axial images of lower chest in different slices before (*upper*) and after (*lower*) injection of gadolinium-diethylenetriaminepentaacetic acid show contrast-enhanced melanoma involving the left ventricular wall as well as the interventricular septum. Note that the pericardial wall does not exhibit increased effusion

Detection of Primary Lung Cancer and Differentiation of Solitary Pulmonary Lesions

Final diagnosis of lung cancer should be confirmed histopathologically by means of transbronchoscopic lung biopsy (TBLB), CT or ultrasound (US)-guided needle biopsies, mediastinoscopy, and thoracoscopy. Since these diagnostic approaches are all invasive, patients should be carefully selected before these histopathological approaches by using non-invasive imaging modalities. Among various imaging modalities, chest X-ray is a primary modality for detecting a solitary pulmonary nodule suspected of being malignant. CT is a standard non-invasive method to characterize the primary pulmonary lesions, and their extent to hilar and mediastinal lymph nodes. Regarding the detection of a solitary pulmonary

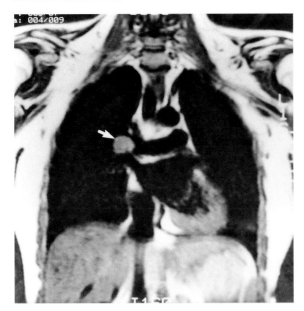

Fig. 9.7. Coronal T$_1$-weighted image of the chest shows a nodular mass (*arrow*) in the right hilum, abutting the right main pulmonary artery. Surgery revealed a squamous cell lung cancer

nodule and the morphological characterization of tumor lesions, the spatial resolution of CT and MRI is superior to that of PET, even if the spatial resolution of recent PET technology has improved. Several papers reported that the detectability of PET with ^{18}F FDG or ^{11}C methionine (CMET) is about 90–100% in sensitivity and 60–100% in specificity (Table 9.3) [23–25]. In other words, FDG shows high sensitivity for detecting primary lung cancer with relatively low specificity because of the false-positive cases from active inflammatory lesions or granulomatous lesions such as sarcoid nodules [25].

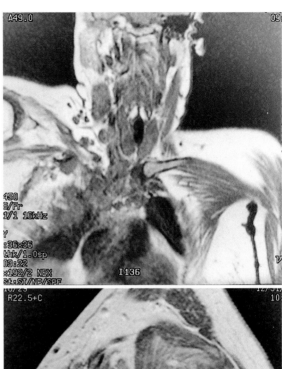

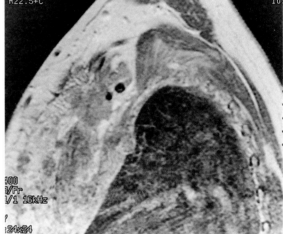

Fig. 9.8. T$_1$-weighted coronal image of the upper chest (*upper*) shows multiple nodular metastatic lesions in the superior mediastinum, right jugular and paraclavicular lymphatic chains

Table 9.3. Positron emission tomography (PET) in the differentiation of solitary pulmonary nodules

Reference	Modality	Sensitivity (%)	Specificity (%)	Accuracy (%)	Positive predictive value (%)	Negative predictive value (%)
[23]	FDG-PET	82/82 (100)	13/25 (52)	95/107 (89)	82/94 (87)	13/13 (100)
[24]	FDG-PET	57/59 (97)	23/28 (82)	80/87 (92)	57/62(92)	23/25(92)
[52]	FDG-PET	29/31 (94)	3/5 (60)	32/36 (89)	29/31 (94)	3/5 (60)
[53]	FDG-PET	8/8 (100)	–	–	–	–
[54]	FDG-PET	19/20 (95)	8/10 (80)	27/30 (90)	19/21 (90)	8/9 (89)
[55]	FDG-PET	26/26 (100)	7/9 (78)	33/35 (94)	26/28 (93)	7/7 (100)
[56]	FDG-PET	42/45 (93)	14/16 (88)	56/61 (92)	42/44 (95)	14/17 (82)
[57]	FDG-PET	14/14 (100)	7/12 (58)	21/26 (81)	14/19 (74)	7/7 (100)
[58]	FDG-PET	29/33 (89)	18/18 (100)	47/51 (92)	29/29 (100)	18/22 (82)
[25]	FDG-PET	10/12 (83)	9/10 (90)	19/22 (86)	10/11 (91)	9/11 (82)
	CMET-PET	13/14 (93)	6/10 (60)	19/24 (70)	13/17 (76)	6/7 (86)

FDG: fluoro-2-deoxy-D-glucose

One of the main applications of PET has been the biochemical characterization of lesions which are unclear on anatomical imaging such as CT or MRI [26]. The differential diagnosis between benign and malignant pulmonary nodules has been done by CT findings, in which the triad of spicular formation, notch sign, and heterogeneous density may strongly suggest malignant tumors, and coarse calcification in the mass lesion may suggest the benign tumor. However, we sometimes encounter the undetermined case with pulmonary solitary nodules by anatomical imaging. Considering the high sensitivity and high negative-predictive value of FDG PET, we can recommend an invasive histopathological diagnostic approach including open lung biopsy, if necessary, to a patient with undetermined pulmonary solitary nodules showing intense FDG uptake. Conversely, when a patient has an undetermined lesion more than 1 cm in diameter with no FDG uptake, we can not recommend histopathological diagnostic procedures. It is possible that a cost-effective diagnostic algorithm for solitary pulmonary nodules may consist of a chest radiograph, followed by a FDG-PET scan which, if positive, then proceeds to a CT-guided transthoracic fine-needle aspiration (TTNA) [26]. The intra-tumoral distribution of FDG may facilitate the TTNA technique because of the location of viable tumor cells showing intense FDG uptake. Illustrative cases are shown in Figs. 9.9 (case 1) and 9.10 (case 2). A patient, case 1, was a 64-year-old male with a huge mass in the lower right lobe of the lung, demonstrated on CT images. TTNA was conducted, but the appropriate tissue specimen could not be obtained because of the sampling error. After the first TTNA, FDG PET was performed to show the doughnut-like FDG distribution with no central tracer uptake by necrosis. The second trial of TTNA was successful in obtaining the suitable tissue specimen on the basis of the information of FDG-PET findings, and squamous cell cancer was confirmed by TTNA procedure. In case 2, the patient was a 66-year-old male with a huge mass in the lower left lobe, demonstrated on CT. FDG-PET revealed homogeneous intense uptake [standardized uptake value (SUV)=14.1] in the tumor, which implies that TTNA is likely to be successful.

One advantage of PET technology is the effectiveness of obtaining the accurate quantitative data of tracer uptake in the lesions, which can be an objective diagnostic criterion. Reproducibility of quantification of FDG uptake in lung-cancer cases was reported to be about 10% mean difference [27]. By using FDG-PET technology, the ab-

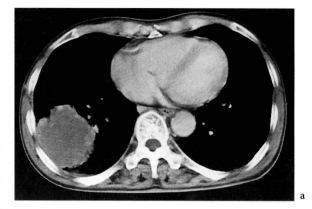

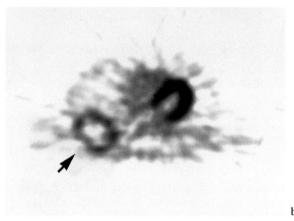

Fig 9.9a,b. Case 1: a 64-year-old male. Computed tomography revealed a huge mass in the lateral or posterior segment of right lower lobe (Fig. 1a). Transthoracic fine-needle aspiration (TTNA) was conducted, but the appropriate tissue specimen could not be obtained because of the sampling error. The sampling site of the first TTNA was near the center of the mass. After the first TTNA, 2-[^{18}F]-fluoro-2-deoxy-D-glucose positron emission tomography (FDG-PET) was performed to show the doughnut-like FDG distribution (standardized uptake value=4.8) with no central tracer uptake by necrosis (*arrow* in Fig. 1b). The second trial of TTNA was successful in obtaining the suitable tissue specimen on the basis of the information from FDG-PET findings, and squamous cell cancer was confirmed by TTNA procedure

solute value of glucose utilization in pulmonary lesions can be quantified on the basis of a three-compartment model in the same way as the measurement of regional brain-glucose utilization. However, the absolute quantification of glucose utilization in lung lesions seems to be not practical clinically, since this technique requires multiple arterial-blood sampling to obtain the plasma tracer concentration as a function of time. There are also some problems such as the unknown lumped constant in lung-cancer lesions and the assumed model configuration. Instead of the quantification of absolute glucose utilization in

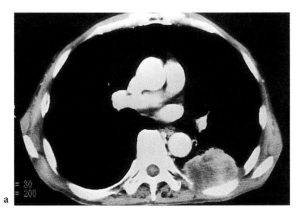

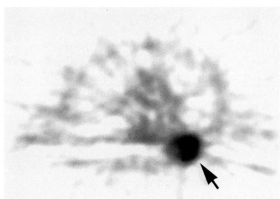

Fig 9.10a,b. Case 2: a 66-year-old male. Enhanced computed tomography showed a huge enhanced mass in the superior segment of the lower left lobe (Fig. 2a). 2-[^{18}F]-fluoro-2-deoxy-D-glucose positron emission tomography revealed homogeneous intense uptake (standardized uptake value=14.1) in the tumor, which implies that transthoracic fine-needle aspiration (TTNA) is likely to be successful (*arrow* in Fig. 2b). The first TTNA was able to demonstrate lung cancer cells

the pulmonary lesion, SUV, a semiquantitative parameter which does not require multiple blood sampling, is now generally used in the field of PET oncology. The term of this semiquantitative parameter is confusing because it is also known as the standardized uptake ratio (SUR), the differential uptake ratio (DUR), or the differential absorption ratio (DAR). The SUV is calculated as the following ratio:

$$SUV = \frac{\text{radioactive concentration in the lesion (mCi/g)}}{\text{injected dose (mCi)/body weight (g)}}$$

If the specific gravity of the human body is assumed to be one, this semiquantitative parameter implies that the amount of tracer concentration exists in the lesion in comparison with the tracer concentration in the body when the total injected tracer is distributed in vivo homogeneously. Although the SUV is criticized by some researchers [28] and it can vary as a function of time [29], it appears to be satisfactory for clinical purposes. In general, FDG uptake in lung-cancer lesions is higher than that in benign pulmonary lesions. It can be expressed objectively by using the SUV method. Duhaylongsod et al. proposed a SUV of 2.5 as the best indicator of malignant lung lesions [24]. As mentioned above, SUV calculation is time dependent and, therefore, standardization of the SUV is necessary to compare results obtained by various institutions. Since FDG uptake is higher in muscle and brain tissue and lower in fat tissue, some modifications of the SUV method using body surface [30] or lean body mass [31] were also proposed.

Miyauchi et al. reported that regional FDG uptake varied in normal lung, and the highest SUV was observed in posterior lower lung with 0.804±0.230 of the maximum value of the mean SUV, which was 41% greater than the mean SUV in the anterior upper lung [32]. Increased blood flow and FDG delivery and also scatter from liver uptake or heart uptake may contribute to this phenomenon. It may cause false-negative lesions located in the posterior lower lung. We need to consider regional differences of FDG uptake in the lung when interpreting FDG-PET images of patients with lung cancer.

Mediastinal Staging

Among various histological types, NSCLC is the most frequent type, and it is possible to cure a patient with this by providing surgical treatment before the lesions spread to mediastinal lymph nodes or systemic organs. If no nodal involvement is present in the mediastinum, 5-year survival after surgical treatment is about 50%. N factor of TNM classification is defined as follows: N0, no nodal metastasis; N1, involvement of ipsilateral hilar node (#11) or peribronchial node (#10); N2, ipsilateral mediastinal nodes (#2,#4,#5) or subcarinal node (#7); N3, contralateral hilar node or mediastinum, or supraclavicular node (Fig. 9.11a). One of the indicators of whether a case is operable is an N factor of less than 2 based on the prognosis data in patients with NSCLC. In other words, the discrimination between the N2 and N3 stage is important clinically in treating lung-cancer patients. Procedures for evaluating mediastinal staging include chest radiography, CT, MRI, mediastinoscopy and transbronchial mediastinal-lymph-node biopsy. Usually, presurgical nodal staging is performed non-invasively by CT on which we assess the nodal size and its location. An enlarged node measuring more than 10 mm between the extremities on the shortest cross section is defined as a lymph node invaded by cancer cells, and its station is localized according to the guideline of the American Thoracic Society mapping system (Fig. 9.11a) [33].

Using nodal size as the criterion for obtaining accurate presurgical evaluation for N staging has limitations. We sometimes encounter cases with cancer cell involvement in normal-sized nodes of adenocarcinoma, and without cancer cell involvement in enlarged nodes caused by anthracosis or reactive inflammatory reaction of obstructive pneumonia resulting from squamous cell cancer invading the main bronchus. The results of multi-institutional Radiologic Diagnostic Oncology Group trials showed that the sensitivity and specificity of CT for mediastinal staging was only 52% and 69%, respectively, whereas MRI was 48% sensitive and 64% specific [34]. The diagnostic accuracy of CT for mediastinal staging seemed to be 40–80% in sensitivity and 70–95% in specificity.

In the past 3 years, many investigators have addressed the utility of FDG-PET mediastinal staging in patients with NSCLC [1, 35, 36]. The diagnostic accuracy of FDG-PET for mediastinal staging is 75–100% in sensitivity and 80–100% in specificity, which seems to be superior to that of CT (Table 9.4). CMET PET has similar diagnostic accuracy for mediastinal staging [36]. Some illustrative cases are shown in Figs. 9.12–9.15.

In case 3 (Fig. 9.12), the patient was a 53-year-old male who suffered from hoarseness for 3 weeks, and left recurrent nerve palsy was observed by otolaryngeal examination. CT revealed a mass lesion located in the AP window invading trachea, and a small lesion in the left upper lobe. FDG-PET revealed intense uptake in the two separate lesions (SUV in the primary lesion was 5.0 and in the mediastinal node was 6.9). Although FDG-PET appears more accurate in staging disease in the mediastinum, the evaluations of tracheal, bronchial, chest-wall, pleural, and vascular invasions are difficult by FDG-PET, and the anatomical imaging by CT or MRI are necessary for operative planning.

In case 4 (Fig. 9.13), the patient was a 56-year-old male who received surgical treatment. CT revealed a small mass in the apical segment of the right lung, and FDG-PET revealed the faint uptake (SUV=1.8) in the primary lesion and no uptake in

Fig 9.11 a, b. Mediastinal staging. a The modified scheme of American Thoracic Society node mapping. b The scheme of N staging. *N0*, no nodal metastasis; *N1*, involvement of ipsilateral hilar node (#11) or peribronchial node (#10); *N2*, ipsilateral mediastinal nodes (#2, #4, #5) or subcarinal node (#7); *N3*, contralateral hilar node or mediastinum, or supraclavicular node

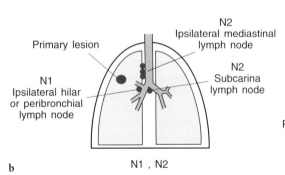

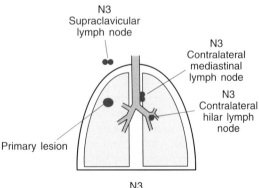

Table 9.4. Mediastinal staging by positron emission tomography (PET) and computed tomography (CT)

Reference	Modality	Sensitivity (%)	Specificity (%)	Accuracy (%)	Positive predictive value (%)	Negative predictive value (%)
[59]	FDG-PET	16/20 (80)	12/12 (100)	28/32 (88)	16/16 (100)	12/16 (75)
	CT	10/20 (50)	9/12 (75)	19/32 (59)	10/13 (77)	9/19 (47)
[36]	FDG-PET	23/26 (90)	21/24 (86)	44/50 (88)	23/26 (88)	21/24 (88)
	CT	15/26 (58)	19/24 (81)	34/50 (68)	15/20 (75)	19/30 (63)
[60][a]	FDG-PET	25/28 (89)	83/84 (99)	108/112 (96)	25/26 (96)	83/86 (97)
	CT	16/28 (57)	79/84 (94)	85/112 (79)	16/21 (76)	79/91 (87)
[61][a]	FDG-PET	13/17 (76)	53/54 (98)	66/71 (93)	13/14 (93)	53/57 (93)
	CT	11/17 (65)	47/54 (87)	58/71 (82)	11/18 (61)	47/53 (89)
[23]	FDG-PET	16/16 (100)	16/16 (100)	32/32 (100)	16/16 (100)	16/16 (100)
	CT	13/16 (81)	9/16 (56)	22/32 (69)	13/20 (65)	9/12 (75)
[35]	FDG-PET	20/24 (83)	49/52 (94)	69/76 (91)	20/23 (87)	49/53 (92)
	CT	15/24 (63)	38/52 (73)	53/76 (70)	15/39 (38)	38/47 (81)
[62]	FDG-PET	7/9 (78)	17/21 (81)	24/30 (80)	7/11 (64)	17/19 (89)
	CT	5/9 (56)	18/21 (86)	23/30 (77)	5/8 (63)	18/22 (82)
[63]	FDG-PET	9/11 (82)	13/16 (81)	22/27 (81)	9/12 (75)	13/15 (87)
	CT	7/11 (64)	7/16 (44)	14/27 (81)	9/12 (75)	13/15 (87)
[64][a]	^{11}C methionine (CMET) PET	28/28 (100)	69/79 (87)	97/107 (91)	28/38 (74)	69/69 (100)

[a] Data indicates number of lymph node; *FDG* fluoro-2-deoxy-D-glucose; *CMET* ^{11}C methionine

the hilar and mediastinal nodes; the TNM classification was T_1,N0,M0, stage I. The primary lesion was squamous cell cancer and the presurgical staging was confirmed after surgical treatment based on the histological examination.

In case 5 (Fig. 9.14), the patient was an 80-year-old male. CT revealed no mediastinal nodal involvement and TNM staging was determined as T_2, N0, M0 in stage I by the conventional imaging, including chest radiography, CT, and bone scan with ^{99m}Tc-hydroxymethylene diphosphonate (HMDP). CT revealed a mass in the lower right lung, without enlarged mediastinal nodes, but FDG-PET showed intense FDG uptake in the primary lesion and faint FDG uptake in the ipsilateral hilar and mediastinal nodes. FDG-PET staging was more than N2 stage, but no metastases were proven histologically after surgical treatment. Anthracosis was proven in these false-positive nodes by histopathological examination on the surgical specimen.

In case 6 (Fig. 9.15), the patient was a 72-year-old male. CT revealed the primary lung lesions in the lower right lobe with ipsilateral-hilar and mediastinal involvement. FDG-PET showed clearly intense uptake of FDG in the primary and ipsilateral-hilar (#11), peribronchial (#10R), mediastinal (#4R), and supraclavicular nodes. N3 stage was proved histopathologically by lymph-node biopsy.

Staging with Whole-Body PET

Recent technological development of PET devices enabled us to obtain whole-body PET images with ^{18}F FDG or fluoride [37]. Lewis et al. retrospectively analyzed 34 patients with operable NSCLC who underwent FDG-PET examination after routine assessment, and found that PET identified unsuspected malignant lesions in 10 patients (29%) and necessitated change in treatment in 14 patients (41%), including 6 patients (18%) whose treatment changed to non-surgical therapy [33]. Valk et al. reported that whole-body FDG-PET showed previously unsuspected distant metastasis in 11 patients (11%), with no demonstrated false-positive results, and clinical imaging follow-up in 14 of 19 patients, who showed negative FDG-PET and positive CT results, showed no evidence of metastasis [35]. Bury et al. also reported that whole-body FDG-PET correctly changed the M stage in six patients (10%) with three false-positive and no false-negative results [36]. Whole-body FDG-PET may be also useful in evaluating the undetermined adrenal mass in patients with lung cancer. Giles et al. reported that the localized FDG-PET helped correctly differentiate between benign and malignant adrenal lesions in 24 adrenal masses in 20 patients, including 10 lung-cancer patients. The SUV in the metastatic adrenal lesions ranged from 2.9 to 16.6 with an average of 7.4, whereas the SUV in the benign adrenal masses ranged from 0.2 to 1.2 with an average of 0.6 [38].

Initial whole-body PET images were emission tomography images such as conventional single-photon-emission tomography (SPECT) images [39], and it was not suitable for quantification because of the lack of attenuation correction. Recent technological developments of PET imaging, such as the simultaneous emission-transmission data-

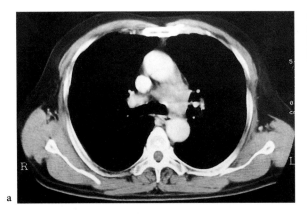
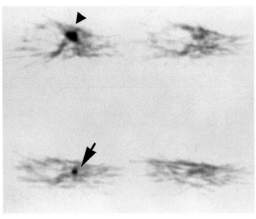
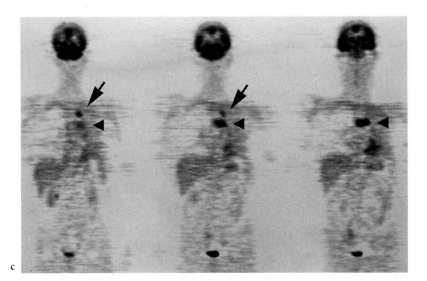
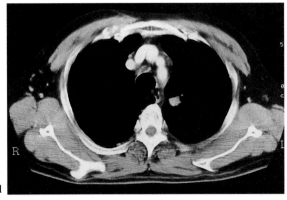

Fig 9.12a–d. Case 3: a 53-year-old male. The patient suffered from hoarseness for 3 weeks, and left recurrent nerve palsy was observed by otolaryngeal examination. **a** Computed tomography (CT) revealed a mass lesion located in the aortopulmonary window invading trachea (#4, #5) and a small lesion in the apical segment of left upper lobe. **b** Consecutive transaxial 2-[^{18}F]-fluoro-2-deoxy-D-glucose positron emission tomography (FDG-PET) images revealed intense uptake in the primary lesion (*arrow*) and mediastinal lymph nodes (#4 and #5) (*arrow head*). The standardized uptake value in the primary lesion was 5.0 and in the mediastinal node was 6.9. **c** Three contiguous coronal slices of whole-body FDG-PET images showed intense uptake in the two separate lesions with no distant metastases. PET staging was defined as Tx, N2, M0. Although FDG-PET appears more accurate in staging disease in the mediastinum, the evaluations of tracheal, bronchial, chest-wall, pleural, and vascular invasions are difficult by FDG-PET, and anatomical imaging by CT or magnetic resonance imaging is necessary for operative planning

acquisition method [40] and the segmented attenuation correction method [41], make it possible to obtain an attenuation-corrected whole-body image with FDG [42].

Whole-body FDG-PET images without attenuation correction in a healthy 45-year-old male volunteer are shown in Fig. 9.16 (case 7). A solution of 185 MBq (5 mCi) ^{18}F FDG was intravenously injected and five sections from the area of the thigh up to the head were imaged with emission-acquisition mode 40–75 min after tracer administration. After 315 transaxial images (63 slices × 5 scans) with 128×128 matrices and 9.6-mm slice thickness were reconstructed, coronal sections from the thigh up to the brain with 10-mm thickness were reconstructed (Fig. 9.16). Since he had been fasting for more than 12 h, no myocardial uptake was observed. It is important to reduce the false-negative results of the pulmonary lesions in the lower left lobe by fasting. Also, since glucose loading may reduce FDG uptake in lung cancer [43], fasting for at least 4 h seems to be necessary. The other preparations for whole-body FDG PET are to avoid vigorous physical activity prior to FDG injection, to remain silent while waiting for the scan, to rinse saliva prior to the scan, and to urinate before imaging. Intense FDG uptakes were observed in brain and urinary bladder.

In a lung-cancer patient with bone metastasis, whole-body FDG-PET images show multiple pathological uptakes in the skeletal system (Fig. 9.17, case 7). Further investigation of the detectability of whole-body FDG-PET in patients with metastatic bone lesions from lung cancer are needed, especially in comparison with the conventional bone scan with ^{99m}Tc-MDP. Even if the detectability of whole-body FDG-PET is less than that of the bone scan, there is no doubt as to the clinical utility of whole-body FDG-PET for surveying the distant metastasis in brain, liver, adrenal gland, skeletal system and other systemic organs.

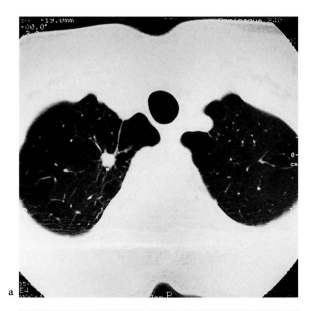

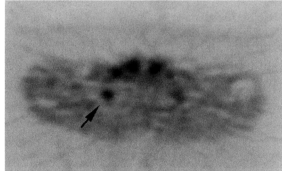

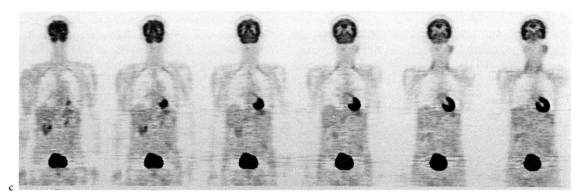

Fig 9.13a–c. Case 4: a 56-year-old male. **a** Computed tomography revealed a small mass (10 mm in diameter) with spicula formation in the apical segment of the right lung. **b** A transaxial slice of fluoro-2-deoxy-D-glucose positron emission tomography (FDG-PET) image showed the faint uptake (standardized uptake value=1.8) in the primary lesion (*arrow*). **c** Six contiguous coronal slices of whole-body FDG-PET demonstrated no uptake in the hilar and mediastinal lymph nodes; namely PET staging was T_1 N0 M0, stage I. The primary lesion was squamous cell cancer and the presurgical staging was confirmed after surgical treatment based on the histological examination

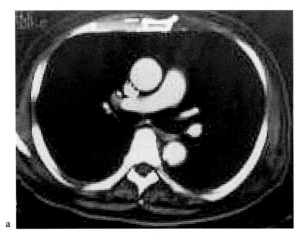

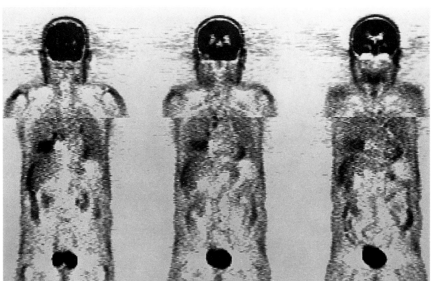

Fig 9.14a,b. Case 5: an 80-year-old male. **a** Computed tomography (CT) revealed no mediastinal nodal involvement and TNM staging was determined as T2, N0, M0 in stage I by the conventional imaging including chest radiography, CT and bone scan with ^{99m}Tc-hydroxymethylene diphosphonate. **b** Three coronal sections of whole-body fluoro-2-deoxy-D-glucose positron emission tomography (FDG-PET) images showed intense FDG uptake in the primary lesion of the lower right lobe and faint FDG uptake in the ipsilateral hilar and mediastinal nodes. PET staging was more than N2 stage. No metastases were proven histologically after surgical treatment. Anthracosis was proven in these false positive nodes by histopathological examination on the surgical specimen

Follow-up FDG Scan After Lung-Cancer Treatment

Non-invasive conventional imaging modalities, such as chest radiography, thoracic CT, and MRI, may provide excellent morphological information for the detection of primary or metastatic lesions at initial diagnosis prior to treatment, but these modalities often cannot provide helpful information in differentiating recurrent or residual tumors from post-treatment changes caused by the lack of existing normal anatomical structure due to surgical treatment or irradiation effects [44]. FDG-PET is useful in the detection of recurrent lung cancer after treatment, but there are limitations in specificity [45]. Although there are few reports of the diagnostic accuracy of FDG PET for differentiation between recurrent or residual lung cancer and benign lesions, FDG-PET shows high sensitivity in detecting recurrent or residual lung cancer (Table 9.5). Slight or no FDG uptake in suspicious lesions indicates no recurrent lung cancer, and follow-up with chest radiography, CT or MRI is required. The threshold SUV for differentiating between recurrent lung cancer and benign lesions varies among investigators, and adequate timing of the FDG-PET scan after the surgical procedure and irradiation to avoid false-positive results by reactive inflammatory process of treatments is still uncertain [46]. Further investigations are needed. An illustrative case is shown in Fig. 9.18 (case 8) [45].

Monitoring Lung Cancer with PET

PET has the unique ability to directly assess changes in tumor metabolism induced by therapy.

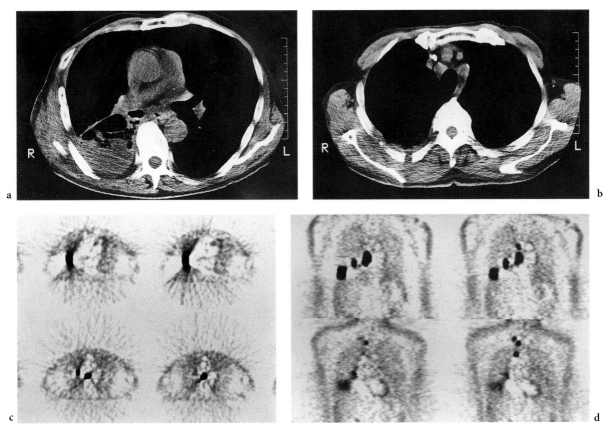

Fig 9.15a–d. Case 6: a 72-year-old male. **a** Computed tomography (CT) revealed the primary lung lesion in the lower right lobe with ipsilateral-hilar and mediastinal lymph nodes involved (#11R, #10R, #7). **b** CT of the upper mediastinum also showed the superior mediastinal lymph-node involvement, and N staging by CT was defined as N3 stage. **c** Transaxial slices of fluoro-2-deoxy-D-glucose positron emission tomography (FDG-PET) revealed clearly intense uptake of FDG in the primary (*upper raw images*) and ipsilateral hilar (#11), peribronchial (#10R), and subcarina node (#7). **d** Coronal slices of thoracic FDG-PET demonstrated intense FDG uptake in the primary lesion, ipsilateral hilar (#11) and peribronchial nodes (#10), subcarina node (#7), pre- and para-tracheal nodes (#4), superior mediastinal nodes (#2) and supraclavicular nodes. N3 stage was proved histopathologically by lymph-node biopsy

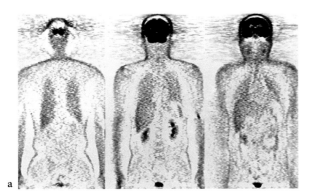
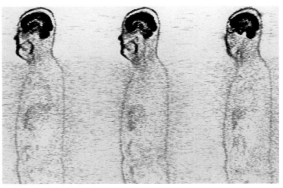

Fig 9.16a,b. Whole-body fluoro-2-deoxy-D-glucose positron emission tomography (FDG-PET) images of a 45-year-old male healthy volunteer. After 315 transaxial images (63 slices × 5 scans) with 128×128 matrices and a slice thickness of 9.6 mm were reconstructed, coronal (Fig. 8a) and sagittal (Fig. 8b) sections from the thigh up to the brain with 10-mm thickness were reconstructed. No myocardial FDG uptake was observed because of patient fasting for more than 12 h. It is important to reduce the false-negative results of the pulmonary lesions in the lower left lobe by fasting. Intense FDG uptake was seen in brain, kidney and urinary bladder, moderate uptake was observed in lung, liver, colon, bone (bone marrow) and skeletal muscle

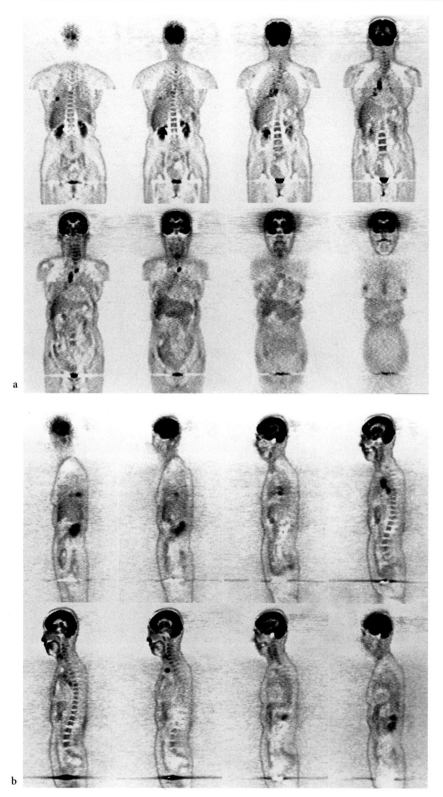

Fig 9.17 a,b. Case 7: a 60-year-old female. A lung-cancer patient with bone metastasis. **a** Six contiguous coronal sections of whole-body fluoro-2-deoxy-D-glucose positron emission tomography (FDG-PET) images. **b** Six contiguous sagittal sections of whole-body FDG-PET images. Whole-body FDG-PET images showed intense FDG uptake of the primary lesion in the lower right lobe, mediastinal lymph nodes, and also multiple pathological uptakes in the skeletal system, suggesting multiple bone metastases

Table 9.5. Detection of the recurrent lung cancer by 2-[^{18}F]-fluoro-2-deoxy-D-glucose positron emission tomography (FDG PET)

Reference	Modality	Sensitivity (%)	Specificity (%)	Accuracy (%)	Positive predictive value (%)	Negative predictive value (%)
[45]	FDG-PET	– (100)	– (89)	– (93)	–	–
[44]	FDG-PET	26/26 (100)	8/13 (62)	34/39 (87)	26/31 (84)	8/8 (100)
[58]	FDG-PET	34/35 (97)	8/8 (100)	42/43 (98)	34/34 (100)	8/9 (89)
[24]	FDG-PET	6/6 (100)	10/10 (100)	16/16 (100)	6/6 (100)	10/10 (100)

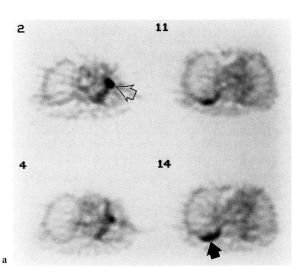
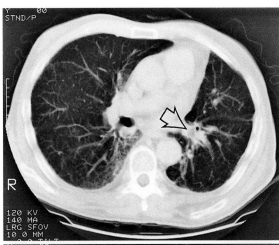
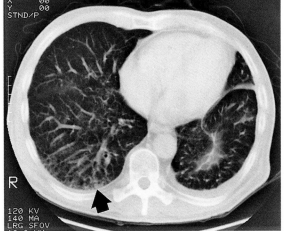

Fig 9.18 a, b. Case 8: a 62-year-old male with an adenocarcinoma. The initial surgical treatment and radiation therapy were conducted 31 months before fluoro-2-deoxy-D-glucose positron emission tomography (FDG-PET) scan. **a** FDG-PET image shows focal uptake (*open arrow*) in the hilar area of the left lung and curvilinear-shaped uptake (*arrow*) in the posterior base of the right lung (the lower number indicates the higher slice level of the lung). **b** Computed tomography demonstrates a possible nodule (*open arrow*) in the left hilar area. The right pleural effusion increased over the next few weeks, but the cultures and cytology were negative. Bronchoscopy of the left bronchus was suggestive of submucosal tumor invasion

Since the FDG tumor uptake in patients with lung cancer is correlated well with the tumor growth rate [47], FDG PET may be a useful tool for monitoring tumor response to therapy. A semiquantitative parameter, SUV, could be used to present objectively the changes of glucose metabolism by treatment [26].

Kubota et al. evaluated treatment response and residual mass in lung cancer with CMET-PET [48]. The evaluation of tumor-volume change with CT was useful in distinguishing the non-recurrence group from the groups in which there was ultimate recurrence, and the assessment of the change of CMET tumor uptake with PET before and after chemoradiation therapy was able to differentiate between the early-recurrence group and the late-recurrence group. When a residual mass is seen on CT, PET seems to be helpful in evaluating tumor viability.

If a hematopoietic growth factor (HGF) is administered to a patient with SCLC, the bone-marrow uptake of FDG on the PET scan for therapy-response monitoring should be taken into consideration because of the sensitive marker of stimulated hematopoiesis [49].

Hypoxic tumor cells are resistant to chemotherapy and radiation therapy. Measuring the hypoxic component in the tumor via ^{18}F fluoromisonidazole (FMISO) may be useful for predicting and monitoring the therapy response of lung-cancer patients. Rasey et al. assessed the tumor fractional hypoxic volume by FMISO-PET in 21 patients with NSCLC and found that the extent of hypoxia varied markedly among tumors of the same histology [50]. This intertumor variance of the volume of hypoxic tumor cells suggests the importance of monitoring oxygenation in individual tumors. ^{18}F erythro-tosyl-misonidazole (ET-MISO), which was developed at the University of Texas M.D. Anderson Cancer Center, Houston, is also a unique water-soluble agent likely to be utilized as a marker for hypoxic tumor cells [51].

In summary, the application of PET technology in the field of lung cancer is now rapidly growing, especially using FDG-PET. However, PET oncology exhibits greater potential via the development of new radiopharmaceuticals based on several tumor characteristics in biochemical and genetic processes. The author believes that it may contribute to the improvement of diagnostic accuracy and prognosis in patients with lung cancer.

References

1. Landis SH, Murray T, Bolden S, Wingo IA (1998) Cancer statistics, 1998. CA Cancer J Clin 48:6–29
2. Parkin DM, Pisani P, Ferlag J (1993) Estimates of the worldwide incidence of eighteen major cancers in 1985. Int J Cancer 54:594–606
3. Garfinkel L, Silverberg E (1991) Lung cancer and smoking trends in the United States over the past 25 years. CA Cancer J Clin 41:137–146
4. Hecht S, Hoffmann D (1988) Tobacco-specific nitrosamines, an important group of carcinogens in tobacco and tobacco smoke. Carcinogenesis 9:97–91
5. Mossman B, Bignon J, Corn M (1990) Asbestos: scientific developments and implications for public policy. Science 247:294–301
6. Harley N, Samet J, Cross F (1986) Contribution of radon and radon daughters to respiratory cancer. Environ Health Perspect 70:17–21
7. Minna J (1993) The molecular biology of lung cancer pathogenesis. Chest 103:449–454
8. Richardson GE, Johnson BE (1993) The biology of lung cancer. Semin Oncol 20:105–127
9. Doyle LA, Marby M, Stahel RA (1991) Modulation of neuroendocrine surface antigens in oncogene-activated small cell lung cancer lines. Br J Cancer Suppl 14:39–42
10. Perez-Soler R, Donato NJ, Shin DM (1994) Tumor epidermal growth factor receptor studies in patients with non-small cell lung cancer or head and neck cancer treated with monoclonal antibody RG83852. J Clin Oncol 12:730–739
11. Prevost G, Bourgeois Y, Mormont C (1994) Characterization of somatostatin receptors and growth inhibition by the somatostatin analogue BIM 23014 in small cell lung carcinoma xenograft SCLC-6. Life Sci 55:155–162
12. Maneckjee R, Minna JD (1991) Nonconventional opioid binding sites mediate growth inhibitory effects of methadone on human lung cancer cell lines. Proc Natl Acad Sci U S A 89:1169–1173
13. Lee JS, Ro JY, Sahin AA (1991) Expression of blood group antigen A: a favorable prognostic factor in non-small cell lung cancer. N Engl J Med 324:1084–1090
14. Zaman GJR, Versantvoort CHM, Smit JM (1993) Analysis of the expression of MRP, the gene for a new putative transmembrane drug transporter in human multidrug resistant lung cancer cell lines. Cancer Res 53:1747–1750
15. Popp W, Rauscher H, Tischka L (1991) Diagnostic sensitivity of different techniques in the diagnosis of lung tumors with the flexible fiberoptic bronchoscope. Cancer 67:72–75
16. Ledermann JA (1994) Serum neuron specific enolase and other neuroendocrine makers in lung cancer. Eur J Cancer 30:574–576
17. Skarin AT (1993) Analysis of long term survivors with small cell lung cancer. Chest 103:440–444
18. Morstyn G, Ihde DC, Lichter S (1984) Small cell lung cancer 1973-1983: early prognosis and recent obstacles. Int J Radiat Oncol Biol Phys 10:515–539
19. Haggar AM, Pearlberg JL, Froelich JW, Hearshen DO, Beute GH, Lewis JW, Schkudor GW, Wood C, Gniewek P (1987) Chest wall invasion by carcinoma of the lung: detection by MRI. AJR Am J Roentgenol 148:1075–1078
20. Cantoni S, Ropolo F, Serrano J, Loria F, Frola C (1995) MR enhancement of pleural effusions on MRI after I.V. administration of Gd-DTPA in patients with bronchogenic carcinoma. Eur Radiol 5[Suppl]:286–291
21. Webb WR (1988) MR imaging in the evaluation and staging of lung cancer. Semin Ultrasound CT MR 9:53–66
22. Glazer GM, Orringer MB, Chenevert TL, Borrello JA, Penner MW, Quint LE, Li KC, Aisen AM (1988) Mediastinal lymph nodes: relaxation time/pathologic correlation and implications in staging of lung cancer with MR imaging. Radiology 168:429–431
23. Sazon DA, Santiago SM, Soo Hoo GW, Khonsary A, Brown C, Mandelkern M, Blahd W, Williams AJ (1996) Fluorodeoxyglucose-positron emission tomography in the detection and staging of lung cancer. Am J Respir Crit Care Med 153:417–421
24. Duhaylongsod FG, Lowe VJ, Patz EF Jr, Vaughn AL, Coleman RE, Wolfe WG (1995) Detection of primary and recurrent lung cancer by means of F-18 fluorodeoxyglucose positron emission tomography (FDG PET). J Thorac Cardiovasc Surg 110:130–139
25. Kubota K, Matsuzawa T, Fujiwara T et al. (1990) Differential diagnosis of lung tumor with positron emission tomography. A prospective study. J Nucl Med 31:1927–1933
26. Hoh CK, Schiepers C, Seltzer MA, Gambhir SS, Silverman DH, Czernin J, Maddahi J, Phelps ME (1997) PET in oncology: will it replace the other modalities? Semin Nucl Med 27:94–106
27. Minn H, Zasadny KR, Quint LE, Wahl RL (1995) Lung cancer: reproducibility of quantitative measurements for evaluating 2-[F-18]-fluoro-2-deoxy-D-glucose uptake at PET. Radiology 196:167–173

28. Keys JW (1995) SUV: standard uptake or silly useless value? J Nucl Med 36:1836–1839
29. Hamberg LM, Hunter GJ, Alpert NM, Choi NC, Babich JW, Fischman AJ (1994) The dose uptake ratio as an index of glucose metabolism: useful parameter or oversimplification. J Nucl Med 35:1308–1312
30. Kim CK, Gupta NC, Chandramouli B, et al. (1994) Standardized uptake values of FDG: body surface area correction is preferable to body weight correction. J Nucl Med 35:164–167
31. Zasadny KR, Wahl RL (1993) Standardized uptake values of normal tissues at PET with 2-[fluorine-18]-fluoro-2-deoxy-D-glucose: variations with body weight and a method for correction. Radiology 189:847–850
32. Miyauchi T, Wahl RL (1996) Regional 2-[18F]fluoro-2-deoxy-D-glucose uptake varies in normal lung. Eur J Nucl Med 23:517–523
33. Tisi GM, Friedman PH, Peters RM, et al. (1983) American Thoracic Society. Medical Section of the American Lung Association: clinical staging of primary lung cancer. Am Rev Respir Dis 127:659–664
34. Webb WR, Gatsonis C, Zerhouni EA, Heelan RT, Glazer GM, Francis IR, McNeil BJ (1991) CT and MR imaging in staging non-small cell bronchogenic carcinoma: report of the Radiologic Diagnostic Oncology Group. Radiology 178:705–713
35. Valk PE, Pounds TR, Hopkins DM, Haseman MK, Hofer GA, Greiss HB, Myers RW, Lutrin CL (1995) Staging non-small cell lung cancer by whole-body positron emission tomographic imaging. Ann Thorac Surg 60:1573–1581
36. Bury T, Dowlati A, Paulus P, Hustinx R, Radermecker M, Rigo P (1996) Staging of non-small-cell lung cancer by whole-body fluorine-18 deoxyglucose positron emission tomography. Eur J Nucl Med 23:204–206
37. Hoh CK, Hawkins RA, Glaspy JA, Dahlbom M, Tse NY, Hoffman EJ, Schiepers, Choi Y, Rege S, Nitzsche E, et al. (1993) Cancer detection with whole-body PET using 2-[18F]fluoro-2-deoxy-D-glucose. J Comput Assist Tomogr 17:582–589
38. Boland GW, Goldberg MA, Lee MJ, Mayo-Smith WW, Dixon J, McNicholas MM, Mueller PR (1995) Indeterminate adrenal mass in patients with cancer: evaluation at PET with 2-[F-18]-fluoro-2-deoxy-D-glucose. Radiology 194:131–134
39. Engel H, Steinert H, Buck A, Berthold T, Böni RAH, von Schulthess GK (1996) Whole-body PET: physiological and artifactual fluorodeoxyglucose accumulations. J Nucl Med 37:441–446
40. Thompson CJ, Ranger N, Evans AC, Gjedde A (1991) Validation of simultaneous PET emission and transmission scans. J Nucl Med 32:154–160
41. Xu EZ, Mullani NA, Gould KL, Anderson WL (1991) A segmented attenuation correction for PET. J Nucl Med 32:161–165
42. Meikle SR, Eberl S, Hooper PK, Fulham MJ (1997) Simultaneous emission and transmission (SET) scanning in neurological PET studies. J Comput Assist Tomogr 21:487–497
43. Langer KJ, Braun U, Kops ER, et al. (1993) The influence of plasma glucose levels on fluorine-18-fluorodeoxyglucose uptake in bronchial carcinoma. J Nucl Med 34:355–359
44. Glazer HS, Lee JKT, Levitt RG, Heiken JP, Ling D, Totty WG, Balfe DM, Emani B, Wasserman TH, Murphy WA (1985) Radiation fibrosis: differentiation from recurrent tumor by MR imaging. Radiology 156:721–726
45. Inoue T, Kim EE, Komaki R, Wong FC, Bassa P, Wong WH, Yang DJ, Endo K, Podoloff DA (1995) Detecting recurrent or residual lung cancer with FDG-PET. J Nucl Med 36:788–793
46. Frank A, Lefkowitz D, Jaeger S, Gobar L, Sunderland J, Gupta N, Scott W, Mailliard J, Lynch H, Bishop J, et al. (1995) Decision logic for retreatment of asymptomatic lung cancer recurrence based on positron emission tomography findings. Int J Radiat Oncol Biol Phys 32:1495–1512
47. Duhaylongsod FG, Lowe VJ, Patz EF Jr, Vaughn AL, Coleman RE, Wolfe WG (1995) Lung tumor growth correlates with glucose metabolism measured by fluoride-18 fluorodeoxyglucose positron emission tomography. Ann Thorac Surg 60:1348–1352
48. Kubota K, Yamada S, Ishiwata K, Ito M, Fujiwara T, Fukuda H, Tada M, Ido T (1993) Evaluation of the treatment response of lung cancer with positron emission tomography and L-[methyl-11C]methionine: a preliminary study. Eur J Nucl Med 20:495–501
49. Knopp MV, Bischoff H, Rimac A, Oberdorfer F, van Kaick G. (1996) Bone marrow uptake of fluorine-18-fluorodeoxyglucose following treatment with hematopoietic growth factors: initial evaluation. Nucl Med Biol 23:845–849
50. Rasey JS, Koh WJ, Evans ML, Peterson LM, Lewellen TK, Graham MM, Krohn KA (1996) Quantifying regional hypoxia in human tumors with positron emission tomography (PET) after injection of hypoxia-binding radiopharmaceutical [18F]fluoromisonidazole ([18FMISO]). Int J Radiat Oncol Biol Phys 36:417–428
51. Yang DJ, Wallace S, Cherif A, Li C, Gretzer MB, Kim EE, Podoloff DA (1995) Development of F-18-labeled fluoroerythronitroimidazole as a PET agent for imaging tumor hypoxia. Radiology 194:795–800
52. Slosmon DO, Spiliopoulos A, Couson F, et al. (1993) Satellite PET and lung cancer: a prospective study in surgical patients. Nucl Med Commun 14:955–961
53. Rege SD, Hoh CK, Glaspy JA, et al. (1993) Imaging of pulmonary mass lesions with whole-body positron emission tomography and fluorodeoxyglucose. Cancer 72:82–90
54. Dewan NA, Gupta NC, Redepenning LS, et al (1993) Diagnostic efficacy of PET-FDG imaging in solitary pulmonary nodules. Potential role in evaluation and management. Chest 104:997–1002
55. Dewan NA, Reeb SD, Gupta NC, et al (1995) PET-FDG imaging and transthoracic needle lung aspiration biopsy in evaluation of pulmonary lesions. A comparative risk–benefit analysis. Chest 108:441–446
56. Gupta NC, Maloof J, Gunel E (1996) Probability of malignancy in solitary pulmonary nodules using fluorine-18-FDG and PET. J Nucl Med 37:943–948
57. Knight SB, Delbeke D, Stewart JR, et al (1996) Evaluation of pulmonary lesions with FDG-PET. Comparison of findings in patients with and without a history of prior malignancy. Chest 109:982–988
58. Patz EF Jr, Lowe VJ, Hoffman JM, et al (1993) Focal pulmonary abnormalities: evaluation with F-18 fluorodeoxyglucose PET scanning. Radiology 188:487–490
59. Guhlmann A, Storck M, Kotzerke J, Moog F, Sunder PL, Reske SN (1997) Lymph node staging in non-small cell lung cancer: evaluation by [18F]FDG positron emission tomography (PET). Thorax 52:438–441
60. Steinert HC, Hauser M, Allemann F, Engel H, Berthold T, von Schulthess GK, et al (1997) Non-small cell lung cancer: nodal staging with FDG PET versus CT with correlative lymphnode mapping and sampling. Radiology 202:441–446
61. Sasaki M, Ichiya Y, Kuwabara Y, et al (1996) The usefulness of FDG positron emission tomography for the detection of mediastinal lymph node metastases in patients with non-small cell lung cancer: a comparative study with X-ray computed tomography. Eur J Nucl Med 23:741–747
62. Chin R Jr, Ward R, Keyes JW, et al (1995) Mediastinal staging of non-small-cell lung cancer with positron emission tomography. Am J Respir Crit Care Med 152:2090–2096

63. Wahl RL, Quint LE, Greenough RL, Meyer CR, White RI, Orringer MB (1994) Staging of mediastinal non-small cell lung cancer with FDG PET, CT, and fusion images: preliminary prospective evaluation. Radiology 191:371–377

64. Miyazawa H, Arai T, Inagaki K, Morita T, Yano M, Hara T (1992) Detection of mediastinal lymph node metastasis from lung cancer with positron emission tomography (PET) using 11C-methionine. Nippon-Kyobu-Geka-Gakkai-Zasshi 40:2125–2130

Breast Cancer

E. E. Kim

Basic Considerations

Breast cancer is still the most common (noncutaneous) cancer afflicting women in the United States and produces considerable anxiety, since controversy surrounds treatment methods and extends to diagnostic and staging techniques.

In 1998, the American Cancer Society estimates that 180,300 women will be diagnosed with breast cancer and that 43,900 women will die of this disease [1]. Until recently, breast cancer was the leading cause of death from cancer among women, but since 1985 it has ranked second after lung cancer [1]. Among women, breast cancer accounts for 32% of all cancers detected and 18% of all cancer deaths [1].

Early detection of breast cancer decreases mortality and facilitates breast-conserving therapy. Studies continue to prove that mammography is the most effective method for early breast-cancer detection [2]. The rate of lesion detection by modern mammography has been significantly improved over the past decade using dedicated units, excellent film-screening combinations and processors. However, mammography lacks adequate specificity for cancer detection and has a low positive-predictive value for detection of breast cancer, which is only 20–30% [3]. One of the major reasons for such low positive-predictive value is that a dense breast obscures the identification of tumors. Approximately 25% of women have dense breasts on mammography [4]. The other problem with the routine use of mammography is its high false-negative rates (26–45%) [5]. Suspicious areas include a mass, a cluster of microcalcification, an asymmetrical area or an area of architectural distortion. More than five microcalcifications in a cubic centimeter and branching calcifications are particularly worrisome. Intra-observer and inter-observer variabilities are also critical. A normal mammogram is obtained in 10% of breasts with clinical cancer. Screening is ideally directed toward the population at greatest risk of developing breast cancer. Evidence of screening benefits in women between 40 years and 50 years of age continues to mount.

Diagnosis, Pathology and Staging

In recent years, the use of fine-needle aspiration (FNA) cytology and a stereotactic core biopsy of the breast have become more available in clinical use. These techniques, although fairly simple, require a trained cytopathologist and costly equipment to perform; nevertheless, they can have an important impact on eliminating some of the excisional biopsies, which are more invasive and costly.

FNA does not allow certain differentiation between invasive and in situ carcinoma. The false-negative rate of core needle biopsies has been greater than that of FNA [6]. As with invasive breast cancer, controversy has long attended discussions of noninvasive breast cancer, which accounts for nearly one-quarter of biopsied breast tumors. The identification of any proliferative lesion is associated with an increased risk of later invasive breast cancer [7].

Carcinoma of the breast is a malignant tumor arising from the epithelium lining of the ducts and lobules of the breast. Histologic types of malignant breast tumors are shown in Table 10.1. The vast majority of them are carcinomas (95% or more), and more than half of them are pure infiltrating duct lesions.

Lobular carcinoma in situ (LCIS) is a microscopic lesion of lobules scattered in normal breast tissue and accounts for 2–3% of breast tumors and one-third to one-half of noninvasive carcinomas. It is most commonly found in pre- or perimenopausal women. The lobular cells are smaller than ductal cells, so that some have referred to LCIS as small cell carcinoma in situ. The process extends beyond the lobule into the adjacent ducts in more than half of the patients. Multicentricity is a hallmark and is reported in two-thirds of patients [8]. LCIS is commonly considered a bilat-

Table 10.1. Histologic types of malignant breast tumors

Carcinoma of mammary ducts
Noninfiltration
Papillary carcinoma
Comedocarcinoma
Infiltration
Papillary carcinoma
Comedocarcinoma
Scirrhous carcinoma
Medullary carcinoma
Colloid carcinoma
Carcinoma of lobules
Noninfiltration
Infiltration
Others
Intercystic carcinoma
Adenoid cystic carcinoma
Squamous cell or epidermoid carcinoma
Spindle cell carcinoma
Sweat gland carcinoma
Carcinoma with osseous & cartilaginous metaplasia
Paget's disease
Inflammatory carcinoma
Sarcoma
Lymphoma

eral process, and contralateral breast biopsy is sometimes recommended to evaluate risk in the opposite breast [9]. The natural history of LCIS is one of bilateral risk with later invasive breast cancer, and the risk is 10–20% in each breast, for a 20–35% total lifetime risk. LCIS should be regarded not as a cancer, but as a marker for genetic instability with a high risk of future carcinoma.

Ductal carcinoma in situ (DCIS), also called intraductal carcinoma, is characterized by malignant ductal cells. Tumors with areas of basement-membrane invasion must be treated as infiltrating-ductal carcinoma. DCIS accounts for 8–22% of biopsied palpable lesions, and the age distribution of DCIS parallels that of invasive breast carcinoma. DCIS often is detected as clustered microcalcifications. In lesions greater than 2.5 cm in diameter, 54% were multicentric; in lesions less than 2.5 cm, 14% were multicentric [10]. DCIS is associated with almost entirely unilateral risk, and the long-term risk of subsequent invasive breast carcinoma is 28% [11].

Invasive ductal carcinoma, which represents 75% of all invasive types, is the most common of all breast cancers. The tumor is usually grayish-yellow with radiating-fibrous trabeculae running toward the periphery of the tumor. The size of the tumor varies, and the degree of hardness depends on the amount of connective tissue present. Intraductal carcinoma grows predominantly within the marrow ducts and is multifocal in about one-third of cases. The malignant cells filling the ducts may be arranged in a solid, papillary or cribriform pattern. Diffuse or scattered microcalcifications are frequent. One-third of the intraductal carcinomas are between 2 cm and 5 cm in diameter, and there is no correlation between the size of the tumor and the degree of infiltration.

Medullary carcinoma often appears in patients under 50 years of age, and the tumor is very well circumscribed with prominent lymphoid infiltrate. The prognosis of medullary carcinoma is more favorable than for invasive ductal carcinoma.

Mucinous (colloid) carcinoma tends to occur in elderly patients and has a slow growth of long duration. Microscopically, the tumor shows epithelial cells floating in a sea of mucin, and the prognosis tends to be good. Papillary carcinoma is rare, and tends to be well circumscribed. The cavity of the cystic type contains necrotic tissue or hemorrhagic fluid. The tumor rarely invades the surrounding stroma. Tubular or well-differentiated adenocarcinoma is usually small and has a lower incidence of axillary metastasis. Epidermoid carcinoma is a tumor of elderly women, and adenoid cystic carcinoma is a rare form of infiltrating carcinoma.

Paget's disease occurs in 1–4% of all patients with breast cancer and is manifested as an eczematoid lesion of the nipple. Its prognosis depends on the histologic type of the associated tumor. Inflammatory carcinoma simulates the appearance of mastitis and is associated with an extremely poor prognosis. There may be a widespread permeation of dermal lymphatics in the absence of the clinical features.

Most stroma or nonepithelial tumors are sarcomas, which are extremely rare and have an ominous prognosis. Cystosarcoma phylloides is an uncommon tumor with both epithelial and nonepithelial elements, and it is mostly benign. There is a direct correlation between tumor size and risk of recurrence, and whether the disease is node-positive or negative [12]. Nuclear or histologic grade describes the degree of tumor differentiation based on nuclear size and shape, number of mitoses and degree of tubule formation. Tumors of low malignancy are designated grade I and are associated with the best prognosis. Grade-III tumors are associated with the worst prognosis [13].

Estrogen- and progesterone-receptor positivity correlate with prolonged disease-free and overall survival. Measurement of hormone-receptor level is valuable for identifying patients likely to benefit from adjuvant endocrine therapy [14]. The degree of cellular proliferation has shown a strong correlation with outcome. Flow cytometry measures both DNA ploidy (content) and S-phase fraction (cells actively cycling or synthesizing

DNA). Aneuploid tumors with a high percentage of cells in S-phase are more likely to recur than tumors with a low S-phase fraction [15].

A relationship between tumor cell kinetics and response to chemotherapy has also been suggested. Patients with an S-phase fraction greater than 10% showed significantly higher response rates to chemotherapy than those with an S-phase fraction less than 5% [16]. Cathepsin D is a lysosomal protein that is synthesized in normal tissues, but is overexpressed and secreted in breast cancers. It may play a role in invasion and metastasis [17]. Overexpression of the HER-2/neu oncogene reflects an increase in the proliferative activity of a tumor and shorter survival [18]. Angiogenesis plays a key role in tumor growth, invasiveness, and progression. Tumor angiogenesis, as manifested by microvessel density, has been shown to be a reliable prognostic marker in node-negative breast cancer [19]. Carcinoembryonic antigen (CEA) levels are elevated in 40–50% of patients with metastasis, and cancer antigen 15-3, which is more sensitive than CEA, is elevated in 70–85% of patients with metastases [20].

Staging

Clinical staging is based on physical examination as well as laboratory and radiological evaluation. Staging is important in the selection of the most appropriate treatment regiment and in prognosis. The most widely used staging system is based on the TNM system (Table 10.2) with the T standing for primary-tumor extent, the N for regional node involvement, and the M for metastases (Table 10.3).

The tumor component (T) of the TNM staging is determined by physical examination and mammography. Not only will the mammogram aid in the preoperative determination of the size and extent of the primary tumor, but it also provides a road map of the breast to guide the surgeon for the biopsy. The initial mammogram can serve as a baseline to measure the progress of therapy. Ultrasonography has detected breast cancers as small as 2 mm [21], but it cannot consistently image small cancers or the clusters of calcifications that might represent minimally invasive or noninvasive carcinoma. Ultrasonography is of particular value in differentiation of cystic from solid masses. Axillary-node involvement is best determined via physical examination and biopsy. The use of lymphoscintigraphy using ^{99m}Tc sulfur colloid is helpful in mapping a lymphatic chain intraoperatively and in performing biopsy of a sentinel node.

Table 10.2. TNM classification for breast cancer

Primary Tumor (T)
Tx = Cannot be assessed
T0 = No evidence
Tis = In situ
T1 ≤ 2 cm
  T1a = No fix to pectoral fascia or muscle
  T1b = Fix to pectoral fascia or muscle
    i ≤ 0.5 cm
    ii = 0.5–1.0 cm
    iii = 1.0–2.0 cm
T2 = 2–5 cm
  T2a = No fix to pectoral fascia or muscle
  T2b = Fix to pectoral fascia or muscle
T3 ≥ 5 cm
  T3a = No fix to pectoral fascia or muscle
  T3b = Fix to pectoral fascia or muscle
T4 = Any size with extension to chest wall or skin
  T4a = Fix to chest wall
  T4b = Edema, ulcer or nodule of breast skin
  T4c = Both of above
Node (N)
Nx = Cannot be assessed
N0 = No metastasis in homolateral axillary node
N1 = Metastasis to homolateral axillary node not fixed
  N1a Micrometastasis
  N1b Gross metastasis
    i = 0.2–2.0 cm in 1–3 nodes
    ii = 0.2–2.0 cm in >4 nodes
    iii = Beyond node capsule (<2 cm)
    iv = ≥2 cm
N2 = Metastasis to homolateral axillary node fixed
N3 = Metastasis to homolateral paraclavicular node
Metastasis (M)
Mx = Cannot be assessed
M0 = No distant metastasis
M1 = Distant metastasis

Table 10.3. Staging of breast cancer

Tis = In situ
X = Cannot be staged
I = T1a or T1b, N0, M0
II = T0, N1a or N1b, M0
  T1a or T1b, N1a or N1b, M0
  T2a or T2b, N0, M0
  T2a or T2b, N1a or N1b, M0
IIIA = T0, N2, M0
  T1a or T1b, N2, M0
  T2a or T2b, N2, M0
  T3a or T3b, N0, M0
  T3a or T3b, N1, M0
  T3a or T3b, N2, M0
IIIB = Any T, N3, M0
  Any T4, any N, M0
IV = Any T, any N, m1

Magnetic Resonance Imaging

The potential of magnetic resonance imaging (MRI) for evaluating breast disease has increased over the past decade concurrently with advances in MRI technology. The intrinsic soft-tissue contrast of MRI and its ability to depict thin contiguous sections throughout the entire breast offered

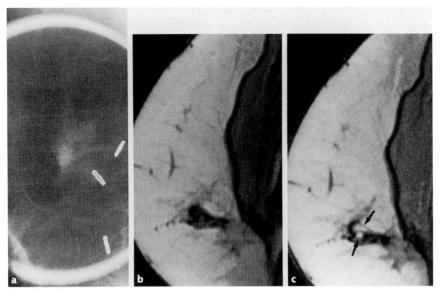

Fig. 10.1a–c. Mammogram shows an ill-defined increased density adjacent to the lumpectomy site for the ductal carcinoma in situ (**a**). Sagittal images of the breast before (**b**) and 1 min after (**c**) injection of gadolinium-diethylenetriaminepentaacetic acid, using a multiplanar spoiled gradient-recalled acquisition sequence, show a rapid, intense enhancement of small nodular lesions, suggesting fibroadenoma or carcinoma (reprinted with permission from [26])

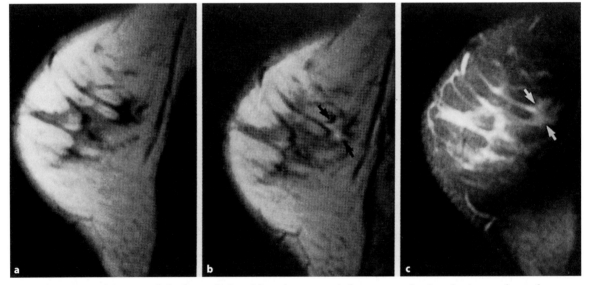

Fig. 10.2a–c. Sagittal images of the breast before (**a**) and 1 min after (**b**) injection of adoteridol, using multiplanar spoiled gradient-recalled acquisition sequence, show an immediate enhancement of a spiculated invasive ductal carcinoma. A fat-suppressed spin-echo image shows the tumor obscured by surrounding enhanced parenchyma (**c**) (reprinted with permission from [26])

the possibility early-on that MRI might better detect malignancies than mammography, particularly in the dense breast. Noncontrast studies did not meet this expectation. However, with the introduction of gadolinium-based contrast agents, the specificity of breast MRI improved and interest was renewed in the application of MRI to breast cancer. The development of surface coils and high-resolution, fast imaging techniques have contributed to improved methods for breast MRI. The role that MRI will play in breast-cancer management is indicated by technical advances in MRI that are currently being used in breast imaging, as well as the specific techniques that show promise for evaluating breast cancer.

Breast MRI is generally performed with the patient in the prone position to minimize image artifacts caused by respiratory motion. Small surface coils mounted within the patient-support device surround one or both breasts to achieve good sensitivity to tissue within the breast. Certain special radiofrequency excitation techniques, such as those used in the fast adiabatic trajectory in the steady state (FATS) and rotating delivery of excitation off-resonance (RODEO) methods, require that the surface coil be used to both transmit and receive the radiofrequency signal, mainly due to their power requirement [22]. The heterogeneous nature of the breast and the overlap in T_1 and T_2 relaxation time between different normal- and abnormal-breast-tissue types frequently renders conventional noncontrast breast MR images confusing and ambiguous. Hybrid imaging approaches combining T_1 and T_2 weighting with fat-suppression techniques as well as multivariate image analysis may be helpful for improving the sensitivity of MRI to breast disease. Carcinoma and fibroadenoma show low-to-medium signals on T_1-weighted images and medium-to-high signals on T_2-weighted images. Fibroglandular tissues also show low-to-medium signals on T_1-weighted images and medium signals on T_2-weighted images. Cysts and other fluid-filled lesions such as necrosis reveal very low signals on T_1-weighted images and very bright signals on T_2-weighted images. Magnetization-transfer (MT) contrast techniques use special radiofrequency pulses to saturate the bound-hydrogen pool (macromolecules) of tissue while not affecting the free-hydrogen pool that contributes signal on MR images. MT contrast has been shown to reduce the image intensity of fibroglandular tissue and may be sensitive for detecting breast lesions [23].

A contrast agent must be used for MRI to be sufficiently sensitive to breast cancer. With the use of contrast agents, GE pulse sequences seem to have largely replaced SE sequences, both two dimensional (2-D) and 3-D. For reliable detection of small (<5 mm) lesions, high-resolution 3-D techniques must be used to provide large area coverage with thin sections and no slice gap. For high-sensitivity imaging, high-resolution 3-D imaging techniques are advocated with approximately 1-mm isotropic spatial resolution [24]. Fat suppression is recommended to distinguish enhancing tumors from fat and to improve the visualization of breast parenchyma. Two-dimensional imaging techniques can provide T_1- or T_2-weighting for excellent soft-tissue contrast, achieve temporal resolutions of 1 min or better and can be used with inversion recovery for fat suppression.

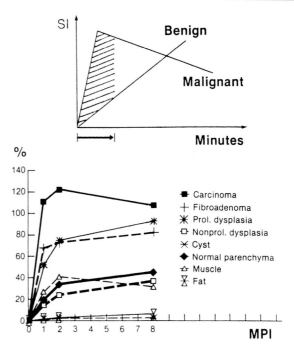

Fig. 10.3. Principle of diagnostic window, 1–2 min after contrast injection can differentiate malignant from benign lesions. Graphic representation of the percentage of signal increase in different breast lesions. MPI, minutes post contrast injection (reprinted with permission from [27])

Overall, the existing data prove a quite high (85%–100%) sensitivity for MRI concerning detection of malignancy. The distinction between in situ carcinoma and proliferative dysplasia is not always possible [25].

Presently, the best strategy for differentiating between benign and malignant breast lesions uses dynamic contrast-enhanced-MRI techniques. The dose of contrast is 0.2 mmol/kg body weight when GE techniques are used because of the increased T_1 sensitivity. The temporal pattern of signal enhancement in the first 1–2 min has been used to differentiate between malignancies and some benign lesions, such as fibroadenomas or fibrocystic changes (Figs. 10.1 and 10.2) [26]. All carcinomas enhanced strongly, 85% focally, and all but 5% rapidly (Figs. 10.3 and 10.4) [27]. More than 70% of benign tissues did not demonstrate significant contrast uptake [28]. The variation in specificity may be attributed to MR technique, diagnostic criteria and patient population. There is doubt that MRI is of greater benefit than biopsy in all masses or microcalcifications. Minimally invasive core biopsy costs less than a contrast-enhanced MRI. Because the sensitivity is so high, it is tempting to use MRI for screening, especially for high-risk patients with mammographically dense breasts. The ability to biopsy lesions under

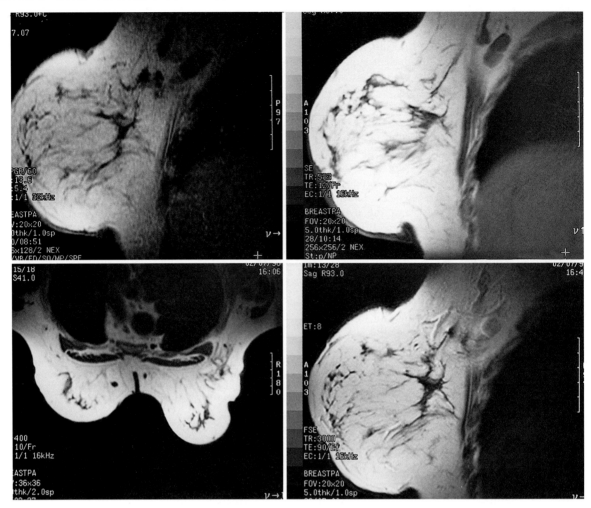

Fig. 10.4. Spiculated enhanced adenocarcinoma of left breast and metastatic nodes in left axilla are on post-gadolinium (Gd) (*upper left*), pre-Gd (*upper right*) sagittal T_1-, sagittal T_2- (*lower right*) and axial T_1- (*lower left*) weighted images

MR guidance currently is under development but not universally available.

Magnetic Resonance Spectroscopy

Any MR scan or spectrum is an actual measurement of biochemical processes and their constituent biomolecules, and depicts the interactions of biomolecules in metabolic pathways, membrane dynamics, the flux of metabolites and how the metabolites affect their solvent, which is water [29]. At the present time, the state-of-the-art for MR spectroscopy (MRS) of the breast can be described in terms of multinuclear spectroscopy using image-guided volume-selection techniques. The majority of MRS experience has been with proton and phosphorus nuclei. Proton (^{1}H) MRS reveals intense water and lipid signals from the glandular and fatty portions of the breast. Most metabolites are present in concentrations that are several orders of magnitude less than those of water and fat. Phosphorus (^{31}P) MRS provides valuable information about high- and low-energy phosphatic intermediaries of metabolism, such as adenosine triphosphate (ATP), adenosine diphosphate (ADP), phosphocreatine (PCr) and phosphorylated sugars (Fig. 10.5) [30]. It is capable of monitoring the energy status of a tissue or tumor and also providing in vivo measurement of pH. Phosphorus sensitivity is significantly less than that of hydrogen (7%), and phosphatic metabolites are generally present in millimolar concentrations in most tissues. The metabolic activity of breast tumors is greater than that of surrounding breast tissue (Fig. 10.6). Fluorine (^{19}F) MRS can be used to observe the distribution and metabolism of 5-fluorouracil, and the fluorine nucleus demonstrates a high MR sensitivity (80%) relative

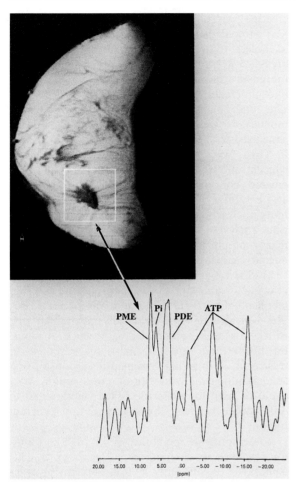

Fig. 10.5. Sagittal T_1-weighted image of a breast (*top*) shows an infiltrating ductal carcinoma with irregular intermediate signal intensity as well as outlining volume for spectroscopic examination. The resultant ^{31}P magnetic resonance spectroscopic profile (*bottom*) is an amplitude vs frequency plot, where the amplitude corresponds to the relative concentration of the detected metabolites and the frequency is characteristic of the detected metabolites. Note elevated phosphomonoesters (*PME*), inorganic phosphate (*Pi*) and phosphodiester (*PDE*) (reprinted with permission from [30])

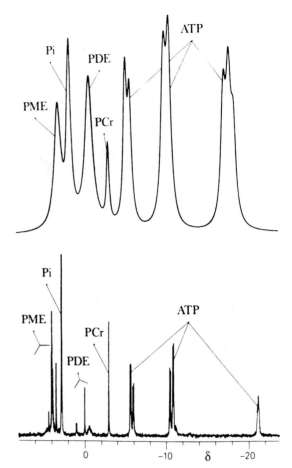

Fig. 10.6. In vivo (*top*) and in vitro (*bottom*) ^{31}P magnetic resonance spectra of a benign breast tumor. Note elevated inorganic phosphate (*Pi*) and phosphocreatine (*PCr*) (reprinted with permission from [30])

to hydrogen. Carbon (^{13}C) MR spectra cover a large range of chemical shifts, but the MR sensitivity of carbon is only 1.6% that of hydrogen.

Performing MRS in vivo requires a number of hardware and software accessories in addition to those necessary to carry out an MRI examination. The majority of clinical MRS has worked on imaging/spectroscopy systems operating with magnetic field strengths of 1.5 T. Resolution and signal-to-noise of MR spectral data improve with increasing magnetic-field strength and homogeneity. The greater the gradient strength, the smaller the volume that may be defined when using an acquisition technique that relies on gradients to define the volume. To achieve a homogeneous magnetic-field distribution and maximize signal-to-noise, a single-breast system is preferable over one that is capable of examining bilateral breasts. A dedicated system encompassing the entire breast (volume-coil design) with transmit-receive and multi-tune (multi-nuclear) capabilities is preferred. The preferred examination is one that is image-guided and volume-selective such that spectral data, whether acquired from single or multiple volume elements, can be correlated with breast MRI. The most common technique uses a surface coil placed over the area of interest, roughly a sphere for a coil with circular shape, in conjunction with volume-selective techniques [31]. Typical volumes range from 0.5 cm^3 to 1.0 cm^3 for ^{1}H MRS and from 2.0 cm^3 to 2.5 cm^3 for ^{31}P MRS. The smallest volumes have been achieved on instruments operating at 4.0 T.

Chemical-shift imaging is a method used to simultaneously acquire spectral data from several volume elements that may be selected from a 1-D column, 2-D plane, or 3-D volume of data. Contrast agents may influence the MR relaxation of spectral elements in unknown ways. Therefore, MRS performed after a contrast infusion cannot be advised. Typical parameters for the acquisition sequence include a repetition time of 3000–6000 ms and 256–512 signal averages.

Even with the present limitations of MRS, promising results have been achieved with ^{31}P MRS. Phosphatic intermediates of metabolism are the principal components of a number of biochemical pathways, including those related to energy metabolism, biosynthesis and cell-membrane metabolism. The phosphorus MR spectrum is divided into several distinct regions on the basis of chemical shift and phosphorus functional group. The first resonance band, located downfield, is called the phosphomonoester resonance band. This includes phosphorus atoms esterified to the residue molecule in a single-ester linkage. These molecules include the phosphorylated sugars. Phosphorylcholine and phosphorylethanolamine are precursors in the metabolism of membranes, neurotransmitters and membrane anchors to cellular antigens. The resonance of inorganic orthophosphate is also included within the phosphomonoester region by virtue of its structure. The phosphodiester region is the region of the spectrum where the breakdown products of membrane metabolism and low molecular weight phosphorylated extramembranous molecules can be found, such as the phosphodiester links in the phosphoglycan side chains of glycoproteins and glycolipids. Phosphocreatine acts as an alternative storage form of energy and is responsible for the phosphorylation of ADP to ATP through the action of creatine kinase. This resonance is followed upfield by ATP and several other energy-storing molecules, such as the dinucleotides and the nucleoside diphosphosugars.

Breast cancers were found to have significantly lower concentrations of phosphomonoesters and inorganic phosphates than normal breast parenchyma [32]. They were distinguishable from both benign tumors and normal breast tissue due to significantly elevated levels of phosphodiesters and phosphorylated glycans. Redmond et al. [33] showed that premenopausal women had reduced phosphocreatine and significantly increased phosphomonoester and βATP. They also demonstrated that the fat-to-water ratio was higher in older women. Also, α- and γATP were significantly higher in breast-cancer tissues, whereas phosphocreatine was significantly reduced. Sijens et al. [34] showed that the fat-to-water ratio was higher in breast tumors than normal tissue and that breast cancers had elevated phosphomonoesters, inorganic phosphate, phosphodiester and little phosphocreatine compared with normal tissues. The total concentration of low-energy phosphomonoesters was increased in malignant tumors compared with benign tumors and normal tissues in vitro [35]. Malignant tissues have increased concentrations of phosphomonoesters and decreased concentrations of phosphocreatine and also exhibit a decrease in the phosphocreatine-to-inorganic-orthophosphate index from tissue-extract analysis [36]. Phosphates are composed primarily of phosphatic metabolites, phosphates in nucleic acids, and phospholipids.

MRS is capable of obtaining useful biochemical information relevant to the energy status and metabolism of a tissue or tumor. MR spectral profiles can also be used to assess intracellular pH, which is a useful parameter with which to monitor both tumor and normal-tissue response to treatment. Monitoring therapeutic response using MRS requires the presence of gross tumor. MRS could be used to assess the tissue viability and to differentiate between the scar and the recurrent tumor.

To demonstrate the ability of ^{31}P MRS to monitor response to chemotherapy, Leach et al. [37] combined ^{31}P MRS and ^{99m}Tc hexamethylpropyleneamine oxide- (HMPAO) perfusion scans, and the total nucleoside triphosphate (NTP)/inorganic phosphate ratio increased while recording an increased uptake of HMPAO in patients receiving chemotherapy. They reported that uptake of HMPAO increased while pH fell, and when the uptake decreased, the pH increased. These findings confirmed others' reports that the ratio of low- to high-energy phosphates decreased as a measure of therapeutic response [33]. MRS data could be used to suggest that maximum response to neoadjuvant therapy has been achieved and that the time for definitive local treatment with surgical resection has arrived. MRS data should be correlated with pathologic and clinical variables to determine their prognostic value in any setting.

Positron-Emission Tomography

Metabolic imaging using ^{18}F-fluorodeoxyglucose positron-emission tomography (FDG-PET) has been introduced as a promising technique for identification of breast cancer [37]. Differentiation between benign and malignant breast abnormalities by means of noninvasive diagnostic procedures still remains a clinical challenge.

Using visual image interpretation, FDG uptake in breast tissue was classified into three categories (negative, probably and definitely positive) (Fig. 10.7). Considering only definite FDG uptake to represent malignancy, a sensitivity of 68% and a specificity of 97% was recorded. Sensitivity increased to 83%, but specificity declined to 84% if probably findings were regarded as positive [38]. In a study by Wahl et al. [39], a relatively low sensitivity of FDG-PET scans was found in the detection of metastatic bony lesions. This may have been due partly to attenuation of tumor activity by bone mass. Recent prospective studies using whole-body FDG-PET reported 93% sensitivity and 79% specificity for the detection of recurrent or metastatic breast cancer when scores of four (probably positive) or five (definitely positive) were considered [40]. The corresponding positive- and negative-predictive values were 82% and 92%. If scores of three (possibly positive) through five were regarded as positive, the sensitivity and specificity were 93% and 61%, respectively. The positive-predictive value for lesions was 62% for a score of four and 90% for a score of five. The negative-predictive values for scores of one to three were 83%, 85% and 83%, respectively. False-negative lesions included five bone metastases and one small breast focus. False-positive lesions were due to muscle uptake in five sites, inflammation in four sites, blood-pool activity in two sites and bowel uptake in one site.

Quantification of FDG uptake in breast tumors provides objective criteria for differentiation between benign and malignant tissue with similar diagnostic accuracy to visual analysis. Comparing all correction and normalization methods, average standard uptake values (SUVs), corrected for partial volume effect and normalized to blood glucose, yielded the highest diagnostic accuracy with 85% sensitivity and 90% specificity [41]. Quantitative analysis of PET studies in oncology is affected by biological and technical factors, i.e., tracer kinetics, composition of tumor tissue, data acquisition and analysis. It cannot be expected that tumors have the same lumped constant (LC), even in the same patient. Fat has a lower FDG uptake than other tissues and, thus, FDG uptake in tumors will be overestimated in heavy patients. Applying the correction method using the lean body mass was not superior to use of SUVs in differentiating between benign and malignant breast tissue. Because of the competition between the transport of endogenous glucose and FDG molecules into the cell, FDG uptake in cancer is sensi-

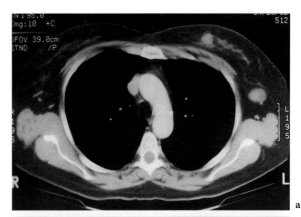

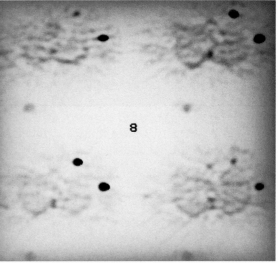

Fig. 10.7. a Contrast-enhanced axial computed-tomography image of the upper chest showing nodular carcinoma in the left breast and a metastatic nodule in the left axilla. b Selected axial positron-emission-tomography images of the left chest show focal areas of markedly increased uptake of ^{18}F-fluoro-2-deoxy-D-glucose, corresponding to the primary left breast cancer and metastatic lesion in the left axilla

tive to variations in blood glucose levels. However, relatively small changes in diagnostic accuracy were found after applying blood-glucose normalization.

We retrospectively investigated the value of FDG-PET for preoperative chemotherapy response in patients with locally advanced breast cancer (Fig. 10.8) [42]. Sensitivity for detection of primary breast cancer before chemotherapy was 100%, 62.5% and 87.5% with FDG-PET, mammography and ultrasonography, respectively. Sensitivity for detection of initial nodal metastasis was 77%, 70% and 87.5%, respectively (Fig. 10.9). The mean SUV of primary cancer was 9.4 (range 2.0–20.7). Improvement was visible with smaller size and less FDG uptake early after chemotherapy (Fig. 10.9), and mean SUV obtained in the follow-

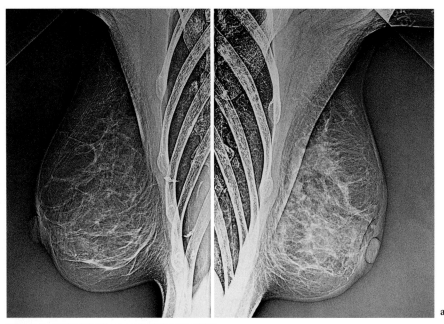

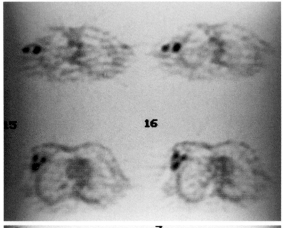

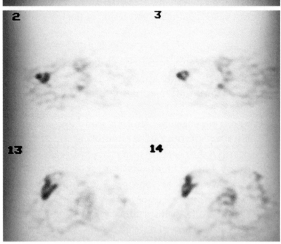

Fig. 10.8. a Lateral views of left and right xeromammograms show spiculated lesions in right breast. Note there is no bilateral nodular metastasis in the axilla. b Selected axial positron-emission-tomography images of the chest before (*upper*) and 1 month after (*lower*) preoperative chemotherapy show a significant interval decrease of ^{18}F fluoro-2-deoxy-D-glucose uptake in three nodular carcinoma lesions in the right breast and two metastatic lesions in the right axilla after chemotherapy

up studies before surgery decreased significantly from those obtained in the first study. FDG-PET was valuable for monitoring preoperative chemotherapy effects with better sensitivity for primary residual tumor and better specificity for nodal metastasis in comparison with ultrasonog-

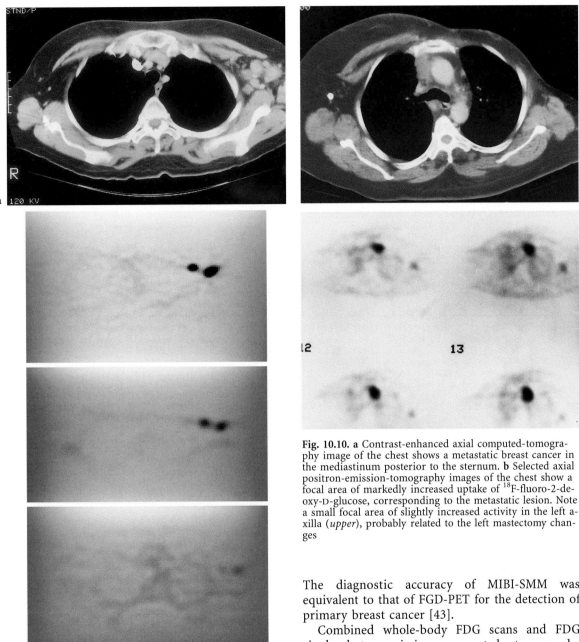

Fig. 10.9. a Contrast-enhanced axial computed-tomography image of the upper chest show several nodular metastatic lesions in the left axilla. **b** Selected axial positron-emission-tomography images before (*top*), 1 month after (*middle*) and 3 months after (*bottom*) preoperative chemotherapy show a significantly decreasing uptake of ^{18}F-fluoro-2-deoxy-D-glucose in two nodular metastatic lesions in the left axilla

Fig. 10.10. a Contrast-enhanced axial computed-tomography image of the chest shows a metastatic breast cancer in the mediastinum posterior to the sternum. **b** Selected axial positron-emission-tomography images of the chest show a focal area of markedly increased uptake of ^{18}F-fluoro-2-deoxy-D-glucose, corresponding to the metastatic lesion. Note a small focal area of slightly increased activity in the left axilla (*upper*), probably related to the left mastectomy changes

raphy. FDG-PET seems to be more sensitive than ^{99m}Tc methoxyisobutylisonitride- (MIBI) scintimammography (SMM) (5 mm) for the detection of in situ lymph-node metastasis of the axilla.

The diagnostic accuracy of MIBI-SMM was equivalent to that of FGD-PET for the detection of primary breast cancer [43].

Combined whole-body FDG scans and FDG single-photon-emission computed tomography (SPECT) with a dual-head gamma camera offers an attractive and practical alternative to FDG-PET. Low FDG uptake in tumors larger than 2–2.5 cm is not usually indicative of malignancy (Fig. 10.10). The lower spatial resolution of SPECT may be of minor importance if the FDG uptake is high even in small lesions [44].

PET was used to assess the clinical usefulness of ^{18}F fluorotamoxifen (FTX) in patients with estrogen-receptor-positive breast tumors. An 80% sensitivity was found for detecting breast cancers with a SUV of 3.0 [45]. Positive lesions on PET in a small number of patients had a good response to tamoxifen therapy, whereas negative lesions showed a poor response.

References

1. Landis SH, Murray T, Bolden S, Wingo PA (1998) Cancer statistics, 1998. CA Cancer J Clin 48:6–29
2. Morrison AS, Brisson J, Khalid N (1988) Breast cancer incidence and mortality in the breast cancer detection demonstration project. J Natl Cancer Inst 80:1540–1547
3. Kopan DB (1992) Positive predictive value of mammography. AJR Am J Roentgenol 158:521–526
4. Jackson VP, Hendrick RE, Karg SA (1993) Imaging of the radiographically dense breast. Radiology 198:297–301
5. Pollei SR, Mettler FA, Barstow SA, Moradian G, Moskowitz M (1987) Occult breast cancer: prevalence and radiographic detectability. Radiol 163:459–462
6. Shabot MM, Goldberg IM, Schick P, Nieberg R, Pilch YH (1982) Aspiration cytology is superior to Tru-Cut needle biopsy in establishing the diagnosis of clinically suspicious breast masses. Ann Surg 196:122–126
7. Dupont WD, Page DL (1985) Risk factors for breast cancer in women with proliferative breast disease. N Engl J Med 312:146–151
8. Schwartz GF, Feig SA, Patchefsky AS (1988) Significance and staging of nonpalpable carcinomas of the breast. Surg Gynecol Obstet 166:6–10
9. Rosen PP, Braun DW Jr, Lyngholm B, Urban JA, Kinne DW (1981) Lobular carcinoma in situ of the breast: preliminary results of treatment by ipsilateral mastectomy and contralateral breast biopsy. Cancer 47:813–819
10. Lagios MD, Westdahl PR, Margolin FR, Rose MR (1982) Duct carcinoma in situ: relationship of extent of noninvasive disease to the frequency of occult invasion, multicentricity, lymph node metastases, and short term failures. Cancer 50:1309–1314
11. Gump FR, Jicha DL, Ozzello L (1987) Ductal carcinoma in situ (DCIS): a revised concept. Surgery 102:190–195
12. Rosen PP, Groshen S, Saigo PE (1989) A long-term follow-up study of survival in stage I (T_1N0M0) and stage II (T_1N1M0) breast carcinoma. J Clin Oncol 7:355–366
13. McGuire WL, Clark GM (1992) Prognostic factors and treatment decisions in axillary-node-negative breast cancer. N Engl J Med 326:1756–1761
14. McGuire WL (1988) Estrogen receptor versus nuclear grade as prognostic factors in axillary node negative-breast cancer. J Clin Oncol 6:1071–1072
15. Clark GM, Mathieu M-C, Owens MA (1992) Prognostic significance of S-phase fraction in good-risk, node-negative breast cancer patients. J Clin Oncol 10:428–432
16. Remvikos Y, Beuzeboc A, Zajdela N (1989) Correlation of pre-treatment proliferation activity of breast cancer with the response to cytotoxic chemotherapy. J Natl Cancer Inst 81:1383–1387
17. Rav PM (1993) Evaluation of cathespin D as a prognostic factor in breast cancer. Breast Cancer Res Treat 24:219–226
18. Toikkanen S, Helin H, Isola (1992) Prognostic significance of HER-2 oncoprotein expression in breast cancer: a 30-year follow-up. J Clin Oncol 10:1044–1048
19. Weidner N, Folkman J, Pozza F (1992) Tumor angiogenesis is an independent prognostic indicator in early-stage breast carcinoma. J Natl Cancer Inst 84:1875–1887
20. Tondini C. Hayes DF, Gelman R (1988) Comparison of CA 15-3 and CEA in monitoring the clinical course of patients with metastatic breast cancer. Cancer Res 48:4107–4112
21. Cole-Beuglet C (1982) Sonographic manifestations of malignant breast disease. Semin Ultrasound CT MR 3:51–57
22. Harms SE, Flamig DP, Hesley KL (1993) MR imaging of the breast with rotating delivery of excitation off resonance: clinical experience with pathologic correlation. Radiology 187:493–501
23. Pierce WB, Harms SE, Flamig DP (1991) Three-dimensional gadolinium-enhanced MRI of the breast: pulse sequence with fat suppression and magnetization transfer contrast. Radiology 181:757–763
24. Harms SE, Flamig DP (1993) MR imaging of the breast. J Magn Reson Imaging 3:277–283
25. Heywang-Koebrunner SH, Viehweg P (1994) Sensitivity of contrast-enhanced MR imaging of the breast. Magn Reson Imaging Clin N Am 2:527–538
26. Piccoli CW (1994) The specificity of contrast-enhanced breast MR imaging. Magn Reson Imaging Clin N Am 2:557–571
27. Kaiser WA (1994) False-positive results in dynamic MR mammography. Magn Reson Imaging Clin N Am 2:539–555
28. Heywang-Koebrunner SH, Beck R, Lomatzsch B (1992) Contrast-enhanced MR imaging of the breast: survey of 1200 patient examinations. Radiology 1185:246
29. Glonek T (1978) Evidence supporting potassium ion-induced lengthening of phosphorus-31 nuclear magnetic resonance T_1 relaxation times in malignant tumors. Biochem Med 19:246–251
30. Merchant TE (1994) MR spectroscopy of the breast. Magn Reson Imaging Clin N Am 2:691–703
31. Ordidge RF, Connelly A, Lohman JAB (1986) Image-selected in vivo spectroscopy (ISIS). A new technique for spatially selective NMR spectroscopy. J Magn Reson 66:283–294
32. Merchant TE, Thelissen GRP, deGraaf PW (1991) Clinical magnetic resonance spectroscopy of human breast disease. Invest Radiol 26:1053–1059
33. Redmond OM, Stack JP, O'Conner NG (1991) In vivo phosphorus-31 magnetic resonance spectroscopy of normal and pathological breast tissues. Br J Radiol 64:210–216
34. Sijens PE, Wijrdeman Moerland MA, Bakker CJG (1988) Human breast cancer in vivo: H-1 and P-31 spectroscopy at 1.5 T. Radiology 169:615–620
35. Merchant TE, Characiejus D, Kasimos JN (1992) Phosphoryldiesters in human breast and colon cancer using ^{31}P magnetic resonance spectroscopy. Magn Reson Med 26:132–140
36. Merchant TE, Gierke LW, Meneses P (1988) ^{31}P magnetic resonance spectroscopic profiles of neoplastic human breast tissues. Cancer Res 48:5112–5118
37. Nieweg ON, Kim EE, Wong W-H (1993) Positron emission tomography with fluorine-18-deoxyglucose in the detection and staging of breast cancer. Cancer 71:3920–3925
38. Avril N, Dose J, Jänicke F (1996) Metabolic characterization of breast tumors with positron emission tomography using F-18 fluorodeoxyglucose. J Clin Oncol 14:1848–1857
39. Wahl RL, Zasadny K, Helvie M, Hutchins GD, Weber B, Cody R (1993) Metabolic monitoring of breast cancer chemohormonetherapy using positron emission tomography: initial evaluation. J Clin Oncol 11:2101–2111
40. Moon DH, Maddahi J, Silvermann DHS, Glaspy JA, Phelps ME, Hoh CK (1998) Accuracy of whole-body fluorine-18-FDG PET for the detection of recurrent or metastatic breast carcinoma. J Nucl Med 39:431–435
41. Avril N, Bense S, Ziegler SI, Dose J, Weber W, Laubenbacher C, Römer W, Jänicke F, Schwaiger M (1997)

Breast imaging with fluorine-18-FDG PET: quantitative image analysis. J Nucl Med 38:1186–1191

42. Bassa P, Kim EE, Inoue T, Wong FCL, Korkmaz M, Yang DJ, Wong WH, Hicks KW, Buzdar AU, Podoloff DA (1996) Evaluation of preoperative chemotherapy using PET with fluorine-18-fluorodeoxyglucose in breast cancer. J Nucl Med 37:931–938

43. Palmedo H, Bender H, Grünwald F, Mallmann P, Zamora P, Krebs D, Biersack HJ (1996) Comparison of fluorine-18-fluorodeoxyglucose positron emission tomography and technetium-99 m methoxyisobutylisonitrile scintimammography in the detection of breast tumors. Eur J Nucl Med 24:1138–1145

44. Holle L-H, Trampert L, Lung-Kurt S, Villena-Heinsen CE, Püschel W, Schmidt S, Oberhausen E (1996) Investigations of breast tumors with fluorine-18-fluorodeoxyglucose and SPECT. J Nucl Med 37:615–622

45. Inoue T, Kim EE, Wallace S, Yang DJ, Wong FCL, Bassa P, Cherif A, Delpassand E, Buzdar A, Podoloff DA (1996) Positron emission tomography using ^{18}F-fluorotamoxifen to evaluate therapeutic responses in patients with breast cancer: preliminary study. Cancer Biother Radiopharm 11:235–245

Gastrointestinal Carcinomas

E. E. Kim

Basic Considerations

Hepatocellular Carcinoma

Hepatocellular carcinoma (HCC) is one of the most common malignancies; it causes an estimated 1,250,000 deaths worldwide every year. Countries and populations are grouped according to incidence rates, i.e., high (20 or more per 100,000 males per year) in China and low (fewer than 5 per 100,000 males per year) in the United States [1]. The estimated new cases and deaths in the United States are 13,900 and 13,000, respectively, in 1998 [2]. Worldwide, HCC occurs in approximately three times as many males as females. The incidence increases with age. HCC is almost always associated with hepatitis B and C. Studies have shown integrated hepatitis-B-virus DNA in the livers of patients with chronic hepatitis and hepatocellular carcinoma [3]. Aflatoxin, a mycotoxin resulting from Aspergillus fungi, appears to be an important cocarcinogen in rural Africans [4]. In the West, HCC generally occurs in the setting of cirrhosis; 80–90% of cases are related to ethanol-induced cirrhosis.

Gastric Cancer

Despite an overall rise in the incidence of gastrointestinal malignancies in the United States, there has been a significant decrease in the incidence of gastric cancer over the past few decades. Gastric cancer remains the eighth leading cause of cancer death in the United States [2]. In 1998, an estimated 22,600 new cases of gastric cancer will occur in the United States, 14,300 of which will occur in males; approximately 13,700 patients will die of this cancer. The 5-year survival rate of less than 20% has not changed significantly during the past 30–40 years [2]. Countries such as Japan and Chile have incidence rates as high as 70–78 per 100,000 population, while the rate is only 10 per 100,000 persons in the United States [5]. Over the past 30 years, the incidence of gastric cancer in the United States has decreased by approximately 20%, whereas the mortality rate has decreased by 30% [5]. Chemical carcinogens have been thought to represent a major environmental etiological factor in the pathogenesis of gastric cancer. Increased consumption of processed, smoked, or salted meat and fish, which are high sources of N-nitroso compounds, is not consistently associated with an increased risk of gastric cancer [6]. Diets low in vegetables, fruits, milk and vitamin A, and high in fried food, processed meat, fish and alcohol have been associated with an increased risk of gastric cancer [7]. Studies have linked cigarette smoking with an increased risk of this cancer [8]. Gastric resection has been implicated as a predisposing factor for gastric cancer, probably due to duodenogastric bile reflux [9]. Intestinal metaplasia has a higher incidence of gastric cancer, and the risk is 20 times higher in patients with pernicious anemia [10]. It is hypothesized that early-life acquisition of Helicobacter pylori increases the risk of developing both gastric cancer and gastric ulcer [11].

Pancreatic Cancer

Pancreatic cancer is the second most common gastrointestinal cancer and the fourth leading cause of cancer death in the United States. It is estimated that 29,000 cases of pancreatic cancer will be diagnosed in the United States during 1998 [2], and 28,900 patients will die of this cancer. The median survival of patients is 3–4 months, and the 5-year survival rate is only 3% [5]. This cancer is usually advanced with obvious or occult metastases before a diagnosis is ever made. Risk increases after the age of 30 years, with most cases occurring between the ages of 65 years and 79 years [2]. The ratio of males to females affected differs according to age, varying from 2 for patients younger than 40 years of age, to 1, for patients older than 80 years. Pancreatic cancer is more common in Hispanic and African-American than in white populations. There is also an increased incidence among Jews and a lower mortality rate among Mormons [12]. Cigarette smoking has been associated with an increased risk of pancreatic carcinoma [13]. It has been postulated that the postgastrectomy achlorhydric environment favors the colonization of bacteria that reduce nitrate-containing compounds to carcinogenic N-nitroso compounds [14]. Calcifications associated with chronic pancreatitis have been found in 3% of patients with pancreatic cancer, and about 15% of pancreatic cancer patients are also diabetic [15].

Colorectal Cancer

In the United States, colorectal cancer is the second most common cause of cancer deaths after lung cancer [2]. Overall incidence for colorectal cancer has begun to drop [16], and the mortality rate has also begun to decline in whites [17]. Colorectal-cancer occurrence is nearly identical in males and females, with colon cancer seen slightly more often in females and rectal cancers seen slightly more in males. For persons under the age of 65 years, the incidence of colorectal cancer is 19.2 per 100,000; for those 65 years or older, it is 337 per 100,000 [2]. Colon carcinomas now constitute approximately 70% of all cancers in the large bowel, with the right side of the proximal colon the most common site [18]. The incidence of colon carcinomas in blacks has increased by 30% since 1973 and is now higher than in whites [2].

Research found that roughly 10% of large-bowel tumors may arise in persons with a genetic susceptibility to them [19]. Familial adenomatous polyposis (FAP) syndrome appears to be due to defects in a single gene, whereas defects in the hereditary nonpolyposis colorectal cancer (HNPCC) syndrome seem genetically heterogeneous. The most commonly affected oncogenes in the genesis of large-bowel tumors are c-myc and c-Ki-ras; those less frequently affected include c-src, c-myb, and c-erb-b2 [20]. FAP syndrome is the result of point mutations in the adenomatous polyposis coli (APC) tumor-suppressor gene, which is localized on chromosome 5 (5q21) [21]. Deletions and point mutations have been identified in a second gene on chromosome 5 – the mutated gene in colorectal carcinoma (MCC) [22] – and the deleted gene in colorectal cancer (DCC) on chromosome 18 is activated in 73% of colorectal cancers [23]. A deletion on chromosome 17 was also associated with point mutations in the p53 allele on the homologous chromosome [24]. A candidate for the HNPCC gene, called MSH-2, has been identified on chromosome 2 [25]. The incidence of colorectal carcinoma is higher in industrialized countries, and diets rich in fats and cholesterol have been linked to an increased risk of colorectal tumors [26]. Excess lipids in the colon may lead to an increase in the concentration of secondary bile acids, which may stimulate protein kinase C, a major cellular communication pathway, resulting in the promotion of cancer [27]. Human tumors have been shown to produce large amounts of prostaglandins, particularly E, which has been implicated in blocking natural killer-cell cytotoxicity; nonsteriodal anti-inflammatory drugs (NSAIDs) are known to inhibit the synthesis of prostaglandins and thus decrease the development of colonic polyps [28]. There is an approximate 5% probability that carcinoma will be present in an adenoma; the risk correlates with the histology and size of the polyp. Adenomatous polyps smaller than 1 cm have a less than 1% chance of being malignant compared with adenomas larger than 2 cm, which have up to a 40% likelihood of malignant transformation [29].

Pathology, Diagnosis and Staging

HCC occurs in two gross patterns – diffuse and nodular forms. The fibrolamellar variant is more frequent in females and has a better prognosis [30]. Invasion of the portal vein has been found in 14% of patients when the cancer was smaller than 2 cm and in 71% when the cancer was larger than 5 cm. These thrombi may involve the hepatic vein, vena cava, and portal vein [31].

About one-third of HCC patients are asymptomatic, and the most common symptoms are abdominal pain (90%), ascites, weight loss, weakness, fullness and anorexia, vomiting, and jaundice (7%). Metastatic disease can present as malignant ascites, skeletal pain, dyspnea, and neurological abnormalities [32]. Hepatomegaly occurs in 50–90% of HCC patients. A number of paraneoplastic syndromes have been reported in association with HCC. They include hypoglycemia, erythrocytosis, hypercalcemia, hypercholesterolemia, carcinoid syndrome, dysfibrinogenemia, sexual changes, and increased thyroxin-binding globulin. Elevated levels of alkaline phosphatase, transaminases, and bilirubin are present in about 50% of patients and predict a short survival [33]. Although alpha fetoprotein (AFP) levels are elevated in germ-cell tumors and during pregnancy, the immunoassay will detect 70–90% of all HCCs [34]. Reports have associated normal levels of AFP with improved survival [34].

Hepatocellular carcinomas are best visualized on computed tomography (CT), which can de-

Table 11.1. TNM evaluation for hepatic cancer

T (primary tumor)	
Tx	Cannot be assessed
T0	No evidence
T1	≤2 cm without vascular invasion
T2	≤2 cm with vascular invasion, or >2 cm solitary without vascular invasion, or ≤2 cm multiple in one lobe
T3	>2 cm with vascular invasion, or £2 cm multiple in one lobe with vascular invasion, or >2 cm multiple with or without vascular invasion
T4	Multiple in more than one lobe or involving portal or hepatic vein
N (lymph node)	
NX	Cannot be assessed
N0	No metastasis
N1	Regional node metastasis
M (distant metastasis)	
MX	Cannot be assessed
M0	No metastasis
M1	Distant metastasis
M1a	Nonregional node
M1b	Bone
M1c	Other sites

Table 11.2. TNM staging for hepatic tumors

Stage I	T1, N0, M0
Stage II	T2, N0, M0
Stage III	T1 or T2, N1, M0
	T3, N0 or N1, M0
Stage IVA	T4, any N, M0
Stage IVB	any T, any N, M1

Table 11.3. TNM staging for gastric cancer

T (primary tumor)	
Tx	Cannot be assessed
T0	No evidence
Tis	In situ
T1	Lamina propria or submucosa
T2	Muscularis or subserosa
T3	Muscularis propria
T4	Adjacent structures
N (regional node)	
NX	Cannot be assessed
N0	No metastasis
N1	Perigastric mode within 3 cm
N2	Perigastric node more than 3 cm, or left gastric, common hepatic, splenic or celiac
M (distant metastasis)	
MX	Cannot be assessed
M0	No metastasis
M1	Distant metastasis
Stage 0	Tis, N0, M0
Stage IA	T1, N0, M0
Stage IB	T1, N1, M0
	T2, N0, M0
Stage II	T1, N2, M0
	T2, N1, M0
	T3, N0, M0
Stage IIIA	T2, N2, M0
	T3, N1, M0
	T4, N0, M0
Stage IIIB	T3, N2, M0
	T4, N1, M0
Stage IV	T4, N2, M0
	Any T, any N, M1

monstrate tumors larger than 1 cm and may identify compression or invasion of the portal or hepatic veins. Ultrasonography (US) is inexpensive, but the hyperechoic HCC may lead to confusion with benign as well as metastatic tumors. Laparoscopy is more invasive, but it allows for a percutaneous needle biopsy under direct vision. Fine-needle aspiration cytology and core-needle biopsy may be performed, directed by US or CT.

The staging (Table 11.2) of hepatic tumors follows the TNM system (Table 11.1). More than 95% of gastric cancers are adenocarcinomas; the remaining 5% consist of lymphomas, leiomyosarcomas, and carcinoid tumors [35]. Gastric cancer is characterized by intestinal and diffuse histopathologic patterns. It tends to invade through the gastric wall early and can involve adjacent structures. The commonly involved lymph nodes are those in the gastrohepatic ligament, celiac, and gastroduodenal region. A common site of peritoneal seeding is Blumer's rectal shelf. The liver is the most common site of hematogenous metastasis, followed by the lungs and bones.

More than one-third of *gastric cancers* present as ulcers and show extensive submucosal infiltration that often involves the serosa. One-quarter of the tumors are scirrhous, with diffuse infiltration, leading to a marked fibrotic reaction. The 5-year survival rate for patients with scirrhous cancer after resection is only 2% [36].

TNM staging for gastric cancer (Table 11.3) has been the most important guide to prognosis. Lesions in the cardia or esophagogastric junction have a poorer prognosis than more distal lesions [37]. Speculation is that the decrease in distal gastric cancer might be linked to a decrease in the rate of H. pylori gastritis. The histologic grade provides no additional prognostic information to the TNM stage.

Pancreatic cancer arises from both the exocrine and endocrine parenchyma of the pancreas, and approximately 95% of pancreatic cancers occur within the exocrine portion of the pancreas. The most common pancreatic cancer is a ductal adenocarcinoma which accounts for about 80% of all pancreatic cancers. Most carcinomas arise in the proximal portion of the pancreas, 20% arise in the body and 5–10% in the tail [37].

Up to 85% of patients with pancreatic cancer have clinically obvious metastases or micrometastases upon presentation. The common sites of metastases are the liver, peritoneum, lymph nodes, and lungs. Two-thirds of patients experience

Table 11.4. TNM staging of pancreatic cancer

T (primary tumor)	
Tx	Cannot be assessed
T0	No evidence
T1	Limited to pancreas
T1a	≤2 cm
T1b	>2 cm
T2	Extends to duodenum, bile duct or peripancreatic tissue
T3	Extends to stomach, spleen, colon, or large vessel
N (regional node)	
NX	Cannot be assessed
N0	No metastasis
N1	Regional nodal metastasis
M (distant metastasis)	
MX	Cannot be assessed
M0	No metastasis
M1	Distant metastasis
Stage I	T1 or T2, N0, M0
Stage II	T3, N0, M0
Stage III	Any T, N1, M0
Stage IV	Any T, any N, M1

symptoms for at least 2 months before the diagnosis is made. Weight loss, often gradual and progressive, is one of the earliest and most frequently unappreciated symptoms. Abdominal pain, the most common symptom, is due to local tumor infiltration into the retroperitoneum and splanchnic nerve plexus. Biliary, gastric-outlet or duodenal obstruction are secondary to local-tumor invasion. Other findings include a palpable gall bladder (Courvoisier's sign), splenomegaly, venous thrombosis and migratory thrombophlebitis (Trousseau's sign). CT of the abdomen is the most useful procedure for diagnosis and staging. However, not all pancreatic carcinomas are observed as masses, and not all masses are pancreatic carcinomas. A review of 100 cases of pancreatic carcinoma showed a false-negative range for CT of only 5% [38]. US may be more accurate than CT in distinguishing obstructive from nonobstructive jaundice for the patient presenting with jaundice. Endoscopic retrograde cholangiopancreatography (ERCP) has high sensitivity (94%) in diagnosing pancreatic cancer and also permits the aspiration of pancreatic secretions for cytologic examination or the measurement of K-ras oncogene from the bile.

The most commonly used staging for pancreatic cancer is the TNM system (Table 11.4) and only stage I, localized within the pancreatic capsule, is amenable to resection.

In *colorectal cancer*, the tumor's gross appearance is ulcerative and/or stenosing in about 75% of the cases (left-sided) and fungating in 25% of the cases (right-sided). Adenocarcinomas make up 90–95% of all large-bowel tumors [39]. Mucinous adenocarcinoma is a histologic variant which occurs more often in males and is more frequently diagnosed when the disease is advanced [40]. Signet-ring cell carcinoma is another variant which is more common in young females and tends to have a particularly poor prognosis [40]. Carcinoid tumors, squamous cell carcinomas, adenosquamous, undifferentiated carcinomas, sarcomas, and lymphomas have been reported [41, 42]. Broders and Dukes classify colorectal carcinomas based on the degree of differentiation. Broder's system has four grades, and Dukes' system considers the arrangement of the cells rather than the percentage of differentiated cells. Dukes' system has three grades, with grade I the most differentiated tumors and grade III the least differentiated [39]. Five-year survival rates of 56–100%, 33–80%, and 11–58% have been reported for grades I, II, and III colorectal tumors, respectively [41]. Colorectal cancer has a tendency for local invasion by circumferential growth and for lymphatic, hematogeneous, transperitoneal, and perineural spread. The common metastatic sites are liver, lungs, bones, kidneys, adrenals, and brain. During the early stages, patients may complain of vague abdominal pain and flatulence. Minor changes in bowel movements with or without rectal bleeding are seen. Cancers on the left side of the colon generally cause constipation; anemia resulting from chronic blood loss may accompany right-sided colon carcinoma. Patients presenting with obstruction and perforation have a poorer prognosis [43]. Many fecal occult blood tests (FOBTs) use guaiac, which detects the peroxidase-like capacity of hemoglobin. Digital rectal examination can detect lesions up to 7 cm from the anal verge.

Almost 50% of all colorectal tumors are within reach of a 60-cm sigmoidoscope. Colonoscopy can be used to obtain biopsy specimens of adenomas and carcinomas, and allows excision of adenomatous polyps. Barium enemas are accurate in detecting colorectal carcinoma and viewed as complementary to colonoscopy. Endoscopic US has improved the accuracy of preoperative tumor and node staging in rectal cancer. In a study of 155 patients with colorectal cancer, immunoscintigraphy using ^{111}In CYT-103 or ^{99m}Tc-anti-carcinoembryonic antigen (CEA) and CT demonstrated similar sensitivities (69% and 68%, respectively) and specificity (77%). Although CT was able to detect a great proportion of liver metastasis (84% vs 41%), immunoscintigraphy showed greater sensitivity in detecting pelvic tumors and extrahepatic abdominal metastases (84% vs 41%) [44].

Of the three staging systems, the modified Astler-Coller (MAC) system is the most widely used

Table 11.5. Staging for colorectal cancer

Modified Astler-Coller (MAC)	Dukes	TNM	
A	A	I:	Tis, N0, M0
B1			T1 or 2, N0, M0
B2	B	II:	T3 or 4a, N0, M0
B3			T4b, N0, M0
C1	C	III:	T1 or 2, N1 or 2 or 3, M0
C2			T3 or 4a, N1 or 2, or 3, M0
C3			T4b, N1 or 2 or 3, M0
D	D	IV:	Any T, any N, M1

Tis, in situ; T1, submucosa; T2, muscularis propria; T3, subserosa or nonperitoneal pericolic or perirectal tissue; T4a, visceral peritoneum; T4b, other organs; N0, no node metastasis; N1, 1~3 pericolic or perirectal nodes; N2, >4 nodes; N3, node along the trunk; M0, no distant metastases; M1, distant metastasis

in the United States (Table 11.5). The prognosis for early (I and II) stages is favorable overall, in contrast to the prognosis for advanced (III and IV) stages [41]. Patients without symptoms tend to have better prognoses, but rectal bleeding has been associated with better survival [45]. Rectal tumors have a poorer prognosis than colon tumors. The 18q chromosome deletion has also been associated with a poorer prognosis [41].

Clinical Applications

In view of the many imaging modalities, each with its own strengths and weaknesses, oncologists can be overwhelmed by the choices in a particular clinical setting and find it difficult to determine what significance to place on the data obtained. Arguments over the relative merits of imaging techniques have tended to be overstated. Parallel use of different diagnostic modalities is costly and inefficient.

US is well established as an invaluable technique that is cheap, quick, and portable. Aided by color and duplex Doppler, vascular involvement and hemodynamic information can be obtained. US also provides a simple method for biopsies and drainage procedures. Its limitations are its nonspecificity for focal lesions and a lack of sensitivity for diffuse liver lesions and extrahepatic disease.

Helical-CT techniques have improved small-lesion detection and also have enabled some degree of lesion characterization with its multiphase scanning capability. Volumetric data acquisition enables three-dimensional (3D) reconstruction, both of vascular anatomy and for demonstrating lesion location, but is time-consuming. Its superior ability to document extrahepatic disease ensures its vital role in the staging process. Currently, CT arterioportography (CTAP) (along with intraoperative US) seems the most sensitive method of staging patients with focal hepatic metastases, but it is an invasive procedure and has a significant false-positive rate due to inhomogeneous perfusion [46].

Magnetic Resonance Imaging

Magnetic resonance imaging (MRI) represents a powerful imaging tool, with its high inherent soft-tissue contrast resolution, technical versatility for sequence selection and modification, provision of biochemical as well as anatomic information, multiplanar imaging, intrinsic sensitivity to blood flow and blood-breakdown products, and lack of ionizing radiation. MRI has taken longer to find its role in hepatic imaging and has been regarded more as a problem-solving technique, to be used when CT and US are unable to provide a complete answer to a particular clinical problem or when alternative imaging is contraindicated.

It has been suggested that dynamic post-contrast MRI is superior to helical CT in detection of HCC in patients with chronic liver disease [47]. Gadolinium-diethylenetriaminepentaacetic acid does increase the conspicuity of the lesions seen on precontrast scans, but its main role is in helping with lesion characterizations. HCC may have a variety of signal patterns on T_1- and T_2-weighted images. The most frequent appearance is slightly low signal on T_1-weighted images and moderately high signal on T_2-weighted images (Fig. 11.1) [48]. High signal on T_1-weighted images on occasion is due to fat, copper, copper-binding protein or high protein content. HCC is frequently hypervascular and enhances in a diffuse heterogeneous fashion. HCC typically demonstrates enhancing stroma throughout the entire tumor on capillary phase images from dynamic contrast studies, whereas metastasis has a peripheral enhancement [49]. Hypovascular tumors are variable in signal on T_1-weighted images, but near isointense on T_2-weighted images, and these tumors are frequently well differentiated [50]. In patients with cirrhosis, mass lesions with high signal intensity on T_2-weighted images that are not cysts or hemangiomas should be considered HCC (Fig. 11.2). Any mass lesion that enhances in a diffuse heterogeneous fashion immediately following gadolinium injection should be considered as a possible HCC. Large-HCC extension into portal or hepatic veins is ob-

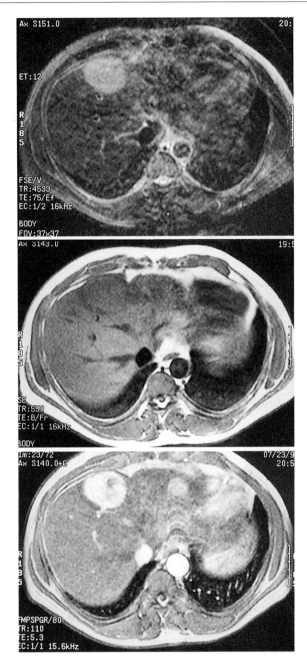

Fig. 11.1. Hepatoma in the superior segment of the right hepatic lobe is noted with slightly low signal intensity on T_1-weighted axial (*middle*), high signal intensity on T_2-weighted axial (*top*) and contrast enhancement on postgadolinium T_1-weighted axial images of the upper abdomen (*bottom*)

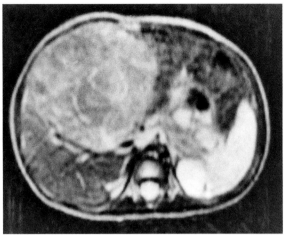

Fig. 11.2. T_2-weighted axial image of the upper abdomen shows a large hepatoblastoma with heterogeneous intermediate and high signal intensity in the right hepatic lobe

served in less than 50% of cases, and pseudocapsules observed in early or well-differentiated HCC have an increased enhancement on delayed images of dynamic study [51]. Well-differentiated HCC may take up more manganese-dipyridoxyl diphosphate (Mn-DPDP) than surrounding liver, reflecting persistent hepatocellular function with decreased biliary clearance [52].

Metastatic liver lesions vary in appearance on T_1- and T_2-weighted images and are frequently irregular (Fig. 11.3). They do not have the classical enhancement patterns of benign lesions [no enhancement with cysts, peripheral nodular enhancement with hemangioma, transient immediate blush with focal nodular hyperplasia (FNH) or adenoma]. The most common enhancement pattern is an immediate peripheral ring of enhancement, and it often progresses centrally [53]. Metastasis from colorectal cancer typically shows a cauliflower-type appearance, and perilesional enhancement is common with colon- and pancreatic-cancer metastasis. Metastases may undergo hemorrhaging, and central coagulation necrosis in colorectal metastasis produces a low signal on T_2-weighted images. Melanoma metastases are usually a mixture of high and low signals on T_1- and T_2-weighted images due to paramagnetic melanin or hemorrhaging (Fig. 11.4). Mucin-producing tumors also produce a high signal on T_1-weighted images due to protein content. Hypovascular metastases from colorectal cancer, transitional cell cancer, and lymphoma are generally low in signal on T_1- and T_2-weighted images, and most conspicuous on the portal phase images of dynamic contrast studies. Hypervascular metastases from renal cancer, carcinoid, islet cell tumor, leiomyosarcoma and melanoma are generally high in signal on T_2-weighted images and possess a peripheral immediate enhancement with a thick irregular rim [54] (Fig. 11.5).

Hemangiomas are low in signal intensity on T_1-weighted images, high in signal on T_2-

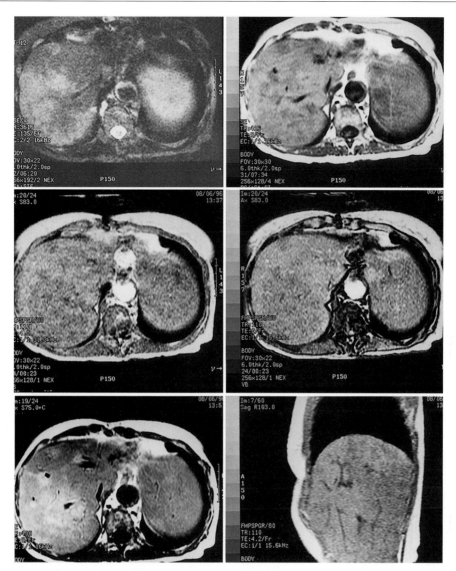

Fig. 11.3. Axial T_2- (*top left*), T_1- (*top right*), gradient echo- (*middle*) and post-gadolinium (*bottom*) T_1-weighted images show multiple hepatic metastases of primary unknown cancer with irregular focal areas of intermediate-signal intensity on T_1-weighted images, heterogeneous high signal intensity on T_2-weighted images and also contrast enhancement

weighted images and maintain signal on long (>120 ms) echo time. Three types of enhancement patterns are observed: uniform immediate enhancement (type I), peripheral nodular enhancement with centripetal uniform progression (type II), and peripheral nodular enhancement with centripetal progression with central scar (type III). Type I is usually observed only in small (<1.5 cm) hemangiomas, and type III is seen in large tumors [55]. MRI of hepatic adenoma shows a variable signal intensity due to fat or hemorrhage on T_1-weighted images and mild hyperintensity on T_2-weighted images. Tumors may lose signal on out-of-phase or fat-suppressed images because of the fat. They have a transient immediate blush with contrast agents which fades by 1 min and they take up Mn-DPDP. FNH shows slight hypointensity on T_1-weighted images and slight hyperintensity on T_2-weighted images. High-signal central scar on T_2-weighted images is observed in 10–49% of patients [56]. FNH has an intense uniform immediate blush, which rapidly (usually at 1 min) fades, and the central scar gradually enhances to hyperintensity. Many gastric cancers are higher in signal than the background stomach on T_2-weighted images, but scirrhous cancers are low-signal because of desmoplastic hypovascularity. Irregularity or loss of the

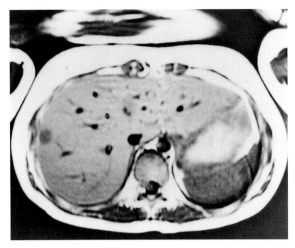

Fig. 11.4. Axial T_1-weighted image of the upper abdomen following the injection of manganese agent shows a small metastatic lesion of breast cancer in the periphery of right hepatic lobe with intermediate signal intensity

fying contiguous spread and intraperitoneal metastasis.

Pancreatic adenocarcinomas on T_1-weighted images are masses with low signal intensity. Contrast between tumor and normal pancreas is accentuated on images with fat suppression. The cancer is depicted as a low-signal defect within the pancreas. The cancers are less vascular than normal pancreas in capillary-phase images of dynamic studies. Many adenocarcinomas enhance greatly on MR images 1 min or more after injection of gadolinium, and enhance to a lesser extent than normal on inflamed pancreatic tissue due to the desmoplastic fibrotic composition. Chronic pancreatitis enhances more than carcinoma [58].

On MRCP images, dilated common bile and pancreatic ducts are demonstrated. Vascular patency may be evaluated by a flow-sensitive gradient-echo technique or dynamic contrast imaging. Pancreatic cancer has a tendency to invade along perivascular, lymphatic, and perineural pathways. While pancreatitis usually spares the fat surrounding these vessels, superior mesenteric artery and celiac axis fat may be obliterated by pancreatic cancers. Pancreatic islet-cell tumors are low in signal intensity on T_1-weighted fat-suppressed images and high in signal intensity on T_2-

low-signal-intensity band that normally surrounds the stomach implies extraserosal disease. This finding had a 97% sensitivity, a 79% specificity, and an accuracy of 92% [57]. Fat suppression with intravenous gadolinium is useful for identi-

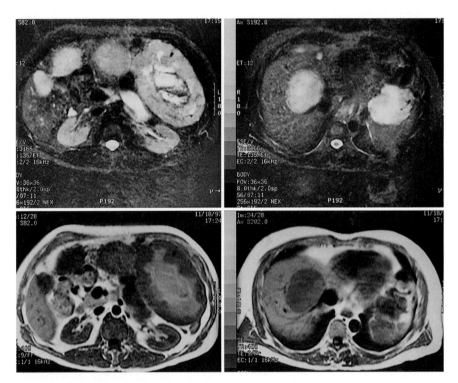

Fig. 11.5. T_2- (*upper*) and T_1- (*lower*) weighted images of the upper abdomen show a large metastatic lesion in the hepatic dome indenting the hepatic vein. Note also multiple peritoneal implants of leiomyosarcoma of the small bowel. Tumors show heterogeneous intermediate signal intensity on T_1-weighted images and high signal intensity on T_2-weighted images

weighted fat-suppressed images; they show ring or homogenous enhancement on immediate post-gadolinium images.

Studies have reported good correlation between gadolinium-enhanced, fat-suppressed MRI and surgical findings of colon-cancer size, bowel-wall involvement, peritumoral extension, and lymph-node involvement [59]. It has been shown that MRI outperforms conventional CT and is more specific than transrectal US for identifying recurrent rectal cancers (83.2% vs 41.6%) [60]. Recurrent cancer is low in signal intensity on T_1-weighted images and brighter in signal intensity on T_2-weighted images. It demonstrates a contrast enhancement, whereas post-treatment fibrosis 12 months postsurgery remains low in signal intensity and negligible in contrast enhancement. Granulation tissue and inflammation may parallel the signal intensity of recurrent cancer, which may be considered if the patient presents with presacral pain or elevated CEA level.

Magnetic Resonance Spectroscopy

A ^{31}P MR spectrum from a healthy liver exhibits resonances from nucleotide triphosphates (primarily ATP), inorganic phosphate (Pi), phosphomonoesters (PME) and phosphodiesters (PDE) (Fig. 11.6) [61]. The major contributors to the PME peak are phosphorylcholine (PC) and phosphorylethanolamine (PE), followed by sugar phosphates, such as fructose-1-phosphate and 3-phosphorylglycerate. The a-adenosine triphosphate (ATP) resonance has about a 20% contribution from nicotinamide adenine dinucleotides (NAD/NADH and their phosphates). Liver, in contrast to brain and muscle, has no phosphocreatine (PCr) because it lacks creatine kinase. Thus, the absence of a PCr peak at 0 ppm, characteristic of muscle, confirms good localization within the liver. Intracellular pH in normal hepatic tissue, calculated from the chemical shift of Pi, varies between 7.2 and 7.4 [62]. Intracellular [Mg^{2+}], estimated from the difference in chemical shift between the a- and β-ATP resonances, is about 0.6 mM [63]. T_1 of ^{31}P measured in healthy livers at 1.5 to 2.1 Tesla strengts vary between 0.8 s and 3 s for PME, 1.4 s and 6 s for PDE, 0.3 s and 0.4 s for ATP and are about 1 s for Pi. These figures were used to calculate molar concentrations of hepatic metabolites [64]. The metabolite concentrations in mmol/kg wet weight are as follows: ATP=2.0±0.1, Pi=2.22±0.4, PME=0.8±0.4 and PDE=5.3±1.9 (mean±SD). Liver-biopsy data tend to overestimate Pi content due to hydrolysis prior to freezing. The calculation of metabolite concentrations

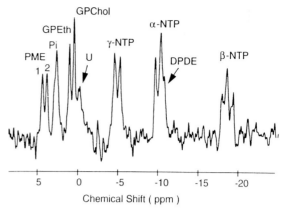

Fig. 11.6. ^{31}P nuclear magnetic resonance spectrum using 3-D chemical-shift imaging of liver of a fasting normal human subject. Peak 1 in the phosphomonoester (PME) region contains phosphoethanolamine (PEth) and adenosine monophosphate (AMP) at 4.2 ppm. Peak 2 contains phosphocholine (PChol) and diphosphoglycerate (DPG) at 3.9 ppm. The inorganic-phosphate (Pi) peak at 2.7 ppm corresponds to an intracellular pH of 7.36. The peaks in the phosphodiester (PDE) region are glycerophosphoethanolamine (GPEth) at 1.0 ppm, glycerophosphocholine (GPChol) at 0.5 ppm, and an unknown peak (U) at 0 ppm. Phosphocreatine (PCr) is not present in the liver. The nucleoside triphosphates (NTP) include adenosine-, cytosine-, guanosine-, thymidine-, and uridine-triphosphates, all of which overlay one another. Diphosphodiesters (DPDE) appear on the upfield side of the a-NTP peak (reprinted with permission from [61])

depends critically upon the determined T_1 and often also T_2 relaxation times of the metabolites. Metabolite concentrations measured in viral hepatitis B were normal except for very high PME [64, 65]. The high PME levels detected in diffuse liver disease are probably due to relatively high concentrations of PE and/or PC, compounds involved in phospholipid biosynthesis, and indicate structural damage. In a patient with glycogen-storage disease, hepatic ^{31}P spectra displayed reduced Pi and ATP levels, and a relatively strong resonance in the PME region due to sugar phosphates [66]. High sugar phosphates indicate a metabolic disorder. Alcoholic cirrhosis patients showed a comparatively high concentration of PC to the PME resonance, while alcoholic hepatitis patients showed a significant sugar-phosphate contribution to the PME peak. A large reduction of absolute signal intensity in all image-selected in vivo spectroscopy (ISIS) spectra from patients with alcoholic liver disease was noted [64].

Calculated hepatic phosphorus metabolite concentrations in alcoholic hepatitis patients were significantly decreased by 31–46%, whereas the decrease in the alcoholic cirrhosis group was between 18% and 50%. The most likely reason for such a decrease is loss of hepatocytes due to ne-

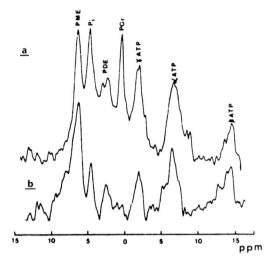

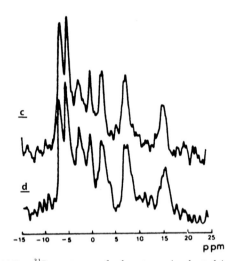

Fig. 11.7 a ^{31}P spectrum of a hepatoma implanted in a rat shows a strong phosphocreatine (PCr) signal. **b** The spectrum after stripping the skin shows the loss of PCr, probably due to the ischemia by the process. **c, d** In a similar experiment with a prolactinoma, skin stripping did not remove the PCr signal (reprinted with permission from [69])

crosis, and/or diffuse replacement of hepatocytes with fat or collagen. Hepatic pH was significantly higher in alcoholic hepatitis and lower in alcoholic cirrhosis compared with normal controls. The elevated hepatic pH in alcoholic hepatitis may indicate cell regeneration, impaired urea synthesis and/or low rate of glycolysis, producing less lactate [67]. The low pH in a cirrhotic liver may reflect the loss of capability of a great portion of the liver to regenerate and may be due to decreased oxidative metabolism and/or increased glycolysis leading to lactic acidosis [68]. Quantitative ^{31}P MRS may be used to distinguish between viral and alcoholic hepatitis since viral hepatitis B has been shown to be characterized by elevated PME [66]. Increased PME/ATP ratio in cirrhotic liver patients may indicate the proportion of fibrous tissue relative to functioning hepatocytes.

^{31}P MRS has a relatively poor spatial resolution (8–27 cm^3) which has limited its application to large tumors. The higher sensitivity of water-suppressed ^{1}H MRS provides a considerable advantage for tumor application at a spatial resolution of as small as 0.2 cm^3 using multivoxel chemical-shift imaging (Fig. 11.7) [69].

^{13}C MRS was used to observe hepatic glycogen formation in men after oral and intravenous glucose administration [70]. While the administration of ^{13}C-enriched glucose increased the signal-to-noise ratio of ^{13}C spectra, it was shown that unlabeled glucose can be used to measure the average liver glycogen concentration in fasted volunteers.

Wolf et al. [71] documented that ^{19}F NMR spectroscopy allows a determination of the metabolic time course of fluorinated drugs in patients with hepatic cancer (Fig. 11.8).

Positron Emission Tomography

Several authors have demonstrated the high sensitivity and specificity, usually greater than 90%, of 2-[^{18}F]-fluoro-2-deoxy-D-glucose positron emission tomography (FDG-PET) in detection of a variety of tumors, including primary and metastatic hepatic cancers (Fig. 11.9) [72, 73]. FDG-PET using modern scanners has the ability to depict small (5–7 mm in diameter) tumors by virtue of increased metabolic rate. Whole-body FDG-PET in a recent report [73] depicted all known intraluminal carcinomas in 37 patients, including two in situ carcinomas (100% sensitivity), but four false-positive findings (three with inflammatory bowel disease, one after recent polypectomy) were noted. In these studies they obtained specificity of 43% (three of seven patients), and 90% positive-predictive value (37 of 41 patients) as well as 100% negative-predictive value (three of three patients). No FDG accumulation was noted in 35 hyperplastic polyps. FDG-PET depicted lymph-node metastases in 4 of 14 patients (29% sensitivity) and hepatic metastases in 7 of 8 patients (88% sensitivity). CT sensitivities for detecting lymph-node and hepatic metastases were 29% and 38%, respectively. FDG-PET and CT correctly depicted the absence of hepatic metastases in 35 and 32 patients, respectively (100% and 97% specificity, respectively). These results are in agreement with those reported previously by others [74]. The low sensitivity of FDG-PET to accurately detect lymph-node metastases is not sig-

Fig. 11.8. Serial ^{19}F magnetic resonance spectra with a surface coil over the liver in a patient receiving 5-fluorouracil (FU) chemotherapy show increasing amounts of α-fluoro-β-alanine (FBAL), a major catabolite of 5-FU at -18.84 ppm (reprinted with permission from [71])

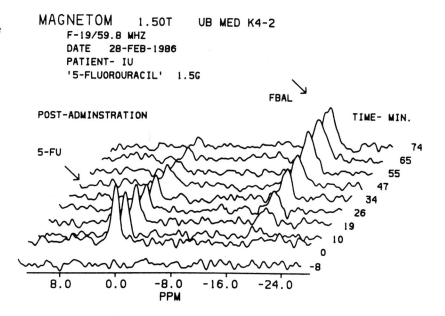

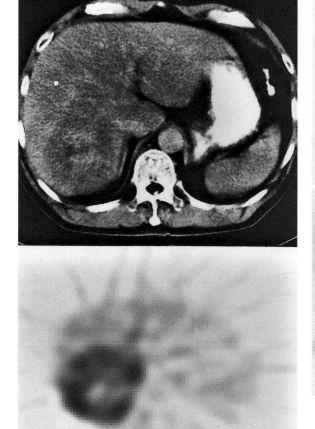

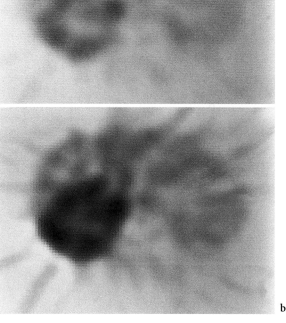

Fig. 11.9. a Contrast-computed-tomography axial image of the upper abdomen (*upper*) shows an ill-defined hepatoma in the posterior segment of right hepatic lobe. Comparable positron-emission tomography (PET) axial image (*lower*) following the injection of ^{18}F-fluoro-2-deoxy-D-glucose (FDG) through the intrahepatic arterial catheter shows a markedly increased activity in the rim of necrotic hepatoma. **b** Axial PET images of the upper abdomen following the injection of ^{18}F FDG in the rim of necrotic hepatoma by intravenous (*upper*) and intra-arterial (*lower*) injections. This patient had a good response to the intra-arterial chemotherapy

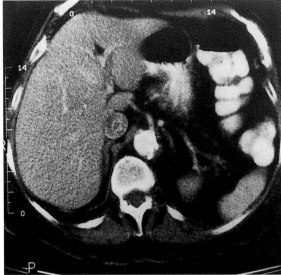

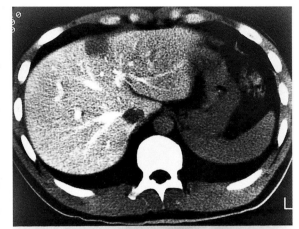

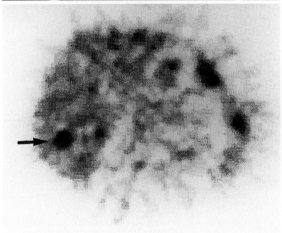

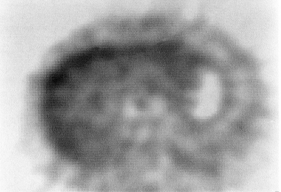

Fig. 11.11. Contrast-computed-tomography axial image of the upper abdomen (*upper*) shows a focal fat deposit in the right hepatic lobe in a patient with colon cancer. Comparable positron-emission tomography image (*lower*) shows no focal area of abnormally increased uptake of ^{18}F-fluoro-2-deoxy-D-glucose. No metastasis was found by subsequent magnetic resonance imaging or ultrasound examinations

Fig. 11.10. a,b Axial contrast computed-tomography image was interpreted as normal. Comparable positron-emission tomography image shows a metastatic lesion (*arrow*) with markedly increased uptake of ^{18}F-fluoro-2-deoxy-D-glucose in the right hepatic lobe (reprinted with permission from [75])

nificantly different from the CT sensitivity, and the limited resolution of FDG-PET is probably a problem for small metastatic nodes. The ability of FDG-PET to detect subclinical hepatic metastases not appreciated at preoperative CT and undetected during surgical exploration could have a direct effect on surgical approach and patient management. If confirmed in a large number of patients, FDG-PET could replace CT as the first screening procedure in routine liver evaluation, and save at least $445 per patient [74]. ^{18}F FDG-PET was more accurate (92%) than CT and CT portography (78% and 80%, respectively) in detecting hepatic metastases and more accurate than CT for extrahepatic metastases (92% and 71%, respectively) in 52 colorectal-cancer patients with 166 suspicious lesions (Figs. 11.10 and 11.11) [75]. Outside the liver, FDG-PET was especially helpful in detecting nodal metastases and differentiating local recurrence form post-treatment changes.

Many studies conclude that FDG-PET should be considered as a screening method in staging patients considered for resection of metastases. The PET findings should guide the performance, increase specificity of CT and CT portography and help to identify patients with resectable disease. PET may also be useful in the evaluation of therapeutic responses for malignant tumors in the abdomen (Figs. 11.9, 11.12–11.16). The limitations of PET include the lack of detection of some tiny metastases and possible false positives in lesions containing activated macrophages. Although PET has been increasingly used to obtain quantitative data about the metabolism of malignant lesions,

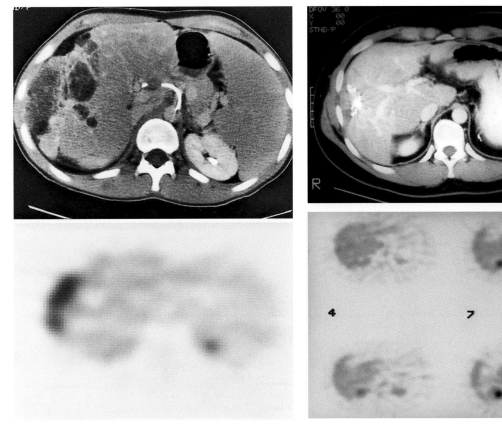

Fig. 11.12. Contrast-computed-tomography axial image of the upper abdomen (*upper*) shows a large irregular necrotic hepatoma after intra-arterial chemotherapy. Comparable positron-emission tomography image (*lower*) shows a slightly increased uptake of ^{18}F-fluoro-2-deoxy-D-glucose only in the lateral margin of the tumor

Fig. 11.13. a. Contrast-computed-tomography axial image of the upper abdomen shows a questionable lesion adjacent to the surgical-clip artifacts for metastatic colon cancer in the right hepatic lobe. **b** Selected positron-emission tomography axial image of the upper abdomen shows no significantly increased uptake of ^{18}F-fluoro-2-deoxy-D-glucose. No tumor was subsequently found

little is known about the use of radiolabeled drugs.

PET has been helpful in differentiating recurrent tumor from scar. In 33 patients with recurrent colorectal cancer, all tumors except one showed high FDG uptake, while FDG uptake was low in the scar area (Fig. 11.17). PET accurately characterized areas of residual or recurrent rectosigmoid cancer in 17 patients (Fig. 11.18) [76]. FDG uptake in recurrent rectal cancer does not decrease significantly within 3 months of radiation therapy [77]. FDG uptake resulting from radiation therapy is probably due to an inflammatory reaction. Only 50% of patients who were thought to have a palliative response had a decrease of FDG uptake in 6 months [78]. PET was more sensitive than CEA measurements for determining tumor recurrence.

In contrast to FDG, radiolabeled cytostatic drugs provide a direct measurement of the distribution of a chemotherapeutic agent in the target area. Therefore, chemotherapy management can be optimized either using metabolic studies with FDG or cytostatic agents [76]. Dynamic PET and ^{18}F-fluorouracil (FU) were used in patients with hepatic metastases from colorectal cancer to examine the pharmacokinetics of the drug up to 120 min after intravenous and intra-arterial injection of the same dose of FU. Dynamic PET studies lasting up to 5 min with ^{15}O-labeled water were performed immediately prior to the FU study. Hepatic metastases from colorectal cancer reached the highest ^{18}F FU concentrations after intra-arterial administration, with a maximum standard uptake value of 18.75 for the FU influx and of 5.03 for FU trapping [79]. Cluster analysis revealed a group of metastases with a nonperfusion-dependent FU transport using the intravenous application, and most of them did not show any enhancement of ^{18}F FU after intra-arterial application.

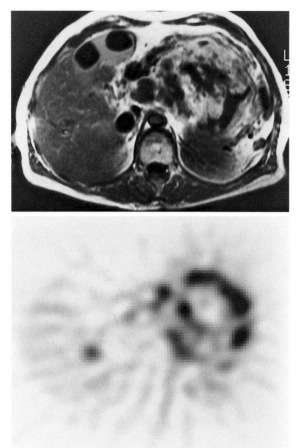

Fig. 11.14. Post-gadolinium T_1-weighted axial magnetic resonance image of the upper abdomen (*upper*) shows irregular contrast enhancement along the thick gastric wall and faint contrast-enhanced lesion in the right hepatic lobe adjacent to the inferior vena cava. Comparable positron-emission tomography image (*lower*) shows a markedly increased uptake of ^{18}F-fluoro-2-deoxy-D-glucose in the wall of active gastric cancer and also metastatic lesion in the right hepatic lobe after chemotherapy

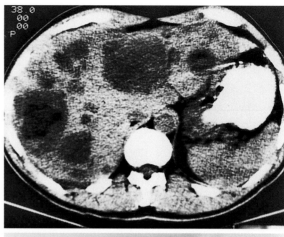

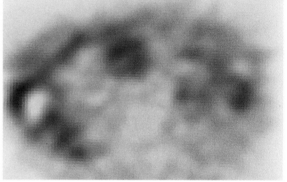

Fig. 11.15. Contrasted-computed tomography axial image of the upper abdomen (*upper*) shows a multiple metastatic leiomyosarcoma in the liver. Comparable positron-emission tomography image (*lower*) also shows an increased uptake of ^{18}F-fluoro-2-deoxy-D-glucose in the walls of necrotic metastatic lesions after chemotherapy

In examination of 106 patients with unclear pancreatic masses by ^{18}F FDG, 63 of the 74 (85%) were identified to have pancreatic carcinoma by PET (Fig. 11.19). PET revealed chronic pancreatitis in 27 of 32 (84%), and it was possible to exclude malignancy. False-negative results (10 of 11) were obtained in patients with elevated serum-glucose levels, and five false positives in patients with pancreatic inflammation. Therefore, PET showed an overall sensitivity of 85%, a specificity of 84%, a negative-predictive value of 71% and a positive-predictive value of 93% (Fig. 11.20) [80].

Accumulation of [1–^{11}C]-acetate by the pancreas allows rapid metabolic imaging using PET, and may be a useful metabolic probe for the study of pancreatic diseases. The normal pancreas demonstrates prompt uptake of [1–^{11}C]-acetate with maximal activity achieved in under 5 min. Moderately reduced [1–^{11}C]-acetate uptake was observed in acute pancreatitis, and pancreatic adenocarcinoma revealed no significant uptake of [1–^{11}C]-acetate [81]. FDG-PET imaging of gastroenteropancreatic (GEP) tumors demonstrated increased glucose metabolism only in less-differentiated GEP tumors with high proliferative activity, and metastasizing medullary thyroid cancer associated with rapidly increasing CEA levels [82]. It was recommended that FDG-PET should be performed for the imaging of neuroendocrine tumors only if somatostatin-receptor scintigraphy is negative.

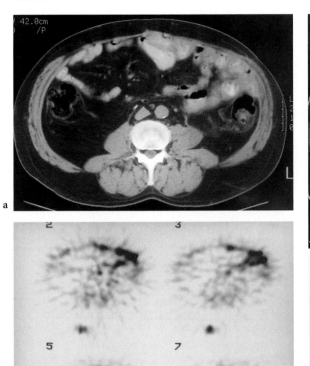

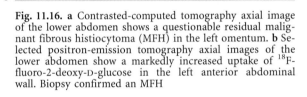

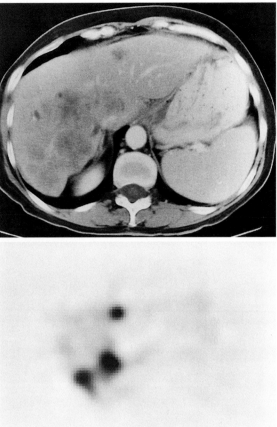

Fig. 11.16. a Contrasted-computed tomography axial image of the lower abdomen shows a questionable residual malignant fibrous histiocytoma (MFH) in the left omentum. **b** Selected positron-emission tomography axial images of the lower abdomen show a markedly increased uptake of ^{18}F-fluoro-2-deoxy-D-glucose in the left anterior abdominal wall. Biopsy confirmed an MFH

Fig. 11.17. Contrast-computed-tomography axial image of the upper abdomen (*upper*) shows multiple metastatic lesions of rectal carcinoma in right and left hepatic lobes. Comparable PET image (*lower*) shows only three metastatic lesions with markedly increased uptake of ^{18}F-fluoro-2-deoxy-D-glucose after chemotherapy

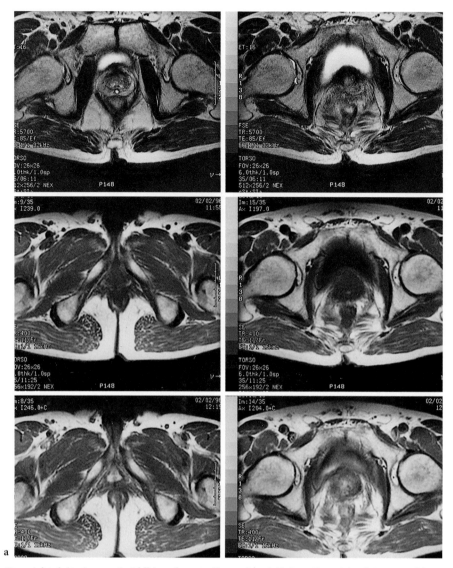

Fig. 11.18. a T_2-weighted (*top*), pre- (*middle*) and post- (*bottom*) gadolinium T_1-weighted images of lower pelvis show a small nodular lesion in the posterior rectum, possibly representing recurrent rectal cancer.

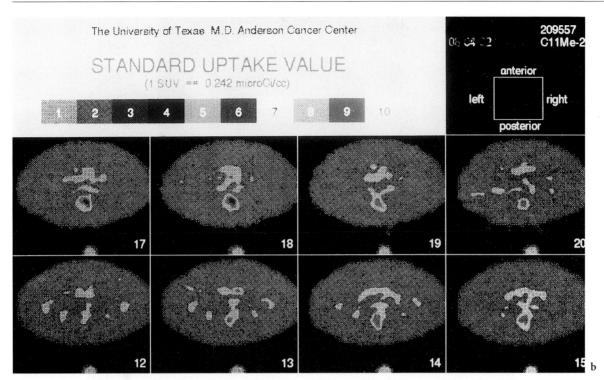

Fig. 11.18 b Selected axial positron-emission tomography images of lower pelvis show a markedly increased uptake of ^{11}C-methionine in the rectum with SUV 5.5. Surgery confirmed a recurrent rectal cancer

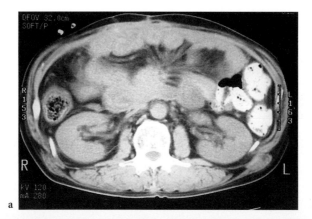
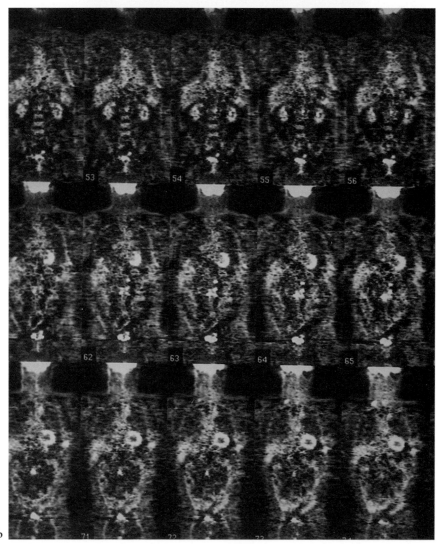

Fig. 11.19. a Contrast-computed-tomography axial image of the abdomen shows a pancreatic cancer in the mesenteric root after chemotherapy using gemcitabine. **b** Selected whole-body positron-emission tomography coronal images show a markedly increased uptake of ^{18}F-fluoro-2-deoxy-D-glucose in the middle of the abdomen (*middle low*), indicating residual active cancer

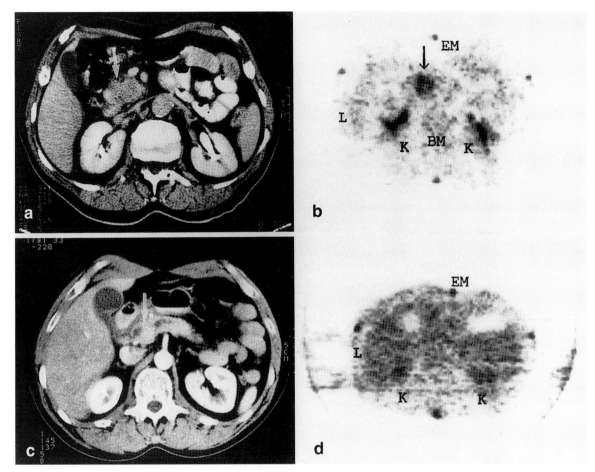

Fig. 11.20a–d. Corresponding contrasted-computed tomography (CT) (*left*) and ^{18}F-fluoro-2-deoxy-D-glucose (FDG) positron-emission tomography (*right*) axial images of the abdomen show nodular contrast-enhanced masses in the pancreatic heads on CTs and proven pancreatic cancer with focal increased ^{18}F-fluoro-2-deoxy-D-glucose (FDG) uptake (**b**). Note the absence of increased ^{18}F FDG uptake in chronic pancreatitis (**d**) (reprinted with permission from [80])

References

1. International Union Against Cancer (1982) Workshop on biology of human cancer. Rep 17: Hepatocellular carcinoma. Geneva
2. Landis SH, Murray T, Bolden S, Wingo PA (1998) Cancer statistics, 1988. CA Cancer J Clin 48:6–29
3. Beasley RP (1983) Prevention of perinatally transmitted hepatitis B virus infections with hepatitis B immune globulin and hepatitis B vaccine. Lancet 2:1099–1122
4. Adamson RC, Corree P (1976) Carcinogenicity of aflatoxin B1 in rhesus monkeys: two additional cases of primary liver cancer. J Natl Cancer Inst 57:67–78
5. Ries LAG, Hankey BF, Miller BA (1988) Cancer statistics review, 1973–1988 (NIH publication no. 91–2789). Bethesda, National Institutes of Health
6. Hall CN, Darkin D, Brimblecombe R (1986) Evaluation of the nitrosamine hypothesis of gastric carcinogenesis in precancerous conditions. Gut 27:491–498
7. Graham S, Haaughey B, Marshall J (1990) Diet in the epidemiology of gastric cancer. Nutr Cancer 13:19–34
8. Hammond EC (1966) Smoking in relation to the death rates of 1 million men and women. Natl Cancer Inst Monogr 19:127–204
9. Weiman TJ, Max MH, Volges CR (1980) Diversion of duodenal contents: its effect on the production of experimental gastric cancer. Arch Surg 115:959–961
10. Sasajima K, Kawachi T, Matsukura N (1979) Intestinal metaplasia and adenocarcinoma induced in the stomach of rats by N-propyl-N-nitro-N-nitrosoguanidine. J Cancer Res Clin Oncol 94:201–206
11. Blaser MJ, Chyou PH, Nomura A (1995) Age at establishment of Helicobacter pylori infection and gastric carcinoma, gastric ulcer, and duodenal ulcer risk. Cancer Res 55:562–565
12. Enstrom JE (1978) Cancer and total mortality among active Mormons. Cancer 42:1943–1951
13. Wynder E (1975) An epidemiologic evaluation of the causes of cancer of the pancreas. Cancer Res 35:2228–2233
14. Pour P, Althoff J, Kruger F (1977) The effects of N-nitroso bis-2-oxopropyl-amine after oral administration to hamsters. Cancer Lett 2:323
15. Robin A, Scott J, Rosenfeld D (1970) The occurrence of carcinoma of the pancreas in chronic pancreatitis. Radiology 94:289–294
16. Hoel DG, Davis DL, Miller AB (1992) Trends in cancer mortality in 15 industrialized countries, 1969–1986. J Natl Cancer Inst 84:313–320

17. Devesa SS, Silverman DT, Young JL (1987) Cancer incidence and mortality trends among whites in the United States, 1947-1984. J Natl Cancer Inst 79:701-770
18. Miller BA, Ries LAG, Hankey BF (1992) Cancer statistics review 1973-1989. National Cancer Institute, NIH Publications N 92-2789
19. Giller T (1994) Advances in genetics and molecular biology of colorectal tumors. Curr Opin Oncol 6:406-412
20. Meltzer SJ, Ahnen DJ, Battifora H (1987) Proto-oncogene abnormalities in colon cancers and adenomatous polyps. Gastroenterol 92:1174-1180
21. Miyoshi Y, Ando H, Nagase H (1992) Germ-cell mutations of the APC gene in 53 familial adenomatous polyposis patients. Proc Natl Acad Sci 89:4452-4456
22. Kinzler KW, Nilbert MC, Vogelstein B (1991) Identification of a gene located at chromosome 5q21 that is mutated in colorectal cancers. Science 25:1366-1369
23. Vogelstein B, Fearon ER, Hamilton SR (1988) Genetic alterations during colorectal development. N Engl J Med 319:525-532
24. Baker SJ, Fearon ER, Nigro JM (1989) Chromosome 17 deletions and p53 gene mutations in colorectal carcinomas. Science 244:217-221
25. Fishel R, Lescoe MK, Rao MRS (1993) The human mutation gene homolog MSH2 and its association with hereditary nonpolyposis colon cancer. Cell 75:1027-1038
26. Steele GD Jr (1994) The national cancer data base report on colorectal cancer. Cancer 74:1979-1989
27. Morotomi M, Guillem JG, LoGerfo P (1990) Production of diacylglycerol, an activator of protein kinase C, by human intestinal microflora. Cancer Res 50:3595-2600
28. Labayle D, Fischer D, Vielh P (1991) Sullindac causes regression of rectal polyps in familial adenomatous polyposis. Gastroenterology 101:635-640
29. Muto T, Bussey HJ, Morson BD (1975) The evolution of cancer of the colon and rectum. Cancer 36:2251-2260
30. Beazley R, Cohn I Jr (1994) Tumors of the pancreas, gallbladder, and extrahepatic ducts. Am Cancer Soc Textbook Clin Oncol 16:219-231
31. Okuda K, Ryn M, Takayoshi T (1987) Surgical management of hepatoma: the Japanese experience. In: Sanebo JH (ed) Hepatic and biliary surgery. Dekker, New York, pp 219-238
32. Okuda K, Obata H (1984) Prognosis of primary hepatocellular carcinoma. Hepatology 4:3-6
33. Chin H, Cheng E, Gellar N (1984) Hepatocellular carcinoma: statistical analysis of 78 consecutive patients (abstract). Proc Am Soc Clin Oncol 3:6
34. Buamah PK, Cornell C, James FW (1986) Serial serum AFP heterogeneity changes in patients with hepatocellular carcinoma during chemotherapy. Cancer Chemother Pharmacol 17:182-184
35. Cont DG, Bremman MF (1990) Gastric neoplasms. In: Moody FG, Carey LC, Jones RS, Kelly KA, Nahrwold DL, Skinner DB (eds) Surgical treatment of digestive diseases. Year Book Medical Publishers, Chicago, pp 212-235
36. Gastrointestinal Tumor Study Group (1982) Controlled trial of adjuvant chemotherapy following curative resection for gastric cancer. Cancer 49:1116-1122
37. Howard JM, Jordan GL (1977) Cancer of the pancreas. Curr Probl Cancer 2-1
38. Ward EM, Stephens DH, Sheedy PR (1983) Computed tomographic characteristics of pancreatic carcinoma: an analysis of 100 cases. Radiographics 3:547-557
39. Hermanek P (1982) Evolution and pathology of rectal cancer. World J Surg 6:502-509
40. Secco GB, Fardelli R, Campora E (1994) Primary mucinous adenocarcinomas and signet-ring cell carcinomas of the colon and rectum. Oncology 51:30-34
41. DeVita V Jr, Hellman S, Rosenberg SA (1993) Cancer principles and practice of oncology, 4th edn. Lippincott, Philadelphia, pp 929-977
42. Evans HL (1985) Smooth muscle tumors of the gastrointestinal tract: a study of 56 cases followed for a minimum of 10 years. Cancer 56:2242-2250
43. Cohen A, Willett C, Tepper JE (1985) Obstructive and perforative colonic carcinoma: patterns of failure. J Clin Oncol 3:379-383
44. Collier BD, Abdel-Nabi H, Doerr RJ (1992) Immunoscintigraphy performed with In-111 CYT-103 in the management of colorectal cancer: comparison with CT. Radiology 185:179-186
45. Steinberg SM, Barkin JS, Kaplan RS (1986) Prognostic indications of colon tumors: the gastrointestinal tumor group experience. Cancer 57:1866-1870
46. Ferruci JT (1994) Liver tumor imaging: current concepts. Radiol Clin North Am 32:39-54
47. Yamashita K, Mitsuzaki K, Yi T (1996) Small hepatocellular carcinoma in patients with chronic liver disease: prospective comparison of detection with dynamic MRI and helical CT of the who liver. Radiology 200:79-84
48. Kadoya M, Matsui O, Takashima T, Nonomura A (1992) Hepatocellular carcinoma: correlation of MRI and histopathologic findings. Radiology 183:819-825
49. Larson RE, Semelka RC, Bagley AS, Molina PL, Brown ED, Lee JK (1994) Hypervascular malignant liver lesions: comparison of various MR imaging pulse sequences and dynamic CT. Radiology 192:393-399
50. Semelka RC, Bagley AS, Brown ED, Krocker MA (1994) Malignant lesions of the liver identified on T_1- but not T_2-weighted MR images at 1.5 T. J Magn Reson Imaging 4:315-318
51. Mahfouz AE, Hamm B, Wolf KJ (1993) Dynamic gadopentatate dimeglumine-enhanced MRI of hepatocellular carcinoma. Eur Radiol 3:453-458
52. Liou J, Lee JI, Borrello JA, Brown JJ (1994) Differentiation of hepatomas from nonhepatomatous masses: use of MnDPDP-enhanced MR images. Magn Reson Imaging 12:71-79
53. Mahfoouz AE, Hamm B, Wolf KJ (1994) Peripheral washout: a sign of malignancy on dynamic gadolinium-enhanced MR images of focal liver lesions. Radiology 190:49-52
54. Outwater E, Tomaszewski JE, Daly JM, Kressel HY (1991) Hepatic colorectal metastases: correlation of MRI and pathologic appearance. Radiology 180:327-332
55. Semelka RC, Brown ED, Ascher SM, Patt RH, Bagley AS, Li W, Edelman RR, Shoenut JP, Brown JJ (1994) Hepatic hemangiomas: a multiinstitutional study of appearance on T_2-weighted and serial gadolinium-enhanced gradient-echo MR images. Radiology 192:401-406
56. Haggar AM, Bree RL (1992) Hepatic focal nodular hyperplasia: MRI at 1.0 and 1.5 T. J Magn Reson Imaging 2:85-88
57. Matushita M, Oi H, Murakami T (1994) Extraserosal invasion in advanced gastric cancer: evaluation with MRI. Radiology 192:87-91
58. Semelka RC, Ascher SM (1993) MRI of the pancreas. Radiology 188:593-602
59. Shoenut JP, Semelka RC, Silverman R, Yaffe CS, Mickflikier AB (1993) MRI evaluation of the local extent of colorectal mass lesions. J Clin Gastroenterol 17:248-253
60. Waizer A, Powsner E, Russo I (1991) Prospective comparative study of MRI vs transrectal US for preoperative staging and follow-up rectal cancer. Dis Colon Rectum 34:1068-1072
61. Negendank WG (1995) MR spectroscopy of musculoskeletal soft tissue tumors. MRI Clin North Am 3:713-725

62. Rajanayagam V, Lee RR, Ackerman Z, Bradley WG, Ross BD (1992) Quantitative P-31 MR spectroscopy of the liver in alcoholic cirrhosis. J Magn Reson Imaging 2:183–190
63. Gupta RK, Moore RD (1980) ^{31}P NMR studies of intracellular free Mg^{2+} in intact frog skeletal muscle. J Biol Chem 255:3987–3993
64. Meyerhoff DJ, Boska MD, Thomas A, Weiner MW (1990) Alcoholic liver disease: quantitative image-guided ^{31}P magnetic resonance spectroscopy. Radiology 173:393–400
65. Radda GK, Oberhaensli RD, Taylor DJ (1987) The biochemistry of human diseases as studied by ^{31}P NMR in man and animal models. Ann N Y Acad Sci 508:300–308
66. Oberhaensli RD, Galloway GJ, Hilton-Jones D (1987) The study of human organs by phosphorus-31 topical magnetic resonance spectrosocpy. Br J Radiol 60:367–373
67. Hassinger D, Gerok W, Stes H (1986) The effect of urea synthesis on extracellular pH in isolated perfused rat liver. Biochem J 236:261–265
68. Oster JR, Perez GO (1986) Acid-base disturbances in liver disease. J Hepatol 2:299–306
69. Griffiths JR, Bhujwalla Z, Coombes RC, Maxwell RJ, Midwood CJ, Morgan RJ, Nias AHW et al. (1997) Monitoring cancer therapy by NMR spectroscopy: from isolated cells to man. In: Cohen SM (ed) Ann New York Acad Sci, New York, pp 183–199
70. Beckmann N, Fried R, Turkalj I, Seelig J, Keller U, Stalder G (1993) Noninvasive observation of hepatic glycogen formation in man by ^{13}C MRS after oral and intravenous glucose administration. Magn Reson Med 29:583–590
71. Wolf W, Silver MS, Albright MJ, Weber H, Reichardt U, Sauer R (1987) A non-invasive study of drug metabolism in patients as studied by 19 F NMR spectroscopy of 5-fluorouracil. In: Cohen SM (ed) Physiological NMR spectroscopy: from isolated cells to man. Ann New York Acad Sci, New York pp 491–493
72. Schiepers C, Penninckx F, DeVadder N (1995) Contributions of PET in the diagnosis of recurrent colorectal cancer: comparison with conventional imaging. Eur J Surg Oncol 21:517–522
73. Abdel-Nabi H, Doerr RJ, Lammonica DM, Cronin VR, Galantowicz PJ, Carbone GM, Spaulding MR (1998) Staging of primary colorectal carcinomas with fluorine-18-fluorodeoxyglucose whole-body PET: correlation with histopathologic and CT findings. Radiology 206:755–760
74. Falk PM, Gupta NC, Thorson AG (1994) Positron emission tomography for preoperative staging of colorectal carcinoma. Dis Colon Rectum 37:153–156
75. Delbeke D, Vitola JV, Sandler MMP, Arildsen RC, Powers TA, Wright JK Jr, Chapman WC, Pinson CW (1997) Staging recurrent metastatic colorectal carcinoma with PET. J Nucl Med 38:1196–1201
76. Strauss LG, Conti PS (1991) The applications of PET in clinical oncology. J Nucl Med 32:623–648
77. Haberkorn U, Strauss LG, Dimitrakopoulou A (1991) PET studies of fluorodeoxyglucose metabolism in patients with recurrent colorectal tumors receiving radiotherapy. J Nucl Med 32:1485–1490
78. Haberkorn U, Reinhardt M, Strauss LG (1992) Metabolic design of combination therapy: use of enhanced fluorodeoxyglucose uptake caused by chemotherapy. J Nucl Med 33:1981–1987
79. Dimitrakopoulou-Strauss A, Strauss LG, Schlag P, Hohenberger P, Irngastinger G, Oberdorfer F, Doll J, van Kaick G (1998) Intravenous and intra-arterial oxygen-15 labeled water and fluorine-15 labeled fluorouracil in patients with liver metastases from colorectal carcinoma. J Nucl Med 39:465–473
80. Zimny M, Bares R, Fab J, Adam G, Cremerius U, Dohmen B, Klever P, Sabri O et al. (1997) Fluorine-18-fluorodeoxyglucose positron emission tomography in the differential diagnosis of pancreatic carcinoma: a report of 106 cases. Eur J Nucl Med 24:678–682
81. Shreve PD, Gross MD (1997) Imaging of the pancreas and related diseases with PET carbon-11 acetate. J Nucl Med 38:1305–1310
82. Adams S, Baum R, Rink T, Schumm-Dräger P-M, Usadel K-H, Hör G (1998) Limited value of fluorine-18 fluorodeoxyglucose positron emission tomography for the imaging of neuroendocrine tumors. Eur J Nucl Med 25:79–83

Urologic Cancers

E. E. Kim

Basic Considerations

Renal Cell Carcinoma

Renal cell carcinoma (RCC) has been rising steadily in the United States; 29,900 new cases are expected to be diagnosed and 11,600 RCC patients will die in 1998 [1]. It occurs most commonly in adults over the age of 40 years [2]. The male-to-female ratio ranges from 2:1 to 3:1 [1]. The most prominent risk factor is tobacco use, and RCC has been reported in patients previously exposed to thorotrast contrast material [3]. RCC has also been associated with acquired renal polycystic disease, xanthogranulomatous pyelonephritis, and phenacetin-related analgesic nephropathy [4]. RCC is known to develop in 40–70% of patients with von Hippel-Lindau disease [5]. These patients are at risk of developing pheochromocytomas or cerebellar and retinal hemangioblastomas. Three tumor-suppressor genes appear to reside in 3p: the VHL gene at 3p25–26 and two more proximal genes, at 3p14 (nonpapillary renal-carcinoma gene or NRC-1) and 3p21. Common presentations of RCC include hematuria, abdominal mass, weight loss, anorexia, or symptoms arising from metastatic sites. A unique aspect of RCC is the frequent occurrence of various panneoplastic symptoms, including hypercalcemia, polycythemia, fever, cachexia, hypertension, and hepatic dysfunction (Stauffer's syndrome) [6]. Metastatic disease is detectable in 25–30% of patients at the time of diagnosis [7]; frequent sites include the lung, bone, lymph nodes, liver, and adrenal glands. Metastases to the brain, contralateral kidney, pancreas, or skin are found in 5–15% of these patients. Advanced local or metastatic disease carries an approximate 15% 5-year survival rate. Aggressive palliative treatment is recommended for patients with a solitary metastasis, and response rates to cytokine therapy remain generally less than 25%.

Bladder Cancer

Bladder cancer is the most common malignant tumor of the urinary tract and accounts for 6.5% of all cancers. The peak age of incidence is the seventh decade, and the male-to-female ratio is 3:1. In 1998, approximately 54,400 new cases will be diagnosed, and 12,500 patients will die of bladder cancer [1]. The incidence is higher in American whites than blacks, higher in Western countries than African and Asian nations, and higher in urban areas than rural areas. Chemical carcinogens, such as benzidine, 2-naphthylamine, and 4-aminobiphenyl have been linked with bladder cancers and associated with occupations in fields related to dye, rubber, textile, painting, leather and hairdressing [8]. Cigarette smoking is responsible for at least 50% of the cases in men. Among smokers, pipe and cigar smokers have a relatively low risk of developing the cancer [9]. Phenacetin-containing analgesics have been implicated in the pathogenesis of urothelial tumors [10]. Chronic cystitis or bladder irritation is also associated with the development of squamous cell carcinoma of the bladder [11]. However, milk and vitamin A have been associated with a decreased risk of bladder cancer [8]. Deletion of part or all of chromosome 9 was found in all stages of bladder cancer [12]. An increasing copy number of chromosome 7 was found to be correlated with high tumor grade and proliferation [13]. Deletion of 3p, 11p, and 17p also occurred predominantly in tumors of advanced stages [14]. The incidence of p53 mutations was 50–60% in bladder tumors, and the presence of p53 mutation correlated with high-grade invasive cancers [15]. Of patients with carcinoma in situ, 48% had overexpression of the p53 protein, and 86.7% of those with p53 overexpression subsequently developed progressive disease [16]. Allelic loss of the retinoblastoma (Rb) gene has been shown in 28 of 94 patients with transitional-cell carcinoma; Rb gene loss was more frequently associated with tumors of high grade and advanced stages [17]. There are no pathognomonic symptoms or signs of bladder cancer; painless, intermittent gross hematuria or microscopic hematuria is the leading sign, occurring in over 75% of patients. About 30% of patients have initial symptoms of bladder cancer, such as dysuria or urinary frequency. Pelvic pain and symptoms of rectal obstruction occur in locally advanced cases, and flank pain often results from ureteral obstruction. Almost 75% of bladder cancers are superficial at diagnosis, but 50–80% of superficial cancers recur. Despite aggressive surgery or irradiation, 50% of patients with muscle-invasive cases ultimately die of cancer [8].

Prostate Cancer

The incidence and mortality of prostate cancer continues to rise, and prostatic cancer has become the most common newly diagnosed cancer in American men. In 1998, about 184,500 men in the United States will be diagnosed with prostate cancer and 3,200 will die of it, a mortality rate second to that of lung cancer [1]. Epidemiologic studies have shown that mortality rates among US whites and blacks continue to rise, with rates increasing more rapidly among males over 74 years old, and reduced in nonwhite young males [18]. Except for an association with chronic prostatitis, no association has been found between prostate cancer and diet, venereal disease, gender, smoking or occupational exposure [19]. It is generally believed that the benign, hypertrophic prostatic cells do not directly transform into malignant cells [20]. It has been observed that prostate cancers are responsive to testosterone suppression, and black men have serum testosterone levels 15% higher than white men on average [21]. The prevalence of latent or incidental tumors is characteristic of the prostate gland. Every decade of aging nearly doubles the incidence of microscopic prostate cancer. It has been estimated that nine of ten men who eventually develop clinically recognized prostate cancer had cancer that remained undetected for decades [22].

Chromosomes 6q, 8p, 9p, 10q, 13q, 16q and 18q are potential sites for genes associated with the initiation of prostate carcinoma, and the most common abnormalities affected sites 8p and 13q [23]. Of the primary prostatic tumors, 74% showed evidence of DNA-sequence-copy-number changes [23]. Although several oncogenes (ras, myc, sis) are expressed with a high frequency in prostatic-cancer cell lines, their overexpression in localized or early prostatic cancers is uncommon [24]. Mutations in the *p53* gene are considered late events in prostatic carcinogenesis, associated with advanced stage, loss of differentiation, and conversion from a hormone-dependent to a hormone-refractory state [25]. Loss of Rb gene appears to be an early event in prostatic carcinogenesis [26]. There is enhanced expression of epidermal growth factor (EGF) and coexpression of the epidermal growth factor receptor (EGFR) in human prostatic tumors [27]. The increased expression of HER 2/neu and c-erbB-3 has also been demonstrated in prostatic intraepithelial neoplasia and in primary prostatic cancers and matching metastases [28]. There is a positive correlation between stage and Gleason grade of tumor, and the immunohistochemical expression of HER-2/neu [29]. The progression of prostatic tumors to a hormone-refractory state is frequently associated with the expression of the anti-apoptotic gene, *bcl-2* [30]. Tumor-induced angiogenesis is an essential step in the progression of malignant tumors and the development of metastases. The production of osteoblastic metastases suggests a bidirectional paracrine interaction between prostate cancer and bone cells. Many patients with localized prostate cancer are curable with local therapy, but treatment of metastatic disease is strictly palliative.

Testicular Cancer

Testicular cancers constitute only 1% of cancers in males, but are the most common malignant tumor in men aged 15–35 years. In 1998, an estimated 7,600 new cases of testicular cancer will be diagnosed in the United States, with an associated 400 deaths [1]. Testicular cancer is most common in white males, who have an incidence more that four times that of black males [31]. The risk is highest in northern Europe, and appears greater if the testis is retained in the abdomen [32]. Trauma, testicular torsion, testicular atrophy from mumps, orchitis, radiation, and exposure to dimethylformamide during leather tanning are possible risk factors [33]. Testicular cancers frequently present at an early stage, are sensitive to chemotherapy, and are variably sensitive to radiotherapy.

Pathology, Staging and Diagnosis

RCC is a solid hemorrhagic and necrotic mass, and reveals numerous vessels and vascular channels. It can be separated into three cellular types: clear, granular and sarcomatoid [34]. Clear cell carcinoma is present in more than 90% of RCCs, and a sarcomatoid component is predictive of a more aggressive behavior. Most RCCs are solid with the blood supply from the sinusoidal vessels, whereas cells aggregate in papillae supplied by a single fibrovascular stalk in the papillary-tumor pattern. A grading scale for RCC based on nuclear size and shape is frequently used. Nuclear grade appears to provide prognostic information, particularly for grade-I and grade-IV tumors [35]. One of the popular staging systems used in clinical practice for RCC is that of Robson (Table 12.1).

The TNM system (Table 12.2) has an advantage in that it will separate patients with tumor thrombi from those with local nodal disease. Local nodal metastasis is associated with shorter survival.

The 5-year survival with Robson's stage I (T_1 or 2, N0, M0) is greater than 90%; stage II (T3a, N0, M0) is 65–70%; stage III (T3b–d or N1–3, M0) is 40%; and stage IV (T4a or M1) is 15–20% [36]. In addition to advanced disease stage, other predictors of poor outcome include high nuclear grade, sarcomatoid element, aneuploidy, and inferior-vena-cava (IVC) thrombus extending into or above the hepatic veins [37]. The overall accuracy of computed tomography (CT) in the staging of RCC is 90–95% [38]. RCC with a papillary tumor pattern or sarcomatoid component appears as a hypovascular mass on renal arteriograms. A chest X-ray should be obtained as part of the initial evaluation, since a significant number of patients have lung metastasis at presentation.

The majority of *bladder cancers* originate in the urothelium, the transitional cell epithelium from the renal pelvis to the proximal urethra. In the United States, 85–95% of bladder cancers are transitional cell carcinomas. Mixed tumors containing squamous cell carcinoma and adenocarcinoma elements are reported in 10–30%. About 70–80% of bladder cancers occur on the lateral or posterior wall of the bladder, and 20% on the trigone. Thirty percent of tumors are multifocal at diagnosis [39]. The grading of transitional cell carcinoma is based on the cellular atypia, nuclear abnormalities, and number of mitoses. Grade-I (low-grade) tumors usually grow superficially with papillary patterns, whereas grade-III (high-grade) tumors are usually solid and invasive [40]. Carcinoma in situ (CIS) is a superficial, nonpapillary, noninfiltrating flat tumor characterized by cellular anaplasia, nonspecific inflammatory changes, and Brunn's nests. About 40% of patients with CIS develop invasive disease within 5 years [41]. There are two staging systems, Jewett-Marshall and TNM (Table 12.3).

The standard procedure for staging of bladder cancer is cystoscopy and bimanual examination under anesthesia (EUA). The accuracy rate of staging EUA is less than 50%, usually because the

Table 12.1. Robson's staging for renal cell carcinoma

Stage I	Confined within renal capsule
Stage II	Invading perinephric fat, within Gerota's fascia
Stage III	Invading renal vein, inferior vena cava (A) or regional lymph-node (B), or both (C)
Stage IV	Invading viscera (excluding ipsilateral adrenal) or distant organ

Table 12.2. TNM staging for renal cell carcinoma

T (Tumor)	
T1	<2.5 cm, confined to kidney
T2	>2.5 cm, confined to kidney
T3	Extension into renal vein, infradiaphragmatic vena cava, adrenal or perinephric fat
T4	Extension beyond Gerota's fascia
N (Nodes)	
N1	Single node <2 cm
N2	Single node >2 cm and <5 cm, or multiple nodes <5 cm
N3	Any node >5 cm
M (Metastasis)	
M1	Distant metastasis

Table 12.3. Staging systems for bladder cancer

Jewett-Marshall	TNM	
0	T0	No tumor
	Tis	Carcinoma in situ
A	Ta	Papillary tumor without invasion
	T1	Lamina propria invasion
B-1	T2	Superficial muscle invasion
B-2	T3a	Deep muscle invasion
C	T3b	Perivesical fat invasion
D-1	T4	Prostate, vagina, uterus or pelvic wall invasion
D-2	N1–3	Pelvic node metastasis
	N1	Single node, <2 cm
	N2	Bilateral nodes, or single node of 2–5 cm
	N3	Any node, >5 cm
D-3	M	Node metastsis beyond pelvis
D-4	M1	Distant metastasis

inflammatory reaction blurs the tumor margin. Multiple biopsies of the bladder wall should be performed. Elevation of serum levels of carcinoembryonic antigen and beta-human chorionic gonadotropin (β-hCG) is not uncommon. CT helps in evaluating the tumor extent and metastasis.

Almost all *prostate cancers* are adenocarcinomas. Sarcomas, transitional cell, small cell, and squamous cell carcinomas are rare. Patients with unusual sites (liver or skin) of metastases, low or normal levels of serum prostate-specific antigen (PSA), and tumors that display hormone resistance should be evaluated for possible anaplastic small cell pathology, which responds better to

Table 12.4. Staging system for prostate cancer

T (primary tumor)		
	Tx	Cannot be assessed
	T0	No evidence
	T1	Not palpable or visible
	T1a	Incidental in 5% or less of tissue resected
	T1b	Incidental in >5% of tissue resected
	T1c	Identified by needle biopsy
	T2	Palpable within prostate
	T2a	Involves <50% of lobe
	T2b	Involves >50% of lobe, not both lobes
	T2c	Involves both lobes
	T3	Extends through prostate capsule
	T3a	Unilateral extracapsular enlargement
	T3b	Bilateral extracapsular extension
	T3c	Invades seminal vesicle(s)
	T4	Fixed or invades other organs
	T4a	Invades external sphincter and/or bladder neck and/or rectum
	T4b	Invades levator muscles and/or pelvic wall
N (lymph node)		
	NX	Cannot be assessed
	N0	No node metastasis
	N1	Single node, ≤2 cm
	N2	Single node, 2–5 cm, or multiple nodes, <5 cm
M (Metastasis)		
	MX	Cannot be assessed
	M0	No metastasis
	M1	Distant metastasis
	M1a	Nonregional node
	M1b	Bone
	M1c	Other sites

Table 12.5. Staging for seminoma

Stage I	Confined to testis
Stage IIa	Retroperitoneal node, <5 cm
Stage IIb	Retroperitoneal node, 5–10 cm
Stage IIc	Retroperitoneal node, >10 cm
Stage III	Lymph node above diaphragm or visceral organs involved

chemotherapy than to hormonal treatments [42]. The Gleason system for histologic grading of prostate cancer is based on morphology and correlates with malignant potential. Patients with well-differentiated lesions (Gleason scores 2–4) usually have early-stage disease and a good prognosis. Gleason scores 8–10 are associated with a poor prognosis. The Gleason score also correlates well with other factors, such as tumor size, pelvic node metastasis, and PSA level [43]. Detection of a high S-phase fraction in a primary tumor may indicate lack of hormonal responsiveness and poor prognosis, and diploid tumors are associated with improved survival [44]. Prostatic cancers typically grow peripherally through the capsule along perineural sheaths that perforate the capsule at the upper outer corner and at the apex. Such tumors often invade the seminal vesicles and the neck of the urinary bladder. Lymphatic spread is usually orderly, first affecting the obturator lymph nodes, then external iliac and hypogastric nodes, and finally common iliac and periaortic nodes. The axial skeleton is involved as the first site of hematogenous metastasis (osseous I). This is followed by spread to the proximal appendicular skeleton (osseous II). The most commonly used staging system for prostatic carcinoma is shown in Table 12.4.

Unfortunately, about 70% of patients present with stage C or D prostate cancer. The 5-year survival rate for patients with stage-D prostate cancer remains less than 20%. A positive bone scan correlates with a high level of PSA and identifies patients with stage-D2 disease. If the bone scan is negative, a CT scan should be performed to look for involvement of the pelvic lymph nodes. Tumor volume in advanced disease appears to influence response to therapy [45].

Testicular cancer is a general term for several distinct but related tumors. Germ cell tumors account for nearly 93% of all primary testicular malignancies. Testicular lymphomas represent about 4–5% of testicular cancers, and sex cord-stromal tumors make up nearly 3%. In 75–99% of testicular cancers, carcinoma in situ is found adjacent to the tumors [46]. Pure seminoma is the most common germ-cell tumor and accounts for approximately 45% of testicular cancers [47]. Low levels of β-hCG are seen in 10–25% of pure seminomas [48]. Seminomas do not secrete alpha-fetoprotein (AFP), and an elevated AFP level should alert the clinician to the presence of nonseminomatous elements. Embryonal carcinoma is the second most common testicular malignancy and in its pure form accounts for 15–30% of nonseminomatous germ-cell tumors. One-third of patients present with metastasis to the para-aortic lymph nodes, lungs, or liver. This tumor secretes both AFP and β-hCG. Yolk-sac carcinoma is the most common testicular tumor in children, accounting for 75% of cases, and is associated with an excellent prognosis. Choriocarcinoma is extremely rare and is found as a component of other testis tumors. Teratoma is a common component of mixed germ-cell tumors. Leydig (interstitial) cell tumors account for 1–3% of all testicular tumors and secrete both androgens and estrogens. Rhabdomyosarcoma is the most common sarcoma in children and can originate in the testis. Primary malignant lymphoma of the testis accounts for 5% of all testicular tumors. This occurs in about 20% of all cases of lymphoma. Leukemic infiltration of the testis usually occurs when the disease is disseminated. Testicular metastases occur in 2.5% of men with malignant tumors. The most common pri-

Table 12.6. TNM classification of testicular tumors

T (Tumor)	
T1	Confined to testis
T2	Extending through tunica albica
T3	Involving rete testis or epididymis, ≥6 involved nodes
T4	Involving scrotal wall
N (Nodes)	
N0	Not involved
N1	Microscopic only
N2A	Largest node ≤2 cm, ≤5 nodes
N3	Nodal extension into adjacent structures
N4	Gross tumor following node dissection
M (Metastasis)	
M1	Supradiaphragmatic or extralymphatic involvement

mary sites are the prostate, lung, skin, colon, and kidney. Staging for seminoma at our institution is shown in Table 12.5.

TNM classification for non-seminomatous germ cell tumors is shown in Table 12.6. The initial staging evaluation should include a chest X-ray, CT of the abdomen and pelvis, bone scan if symptoms indicate, and a magnetic resonance (MR) image of the brain if neurologic symptoms are present.

Magnetic Resonance Imaging

Magnetic resonance imaging (MRI) is establishing its role as a modality complementary to CT and ultrasonography in the evaluation of renal and perirenal pathology (Fig. 12.1). It is used primarily for the staging of renal tumors in patients for whom CT is contraindicated or has yielded equivocal results. MRI is particularly valuable in the evaluation of the intravascular extent of tumor thrombi (Fig. 12.2). It has proven to be effective in the characterization of renal masses. Benign renal tumors are rare, and specific diagnoses can be made for the fat-containing angiomyolipoma or hamartoma. Fat-suppression techniques are helpful to distinguish hemorrhagic masses from fatty lesions with MR. RCCs are usually solitary, although bilateral tumors are encountered in 2% of patients. They commonly metastasize by lymphatic and hematogenous routes, and they may be locally aggressive, extending into the renal veins and the IVC, or invading adjacent soft-tissue structures. Nodal metastases commonly involve pararenal and para-aortic nodes and may also involve mediastinal and hilar nodes. Common sites of hematogenous metastases include bone, liver, and lungs. Renal cell carcinomas demonstrate variable signal characteristics, depending on the degree of tumor vascularity and the presence or absence of hemorrhage, necrosis, calcification, and iron particles in the tumor cells. In the absence of hemorrhage or necrosis, renal cell carcinomas are isointense to normal renal parenchyma on both T_1- and T_2-weighted images. When intratumoral hemorrhage or necrosis is present, signal intensity can be heterogeneous on both T_1- and T_2-weighted images. Hemorrhage may result in deposition of iron and may lower the signal intensity of the tumor on T_1- and T_2-weighted images. The differential diagnosis includes fibroma, milk-of-calcium cysts and other calcified renal lesions. Postcontrast T_1-weighted images are helpful for depiction of small tumors.

Tumors less than 3 cm in diameter have been detected with an accuracy of 60–64% on noncontrast MR images, whereas 99–100% of tumors greater than 3 cm are detected without contrast administration [49]. Gradient-echo (GE) breathhold sequences have shown variable results (47–93%) in the detection of lesions less than 3 cm [50]. Accuracy in the detection of renal cell carcinomas less than 3 cm in size improves to 80–100% when spin-echo T_1-weighted images are obtained after gadolinium-chelate administration [50]. Hemorrhagic lesions may also demonstrate high signal on T_1-weighted images and, therefore, evaluation of scans both before and after contrast injection is necessary. Stage-I lesions have an intact rim of normal renal parenchyma or, if peripheral in locations, have a smooth, convex margin. A tumor is considered stage II when extension through the renal capsule by the lesion is confined within the perirenal fascia. There is also irregularity of the margin between the tumor and the perinephric fat, as well as gross invasion of the perinephric fat or adrenal glands. Perirenal soft-tissue stranding or thickening of the perirenal fascia is not considered a definitive finding of tumor invasion and may represent secondary perirenal inflammatory changes. Stage III_a indicates invasion of the renal vein and/or the IVC (Figs. 12.3 and 12.4). Stage III_b involves extension to local lymph nodes, and stage III_c indicates both venous and local nodal involvement. The accuracy in the determination of IVC thrombus is 100% on MRI, compared with 79–88% for CT and 68% for ultrasonography [51]. MR accuracy in the determination of renal-vein thrombus is lower, at 88%. Tumor thrombus is usually distinguished by its higher signal on GE images, whereas bland thrombi are usually low in signal because of the presence of hemosiderin (Figs. 12.3 and 12.4). Nodes measuring more than 1 cm in diameter on the short axis are considered abnormal. Approximately 66% of nodes measuring

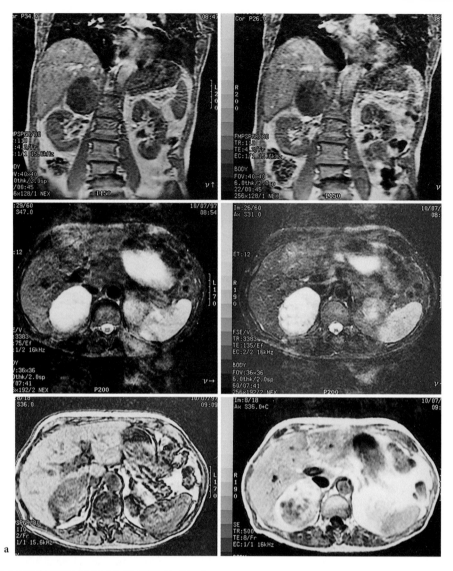

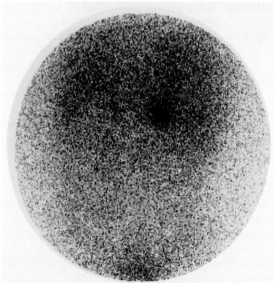

Fig. 12.1. a The pheochromocytoma in the right adrenal gland shows heterogeneous intermediate signal intensity on T_1-weighted coronal images (*top*) and high signal intensity on T_2-weighted images (*middle*). Note also irregular contrast enhancement of the tumor on the post-gadolinium (Gd) T_1-weighted axial image (*bottom right*). b Posterior image of the abdomen using ^{131}I-metaiodobenzylguanidine shows a focal increased activity in the right adrenal gland, indicating active pheochromocytoma

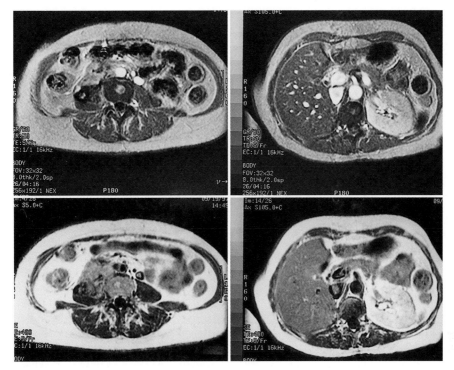

Fig. 12.2. The contrast-enhanced retroperitoneal sarcoma abutting the lumbar spine shows an involvement of the right psoas muscle seen on the post-gadolinium T_1-weighted axial image of the lower abdomen (*lower left*). Gradient-echo axial images of the lower (*upper left*) and upper (*upper right*) abdomen as well as a T_1-weighted axial image of the upper abdomen (*lower right*) show thromboses in the center of the inferior vena cava (IVC) and splenic vein

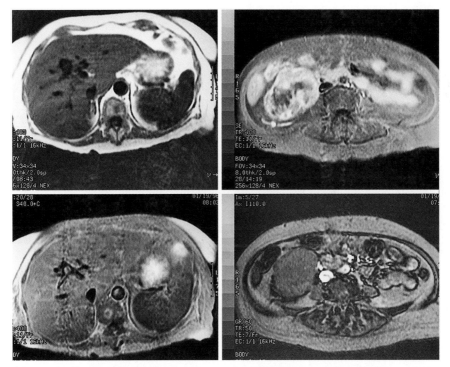

Fig. 12.3. The right renal cell cancer shows a heterogeneous contrast enhancement on the post-gadolinium (Gd) T_1-weighted axial image of the lower abdomen (*upper right*). T_1-weighted axial images of the upper abdomen before (*upper left*) and after (*lower left*) injection of Gd-diethylenetriaminepentaacetic acid show a contrast-enhanced tumor thrombus in the right portal vein. Note also a compression of the right renal vein by adjacent tumor mass on the gradient axial image of the lower abdomen (*lower right*)

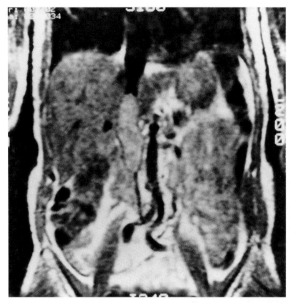

Fig. 12.4. Coronal T_1-weighted image of the abdomen shows a tumor thrombus with heterogeneously increased signal intensity in the inferior vena cava in a patient with renal cell cancer

1–2.2 cm in the setting of renal cell carcinoma have been shown to be inflammatory or hyperplastic rather than metastatic [52]. Stage-IV disease involves either invasion of the adjacent organs (IVa) or distant metastasis (IVb). Renal cell carcinomas tend to be of higher signal on T_2-weighted images than normal liver, pancreas, and muscles. Renal metastasis may present as multiple small masses or, less commonly, as a solitary lesion, and it cannot be distinguished from primary renal carcinoma on the basis of MRI findings, although metastatic lesions usually do not distort the renal contour. Renal lymphoma is variable in appearance and often associated with retroperitoneal lymphadenopathy.

MRI is appropriate for anatomic staging of detected bladder tumors, for radiation therapy planning, and for evaluation of therapeutic response. MRI may be used to determine the feasibility of segmental cystectomy, the desirability of pelvic lymphadenectomy, or the possibility of radical cystectomy (Fig. 12.5). MR can also identify patients with advanced stages who received primary radiation and/or chemotherapy instead of surgery. Bladder carcinomas may demonstrate different patterns of growth: papillary, sessile, infiltrative, or mixed pattern. T_1-weighted images are used to evaluate papillary tumors, extension of tumor through the bladder wall into the perivesical fat, and for evaluation of pelvic nodes. T_2-weighted images allow for evaluation of signal abnormalities of the bladder wall and demonstration of pelvic anatomy. Contrast-enhanced images im-

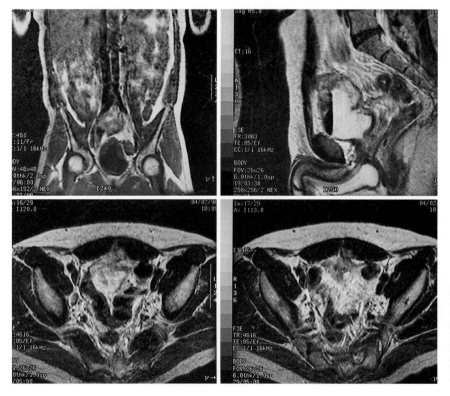

Fig. 12.5. T_1-weighted coronal (*upper left*), T_2-weighted sagittal (*upper right*) and axial (*lower*) images of the pelvis show an irregular mass in the superior and anterior walls of the urinary bladder, involving the rectus abdominis muscle

prove identification of small bladder tumors and allow for differentiation between tumor from blood clot and debris. Dynamic contrast-enhanced images have been shown to improve evaluation of tumor invasion of the bladder wall and to improve staging accuracy. Superficial (stage-T_1) lesions are diagnosed when an intact low-signal-intensity muscular wall is identified. Superficial bladder-wall invasion (T_2) is diagnosed when T_2-weighted images show abnormal high signal intensity within the wall or irregular contrast enhancement of inner bladder wall. Deep invasion (T3a) is diagnosed when full-thickness bladder-wall signal abnormality or contrast enhancement is present. Tumor extension into the perivesical fat (T3b) will cause a focal decrease of signal intensity of the fat on T_1-weighted images. Tumor invasion of the adjacent prostate gland, seminal vesicles, uterine corpus and cervix is best demonstrated on T_2-weighted images. Lymph nodes larger than 1 cm in diameter should be considered pathologic. There are no signal-intensity characteristics that are unique for tumor involvement within lymph nodes. It has been established that microscopic lymph-node metastasis can be expected in 40% of patients with deep muscle invasion and in 60% of patients with adjacent pelvic-visceral invasion or sidewall invasion [53]. Anatomic staging of bladder carcinoma by MRI is complicated in the presence of coexistent cystitis or recent postbiopsy or post-resection change. The accuracy for staging bladder carcinoma by MRI varies from 75% to 93%, and the accuracy by CT is 55% [54].

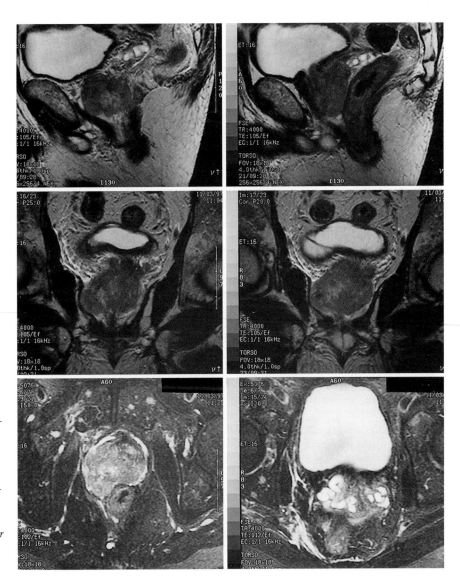

Fig. 12.6. T_2-weighted sagittal (*top*), coronal (*middle*) and axial (*bottom*) images of the lower pelvis show an enlarged prostate with heterogeneous signal intensity in the central and peripheral zones. The prostatic carcinoma arising from the right-posterior periphery involves bladder wall (*upper right*), levator ani muscle (*middle*) and left seminal vesicle (*lower right*)

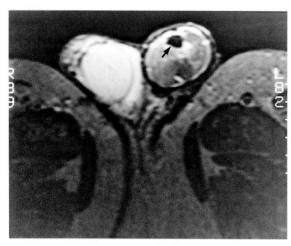

Fig. 12.7. T_2-weighted axial image shows a small nodular malignant fibrous histiocytoma mass (*arrow*) in the left testicle. Note a normal right testis with uniform high signal intensity

MRI has assumed a primary role in the staging of carcinomas of the genitourinary and gynecologic organs (Figs. 12.6 and 12.7). The normal prostate gland measures 4×3×2.5 cm and is surrounded by a thin fibrous capsule. Anatomically, the prostate is divided into five lobes: anterior, median, posterior, and two lateral lobes. A group of nerves, lymphatics and vessels termed the neurovascular bundles or lateral venous plexi perforates the fibrous prostatic capsule. Both carcinoma and prostatitis may be found in either the peripheral or central zones of the outer gland. About 70% of cancers are found in the peripheral zone and 10% in the central zone. While CT may accurately display gland shape and size, it cannot distinguish internal abnormalities within the gland. Endorectal ultrasonography allows more detailed examination of the prostate gland than CT. However, as many as 40% of prostate cancers larger than 5 mm may not be identified by ultrasonography [55].

Body-coil MRI of the pelvis is combined with high-resolution endorectal imaging of the prostate, providing information regarding both local and distant disease. Axial, coronal, and sagittal planes enable a better delineation of prostatic lesions. The prostate, seminal vesicle, and periprostatic veins are of uniform low signal on T_1-weighted images. The periprostatic veins laterally and Santorini's plexus anteriorly may have high signal intensity on T_2-weighted images. As the inner gland enlarges, the outer gland is compressed, and the thin space between the enlarged inner and compressed outer gland is referred to as the surgical capsule. Adenocarcinoma is not distinctly seen on T_1-weighted images. It typically appears as a focus of low signal in the peripheral zone on T_2-weighted images; this finding is nonspecific. However, areas that are larger, poorly differentiated, or located posteriorly are more likely cancers (broken septa sign) (Fig. 12.6) [56].

Rarely, mucinous types of adenocarcinoma may display high signal intensity on T_2-weighted images. Cancers arising in the central gland are isodense to surrounding glandular tissue. Hemorrhagic foci have high signals on T_1-weighted images and may mask a low-signal carcinoma on T_2-weighted images. Capsular penetration occurs most commonly at the posterolateral aspect of the gland, adjacent to the neurovascular bundles. Capsular invasion shows a disruption of periprostatic fat on T_1-weighted images. An irregular capsular bulge is associated with capsular invasion in 75% of cases. [57]. Asymmetry of the neurovascular bundles is also associated with capsular invasion [58]. Early improvement of the seminal vesicles is evidenced by thickening of tubal walls, followed by intraluminal low-signal foci on T_2-weighted images. Postbiopsy hemorrhage and radiation fibrosis may also result in intraluminal low signal. Lymphadenopathy may be identified as rounded, globular, or coalescent nodules in the periprostatic, perivesicle, or iliac areas. Neither MRI nor CT can differentiate between normal-sized and tumor-invaded nodes, nor can they distinguish between enlarged neoplastic and inflammatory nodes. The overall staging accuracy with the endorectal coil ranges from 82% to 90%, and showed up to 16% improvement when compared with the body coil [59]. It has been suggested that the volume of prostatic carcinoma is an important predictor of its clinical behavior. [60].

Magnetic Resonance Spectroscopy and Spectroscopic Imaging

Magnetic resonance spectroscopy (MRS) is a technique that uses magnetic fields and radiofrequency energy to detect chemicals in tissues. MRS may be performed using conventional MRI scanners. ^{31}P MRS was used to investigate renal function in human renal transplants [61]. When adenosine triphosphate (ATP) was present, renal function was higher. Phosphodiester/phosphomonoester (PDE/PME) and inorganic phosphate (Pi)/ATP ratios were elevated in transplant rejection. Recent studies have demonstrated that MR spectroscopic imaging can metabolically enable identification of regions of prostate cancer both before and after therapy [62]. In a three-dimensional proton MRS study in 85 patients with prostate

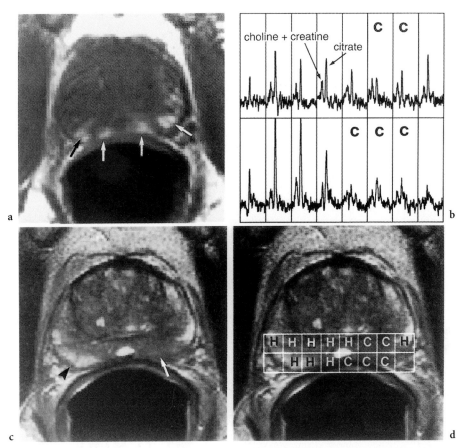

Fig. 12.8. a T_1-weighted axial image of the prostate shows a bilateral postbiopsy hemorrhage as high signal intensity areas in the peripheral zone (*arrows*). **b** T_2-weighted axial images at the comparable level show areas of low (*arrow*) and high (*arrowhead*) signal intensity. A spectral array from three-dimensional ^1H magnetic resonance spectroscopy (MRS) data shows choline, creatine and citrate peaks in a representative healthy voxel (**c**), and cancer (**d**) in five voxels. Superimposition of the MRS grid on (**b**) shows metabolic regions of healthy (H) and cancer (C) tissues (reprinted with permission from [63])

cancer before radical resection, statistically significant higher choline levels and lower citrate levels were observed in regions of cancer than in normal prostatic tissue. The ratio of (choline+creatine)/citrate provided a specific marker for cancer within the peripheral zone, with 98% of cancers having a (choline+creatine)/citrate ratio of greater than three standard deviations above the normal ratio. In addition, MRS was able to help discriminate between residual cancer from necrosis and other residual tissues in a study of 25 patients [63]. Kali et al. [64] have retrospectively assessed whether MR spectroscopic imaging with MRI can improve prostate-cancer localization in 49 post-biopsy hemorrhage cases. On T_2-weighted images, a higher percentage (80%) of hemorrhagic sites demonstrated low signal intensity, which is similar to the signal intensity seen with cancer. The addition of MR spectroscopic imaging to MRI resulted in a significant increase in the accuracy (52–75%) and specificity (26–66%) of tumor detection (Figs. 12.8 and 12.9). They used a 1.5-T system with a body coil to transmit radiofrequency pulses, and an endorectal coil in combination with pelvic phase-array coil to receive signals. Conventional T_1- and T_2-weighted axial as well as coronal images were obtained with a 14- to 16-cm field of view. The point-resolved spatial-selection technique was used to select a volume. Water and lipid suppression were accomplished by using band-selective inversion with gradient dephasing. An 8×8×8 or 16×8×8 phase-encoded array of spectra was acquired in 17 min. To spatially correlate the metabolic data with the prostatic zonal anatomy and MR images, the spectral arrays were overlaid on the corresponding T_2-weighted axial images. The MRI diagnosis of cancer was based on findings of a low-signal-intensity focus on the T_2-weighted images, and the MRS diagnosis of cancer was

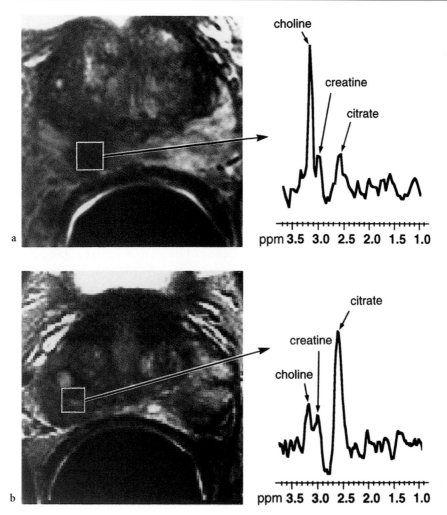

Fig. 12.9a,b. T_2-weighted axial image (*left*) in two different patients (**a** and **b**) show a low signal intensity at the sites of postbiopsy hemorrhage. Corresponding magnetic resonance spectra (*right*) show elevated choline and reduced citrate levels in **a**, proved to be a cancer, and normal choline and citrate levels in **b** (reprinted with permission from [63])

based on the (choline+creatine)/citrate peak-area ratio of more than three standard deviations greater than the normal value in one or more voxels.

Early studies demonstrated the feasibility of obtaining ^{31}P MRS spectra from perfused kidneys [64]. MRS studies suggested that noninvasive measurements of tissue pH and phosphates may provide a predictor of graft function after transplantation, and demonstrated metabolic changes produced by acute ischemic renal failure and the recovery of renal function by infusion of Mg^{2+} ATP [65]. MRS will be used to investigate and diagnose various forms of acute renal failure and to evaluate the metabolism of renal transplants during rejection, acute tubular necrosis, and cyclosporin nephrotoxicity [66]. Neuroblastoma is one of the most common childhood cancers and uniquely suited to in vivo MRS because it grows rapidly and stretches the abdominal wall quite thin. Studies have shown that ^{31}P MRS preceded and predicted the chemotherapeutic response (Fig. 12.10) [67]. Initial PME/ATP was 2.1, as measured on day 3 of the study. Ten days later, it had risen to 2.7, and the tumor increased 6 cm, as measured by abdominal girth. Six hours after chemotherapy using CDDP (cisplatin) and VP-16 (etoposide), the PME/ATP ratio was 2.7 (day 13), and 18 h after treatment it had fallen to 2.2. Six days following treatment, it continued to fall to 1.5. Little optimism remains for ^{31}P MRS as a substitute for histologic diagnosis; however, the proven ability of ^{31}P MRS to monitor cancer therapy implies a link with prognosis and detection of relapse [68].

Chapter 12 Urologic Cancers

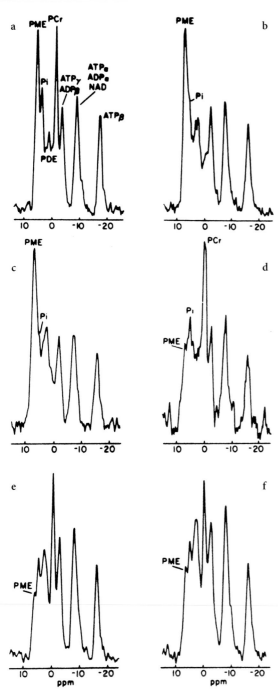

Fig. 12.10 a–f. ^{31}P MR spectral changes of neuroblastoma before (**a**), 4 (**b**), 8 (**c**), 16 (**d**) and 24 (**e, f**) weeks after treatment. A rise of the phosphomonoester (PME) peak seemed to predict tumor growth, while treatment produced an early fall of the PME peak (reprinted with permission from [67])

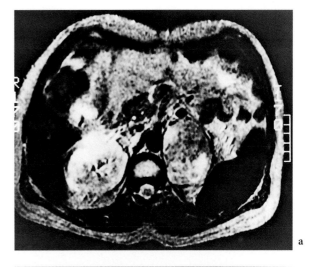

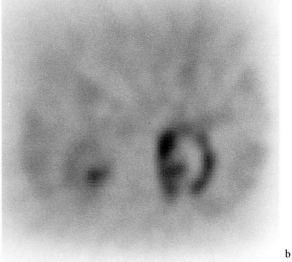

Fig. 12.11. a T_2-weighted axial MR images of the upper abdomen show a left renal-cell carcinoma with heterogeneous signal intensity after chemoembolization therapy. Note the tumor abutting the abdominal aorta. **b** Axial positron-emission tomography image of the upper abdomen shows an increased uptake of ^{18}F fluoro-2-deoxy-D-glucose in the rim of the left renal-cell carcinoma. Note also physiologic activity in the right renal pelvis

Positron Emission Tomography

Metabolic activity of RCCs, neuroblastomas and pheochromocytoma has been characterized by ^{18}F-fluoro-2-deoxy-D-glucose positron-emission tomography (FDG-PET) (Figs. 12.11–12.13) [69]. Uptake of FDG was detected in 16 of 17 patients with neuroblastomas, and primary as well as metastatic lesions avidly concentrated FDG prior to chemotherapy or radiation therapy. FDG uptake in one patient was intense, but ^{131}I metaiodobenzylguanidine (MIBG) failed to accumulate. Prelim-

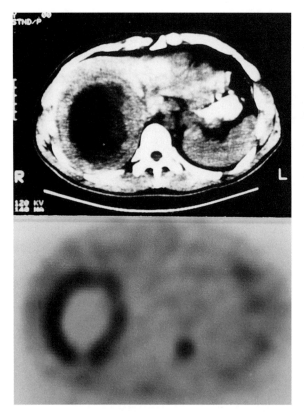

Fig. 12.12. Contrast computed-tomography axial image of the upper abdomen (*upper*) shows a large metastatic renal cancer in the right hepatic lobe with peripheral contrast enhancement. Corresponding positron-emission tomography image (*lower*) shows also a markedly increased uptake of ^{18}F-fluoro-2-deoxy-D-glucose in the rim of the necrotic metastasis

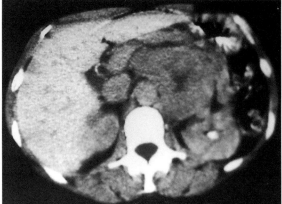

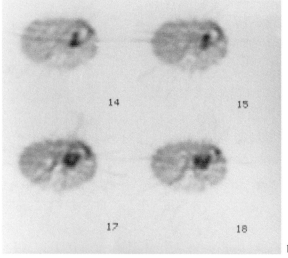

Fig. 12.13. a Axial contrast computed-tomography image of the upper abdomen shows a large mass lesion in the left adrenal gland. **b** Comparable positron-emission tomography axial image shows a markedly increased uptake of ^{18}F-fluoro-2-deoxy-D-glucose in the periphery of necrotic pheochromocytoma in the left adrenal gland

inary studies indicate the feasibility of ^{18}F FDG-PET scans in patients with bladder cancer, although a major remaining pitfall is intense FDG accumulation in the urine, despite retrograde irrigation of the urinary bladder with 1000–3700 ml saline. A FDG-PET scan was true positive in 8 of 12 patients (66.7%), but false negative in 4 (33.3%). Of 20 organs with tumor mass lesions, 16 (80%) were detected by FDG-PET scan. PET detected all of 17 distant metastatic lesions and 2 of 3 proven lymph-node metastases (Fig. 12.14). FDG-PET was capable of differentiating between viable recurrent bladder cancer and radiation-induced changes in two patients [70]. Of 202 untreated prostate-cancer bone metastases, 22 patients had a sensitivity to ^{18}F FDG-PET of 65% (131 of 202 lesions), with a positive-predictive value of 98% (131 of 133 lesions). The estimated standard uptake value (SUV) in metastases was 2.1–5.7 (Fig. 12.14) [71]. Soft-tissue metastases to the lymph nodes or liver were also identified, but evaluation of pelvic lymph nodes was severely limited by the bladder activity [72]. The more global measures of FDG metabolism, such as SUV and metabolic rate of FDG utilization, were not significantly changed in rat-prostate adenocarcinoma after chemotherapy with gemcitabine, while DNA synthesis and cell viability declined (Fig. 12.15) [73]. Tumor differentiation of testicular teratocarcinoma metastases may be assessed by measuring glucose metabolism. Before chemotherapy, the retroperitoneal metastases of a testicular teratoadenocarcinoma predominantly composed of embryonal carcinoma demonstrated heterogeneously increased glucose metabolism, as measured by ^{18}F FDG-PET. After chemotherapy, FDG uptake was reduced to normal values despite increased tumor volume [74].

CHAPTER 12 Urologic Cancers   195

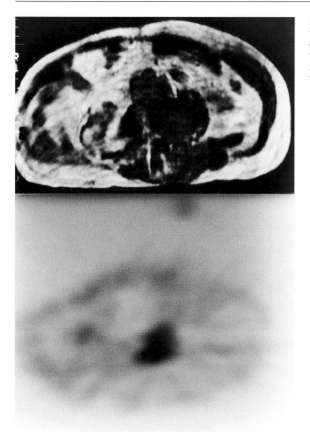

Fig. 12.14. T_1-weighted axial magnetic resonance image of the lower abdomen (*upper*) shows a metastatic bladder carcinoma involving L4 vertebral body and left psoas muscle with low signal intensity. Comparable positron-emission tomography image (*lower*) shows a markedly increased uptake of ^{18}F-fluoro-2-deoxy-D-glucose

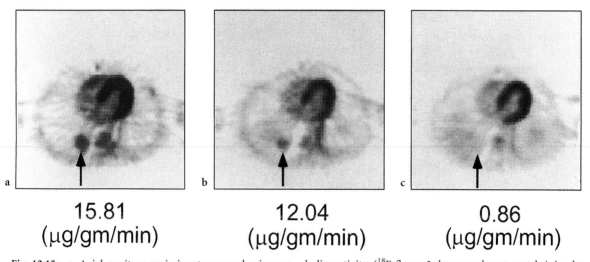

Fig. 12.15a–c. Axial positron-emission tomography images of the lower chest before (**a**), 1 week (**b**) and 8 weeks (**c**) after treatment using Suramin show the decreasing metabolic activity (^{18}F-fluoro-2-deoxy-D-glucose uptake) in the metastatic prostate carcinoma in the right posterior lower lung (*arrows*) (reprinted with permission from [71])

References

1. Landis SH, Murray T, Bolden S, Wingo PA (1998) Cancer Statistics, 1998. CA Cancer J Clin 48:6–29
2. Broecker B (1991) Renal cell carcinoma in children. Urology 38:54–56
3. Kauzlaric D, Barmeir E, Luscieti P (1987) Renal carcinoma after retrograde pyelography with thorotrast. AJR Am J Roentgenol 148:897–898
4. Papadopoulos I, Wirth B, Wand H (1990) Xanthogranulomatous pyelonephritis associated with renal cell carcinoma. Eur Urol 18:74–76
5. Maher ER, Yates JRW (1991) Familial renal cell carcinoma: clinical and molecular genetic aspects. Br J Cancer 63:176–179
6. Altaffer LF, Chenault OW (1979) Paraneoplastic endocrinopathies associated with renal tumors. J Urol 122:573–577
7. Holland JM (1973) Cancer of the kidney: natural history and staging. Cancer 32:1032–1042
8. Silverman DT, Hartge P, Morrison AS (1992) Epidemiology of bladder cancer. Hematol Oncol Clin North Am 6:1–30
9. Burch JD, Rohern TE, Howe GR (1989) Risk of bladder cancer by source and type of tobacco exposure: a case-control study. Int J Cancer 44:622–628
10. Piper JM, Tonocia J, Matanoski GM (1985) Heavy phenacetin use and bladder cancer in women aged 20 to 49 years. N Engl J Med 313:292–295
11. Kantor AF, Hartge P, Hoover RN (1984) Chromosome 9 allelic loss and microsatellite alterations in human bladder cancer. Cancer Res 54:2848–2851
12. Orlow I, Lianes P, Lacombe L (1994) Chromosome 9 allelic loss and microsatellite alterations in human bladder cancer. Cancer Res 54:2848–2851
13. Walman FM, Carroll PR, Kerschmann R (1991) Centromeric copy number of chromosome 7 is strongly correlated with tumor grade and labeling index in human bladder cancer. Cancer Res 51:3807–3813
14. Presti JCV Jr, Reuter VE, Galan T (1991) Molecular genetic alteration in superficial and locally advanced human bladder cancer. Cancer Res 51:5405–5409
15. Esrig DE, Elamjian D, Groshen S (1994) Accumulation of nuclear p53 and tumor progression in bladder cancer. N Engl J Med 331:1259–1264
16. Sarkis AS, Dalbagni G, Gordon-Cardo C (1994) Association of p53 nuclear overexpression and tumor progression in carcinoma in situ of the bladder. J Urol 152:388–392
17. Cairns P, Proctor AJ, Knowles MA (1991) Loss of heterozygosity at the Rb locus is frequent and correlates with muscle invasion in bladder carcinoma. Oncogene 8:2305–2308
18. Hsing AW, Devesa SS (1994) Prostate cancer mortality in the United States by cohort year of birth, 1865–1940. Cancer Epidemiol Biomarkers Prev 3:527–530
19. Zaridze DG, Boyle P (1987) Cancer of the prostate: epidemiology and etiology. Br J Urol 59:493–502
20. Carter HB, Coffey DS (1990) The prostate: an increasing medical problem. Prostate 16:39–48
21. Ross RK, Bernstein L, Judd H (1986) Serum testosterone levels in healthy young black and white men. J Natl Cancer Inst 76:45–48
22. Gitter RF (1991) Carcinoma of the prostate. N Engl J Med 324:236–245
23. Visakorpi T, Kallioniemi AH, Syuvanen A-C (1995) Genetic changes in primary and recurrent prostate cancer by comparative genomic hybridization. Cancer Res 55:342–347
24. Peehl DM (1993) Oncogenes in prostate cancer. Cancer 71:1159–1164
25. Navone NM, Troncoso P (1993) p53 protein accumulation and gene mutation in the progression of human prostate carcinoma. J Natl Cancer Inst 85:1657–1669
26. Phillips SM, Barton CM, Lee SJ (1994) Loss of the retinoblastoma susceptibility gene (Rb 1) is a frequent and early even in prostatic tumorigenesis. Br J Cancer 70:1252–1257
27. Ching KZ, Ramsey E (1993) Expression of mRNA for epidermal growth factor, transforming growth factor-alpha and their receptors in human prostate tissue and cell lines. Mol Cell Biochem 126:151–158
28. Myers RB, Srivastara S, Oelschlager DK (1994) Expression of p 160 $^{erb\ B-3}$ and p185 $^{erb\ B-2}$ in prostatic intraepithelial neoplasia and prostatic adenocarcinoma. J Natl Cancer Inst 86:1140–1145
29. Sadasivan R, Morgan R (1993) Overexpression of HER-2/neu may be an indicator of poor prognosis in prostatic cancer. J Urol 150:126–131
30. Colombel M, Symmans F (1993) Detection of the apoptosis-suppressing of oncoprotein bcl-2 in hormone-refractor human prostate cancer. Am J Pathol 143:390–400
31. Schottenfeld D, Warshauer ME, Sherlock S (1980) The epidemiology of testicular cancer in young adults. Am J Epidemiol 112:232–246
32. Strader CH, Weiss NS, Daling JR (1988) Cryptorchism, orchiopexy and the risk of testicular cancer. Am J Epidemiol 127:1013–1318
33. Mills PK, Newell GR, Johnson DE (1984) Testicular cancer associated with employment in agriculture and oil and natural gas extraction. Lancet 1:207–209
34. O'Toole KM, Brown M, Hoffman P (1993) Pathology of benign and malignant kidney tumors. Urol Clin North Am 20:193–205
35. Fuhrman SA, Lasky LC, Limas C (1982) Prognostic significant of morphologic parameters in renal cell carcinoma. Am J Surg Pathol 6:655–663
36. Sene AP, Hunt L, McMahon RFT (1992) Renal carcinoma in patients undergoing nephrectomy: analysis of survival and prognostic factors. Br J Urol 70:125–134
37. Ljungberg B, Roos G (1990) Value of DNA analysis for treatment of renal cell carcinoma. Eur Urol 18:31–32
38. Benson MA, Haaga JR, Resnick MI (1989) Staging renal carcinoma: what is sufficient? Arch Surg 124:71–73
39. Melicow MM (1974) Tumor of the bladder: a multifaceted problem. J Urol 68:467–478
40. Cooper PH, Waisman J, Johanston WH (1973) Several atypia of transitional epithelium and carcinoma of the urinary bladder. Cancer 31:1055–1060
41. Althausen AF, Prout GR Jr, Daly JJ (1976) Noninvasive papillary carcinoma of the bladder associated with carcinoma in situ. J Urol 116:575–579
42. Amato RJ, Logothetis CJ (1992) Chemotherapy for small cell carcinoma of prostatic origin. J Urol 147:935–937
43. Brown PN, Ayala AG, von Eschenbach AC (1982) Histologic grading study of prostate adenocarcinoma. The development of a new system and comparison with other methods – a preliminary study. Cancer 49:525–532
44. Visakorpi T, Kallioniemi OP, Koivula T (19903) Review of new prognostic factors in prostatic carcinoma. Eur Urol 24:438–449
45. Sella A, Kilbourn R (1994) Phase II study of ketoconazole combined with weekly doxorubicin in patients with androgen-independent prostate cancer. J Clin Oncol 12:683–688
46. Gondos B, Berthelsen JG, Skakkeback NE (1983) Intratubular germ cell neoplasms (carcinoma in situ): a preinvasive lesion of the testis. Ann Clin Lab Sci 13:185–192
47. Ulbright TM, Rorth LM (1987) Should an elevated human chorionic gonadotropin titer after therapy for seminoma? J Urol 131:63–65

48. Yamashita Y, Miyazaki T, Hatanaka Y, Takahashi M (1995) Dynamic MRI of small renal cell carcinoma. J Comput Assist Tomogr 19:759–765
49. Scattoni V, Columbo R, Nava L (1995) Imaging of renal cell carcinoma with gadolinium-enhanced magnetic resonance: radiological and pathological study. Urol Int 54:121–127
50. Kallman DA, King BF, Hattery RR (1992) Renal vein and inferior vena cava tumor thrombus in renal cell carcinoma: CT, US, MRI, and venacavography. J Comput Assist Tomogr 16:240–247
51. Studer UE, Scherz S, Scheidegger J (1990) Enlargement of regional lymph nodes in renal cell carcinoma is often not due to metastasis. J Urol 144:243–245
52. Whitmore WFJ (1983) Management of invasive bladder neoplasm. Semin Urol 1:34–41
53. Kim B, Semelka RC, Ascher SM, Chalpin DB, Carroll PR, Hricak H (1994) Bladder tumor staging: comparison of contrast-enhanced CT, T_1- and T_2-weighted MRI, dynamic gadolinium-enhanced imaging, and late gadolinium-enhanced imaging. Radiology 193:239–245
54. Rifkin MD, Dahner W, Kurtz AB (1990) State of the art endorectal sonography of the prostate gland. AJR Am J Roentgenol 154:691–700
55. Schiebler ML, Schnall MD, Pollack HM (1993) Current role of MR imaging in the staging of adenocarcinoma of the prostate. Radiology 189:339–352
56. Schnall MD, Tomaszewski J, Pollack HM (1991) The bulging prostate gland: a sign of capsular involvement. J Magn Res Imaging 1:279–284
57. Tempany CM, Rhamouni AD, Epstein J (1991) Invasion of the neurovascular bundle by prostatic cancer: evaluation with MR imaging. Radiology 181:107–112
58. Schnall MD, Imai Y, Tomaszewski J (1991) Prostate cancer: local staging with endorectal surface coil MR imaging. Radiology 178:797–802
59. McNeal JE (1992) Cancer volume and site of origin of adenocarcinoma in the prostate: relationship to local and distant spread. Hum Pathol 23:258–266
60. Grist TM, Charles HC, Sostman HD (1991) Renal transplant rejection: diagnosis with 31p MR spectroscopy. AJR Am J Roentgenol 156:105–112
61. Kurhanewicz J, Vigneron DB, Hricak H, Narayan P, Caroll P, Nelson SJ (1996) Three-dimensional H-1 MR spectroscopic imaging of the in situ human prostate with high spatial resolution. Radiology 198:795–805
62. Perivar F, Hricak H, Shinohara K (1996) Detection of locally recurrent prostate cancer after cryosurgery: evaluation by transrectal ultrasound, magnetic resonance imaging, and three-dimensional proton magnetic resonance spectroscopy. Urology 48:594–599
63. Kali Y, Kurhanewicz J, Hricak H, Sokolov D, Huang LR, Nelson SJ, Vigneron DB (1998) Localizing prostate cancer in the presence of postbiopsy changes on MR images: role of proton MR spectroscopic imaging. Radiology 206:785–790
64. Ackerman JJH, Lawry M, Radda GK, Ross BD, Wong GG (1981) The role of intrarenal pH in regulation of ammoniagenesis: ^{31}P NMR studies of the isolated perfused rat kidney. J Physiol (Lond) 319:65–80
65. Siegel NJ, Avison MJ, Reilly HF, Alger JR, Shulman RG (1983) Enhanced recovery of renal ATP with postischemic infusion of ATP-MgCl$_2$ determined by ^{31}P NMR. Am J Physiol 245:F530–F534
66. Wong GC, Ross BD (1983) Application of phosphorus NMR to problems of renal physiology and metabolism. Miner Electrolyte Metab 9:222–289
67. Maris J, Evans A, McLaughlin A, D'Angio G, Bolinger L, Manos H, Chance B (1985) ^{31}P NMR spectroscopic investigation of human neuroblastoma in situ. New Engl J Med 312:1500–1505
68. Chance B, Northrop J (1986) How MR spectroscopy is deployed depends upon intended goals. Diagn Imaging (November) pp 311–320
69. Shulkin BL, Hutchinson RJ, Castle VP, Yanik G, Shapiro B, Sisson JC (1996) Neuroblastoma: PET with 2-F-18-fluoro-2-deoxy-D-glucose compared with metaiodobenzylgeaimidine scintigraphy. Radiology 199:743–750
70. Kosuda S, Kison PV, Greenough R, Grossman HB, Wahl RL (1997) Preliminary assessment of fluorine-18 fluorodeoxyglucose positron emission tomography in patients with bladder cancer. Eur J Nucl Med 24:615–620
71. Hoh CK, Schiepers C, Seltzer MA, Gambhir SS, Silverman DHS, Czernin J, Maddahi J, Phelps ME (1997) PET in oncology: will it replace the other modalities? Semin Nucl Med 27:94–106
72. Shreve PD, Grossman HB, Gross MD, Wahl RL (1996) Metastatic prostate cancer: initial findings of PET with 2-deoxy-2-[F-18] fluoro-D-glucose. Radiology 199:751–756
73. Haberkorn U, Bellemann ME, Altmann A, Gerlach L, Moss I, Oberdorfer F, Brix G, Doll J, Blatter J, van Kaick G (1997) PET 2-fluoro-2-deoxyglucose uptake in rat prostate adenocarcinoma during chemotherapy with gemcitabine. J Nucl Med 38:1215–1221
74. Reinhardt MJ, Müller-Mattheis VGO, Gerharz CD, Vosberg HR, Ackermann R, Müller-Gartner H-W (1997) FDG PET evaluation of retroperitoneal metastases of testicular cancer before and after chemotherapy. J Nucl Med 38:99–101

Gynecologic Cancers

E. E. Kim

Basic Considerations

Ovarian Cancer

Ovarian cancer is the sixth most common cancer, with 25 400 new cases estimated for 1998. It is the fourth most common cause of cancer-related deaths in American women and the most frequent cause of death from gynecologic cancers in the United States; it is predicted that it will account for 14,500 deaths in 1998 [1]. The median age at diagnosis is about 62 years, and incidence rises rapidly after age 60 years [2]. The strongest risk factor for ovarian cancer is a familial pattern of ovarian cancer, which is reported in about 7% of cancer patients [3].

Two factors, an increasing number of pregnancies and the use of oral contraceptives, have been shown to reduce the risk for this cancer, possibly due to excess gonadotropin secretion or incessant ovulation [4]. Estrogen has been shown to stimulate the growth of ovarian cancer cell lines [5]. It has been suggested that the intraperitoneal growth of ovarian cancer may be related to a local deficiency of antitumor immune-effector mechanisms. Levels of interleukin-10 and -6 are particularly elevated in ovarian cancer ascites [6]. Epidermal-growth-factor (EGF) receptors have been detected in a high percentage of ovarian cancer specimens, and their overexpression has been correlated with a poor prognosis. The effects of transforming growth factor beta (TGF-β), which is closely related to EGF, are mediated through the EGF receptor, and TGF-β has been shown to inhibit some ovarian cancer cell lines [5]. HER-2/neu is overexpressed in about 30% of ovarian cancers and appears to indicate poor prognosis and survival [7]. The $p53$ gene located on chromosome 17p has been seen to be overexpressed and mutated in about 30–50% of ovarian cancers [8]. MDR-1 is specifically stimulated by mutant p53 and repressed by wild-type p53, implying an increased drug resistance [9]. Levels of tumor necrosis factor (TNF)-α are also increased in ascites, and TNF has been shown to upregulate $p53$ mRNA expression and to induce apoptosis in an ovarian cancer cell line [10]. The highest carcinoma antigen (CA)-125 levels are seen in the most poorly differentiated tumors, but the absolute level of CA-125 does not relate to the volume of ovarian tumor, tumor grade, DNA ploidy or S-phase fraction [11]. Most invasive cancers are aneuploid and most borderline tumors are diploid. The 5-year disease-free survival for patients with diploid tumors is 90% versus 64% for those with aneuploid tumors [12]. The prognostic factors in early (stage I–IIa) ovarian cancer are stage, histologic grade and type, and age [13]. The high-risk patients are older than 70 years of age, have tumors that are aneuploid, stage IV, clear cell and/or unclassified type, grade III, and have bulky disease. Low-risk patients are younger than 40 years of age, have tumors that are euploid, stage III, serous and/or endometrioid type, grade I, and have no residual tumors [5]. It is now clear that 30–50% of patients with no pathologic evidence of disease will experience a relapse [14]. Pretreatment characteristics used in calculating the prognostic index are performance status, tumor stage, grade and residual size, and presence of ascites [15].

Carcinoma of the Uterine Endometrium

Carcinoma of the uterine endometrium is the most common female pelvic malignancy and the fourth most common cancer in females. In 1998, it is estimated that 36,100 new cases will arise, from which 6,300 related deaths will occur in the United States [1]. The recent rise in the incidence of endometrial carcinoma may be related to the decreased incidence of cervical carcinoma, prolonged life expectancy, and earlier diagnosis. This cancer occurs mostly in postmenopausal women. Clinical evidence indicates that conditions resulting in hyperestrinism predispose patients to endometrial carcinoma. Adipose tissue contains aromatase enzymes that convert the adrenal-derived androstenedione to estrone, which can be converted to estradiol, resulting in endometrial proliferation, hyperplasia and, potentially, carcinoma. Polycystic ovarian syndrome increases the risk of endometrial carcinoma secondary to anovulation. Most studies confirm that tamoxifen may cause potentially malignant changes in the endometrium of postmenopausal women [16]. Tamoxifen and its metabolite, 4-hydroxytamoxifen, stimulate some endometrial carcinoma cell lines but inhibit others, as well as some primary cultures of human endometrial carcinoma cells [17].

Uterine Cervical Cancer

Uterine cervical cancer is the most common cancer among females in some developing countries; in the United States, it is the seventh most common cancer in females. It is estimated that 13,700 new cases will be found and 4,900 deaths will be caused by uterine cervical cancer in 1998 [1]. The incidence and mortality rates for cervical carcinoma have decreased over the past four decades in the United States by as much as 70–75% [18]. Infection with human papilloma virus (HPV) types 16, 18, 45, or 56 has a high correlation with cervical cancer. It is known that the E6 protein produced by high-risk HPV types 16 and 18 can combine with the p53 protein and cause the same functional consequences as a *p53* gene mutation [19]. The E7 protein of HPV-16 was also shown to bind to the p105-RB protein encoded by the retinoblastoma gene (*Rb1*) [20]. A higher rate of recurrent cervical cancer was seen in patients with an S-phase fraction greater than or equal to 20% [21]. The overexpression of the HER-2/neu and c-myc oncogenes has been found to be associated with a poor prognosis [22]. Other factors affecting survival are tumor stage, size and volume, endometrial extension, and bilateral parametrial involvement. Five-year survival ranged from 91% in patients with tumors smaller than 2.5 cm^3 to 48% for patients with tumors larger than 50 cm^3 [23]. A decreased survival rate for patients having bilateral parametrial extension, compared with patients having unilateral involvement, was reported for stage IIB disease [24]. Tanaka et al. [25] reported a 10% 5-year survival for patients with periaortic-lymph-node metastasis, and 49% for those with involved pelvic lymph nodes. Both anemia and thrombocytosis have been associated with decreased survival rates in patients treated with radiation therapy [26].

Pathology, Diagnosis and Staging

The epithelial lining of the ovary and the peritoneum is similar to the coelomic epithelium which gives rise to the fallopian tube, uterus, cervix, and Müllerian duct, and from which approximately 75% of all primary *ovarian tumors* arise. Epithelial ovarian tumors are characterized by varying amounts and activities of the gonadal mesenchyma, and they are classified as benign, borderline malignant, of low malignant potential, or malignant. The major cell types of epithelial tumors are serous, mucinous, endometrioid, clear cell, transitional, and undifferentiated. They show different biologic behaviors, likelihoods of metastasis, and consequent variations in prognosis and treatment. However, identifying the histologic types of invasive epithelial carcinomas has limited prognostic significance. Serous tumors represent 50% of epithelial ovarian tumors, and 10% of them are borderline malignant tumors; 50% occur before the age of 40 years, and the 5-year-survival rate is 80–90%. Malignant psammoma bodies are found in 80% of serous carcinomas. Mucinous tumors make up 8–10% of epithelial ovarian tumors, and the mucinous lesions are intra-ovarian in 95–98% of cases. Pseudomyxoma peritonei is most commonly secondary to mucinous ovarian carcinoma. About 6–8% of epithelial ovarian tumors resemble endometrial adenocarcinoma, and concurrent endometriosis is present in 10% of cases.

Identification of multifocal disease is important. Two histologic grading systems are in common use, the pattern system and Broder's grading system. The pattern system considers the microscopic appearance of a lesion; lesions range from grade I (well-differentiated) to grade II (moderately differentiated) to grade III (poorly differentiated and predominantly solid). Broder's grading system classifies lesions from grade I to grade IV, depending on the cytologic and nuclear characteristics.

The clinical signs of ovarian carcinoma are nonspecific and include pelvic mass, ascites, pleural effusion and occasionally supraclavicular lymphadenopathy. Some patients may present with various types of paraneoplastic conditions, such as hypercalcemia, cerebellar degeneration, seborrheic keratosis, or chronic intravascular coagulation.

A preoperative evaluation should include abdominal/pelvic computed tomography (CT), chest X-ray and CA-125 measurement. Mammography may be helpful in ruling out metastatic breast cancer. Ascitic fluid should be tapped and examined.

Table 13.1. International Federation of Gynecology and Obstetrics staging of ovarian cancer

Stage I	Limited to ovaries
IA	One ovary; capsule intact; no ascites
IB	Both ovaries; capsule intact; no ascites
IC	Tumor on surface; ruptured capsule; or ascites
Stage II	One or both ovaries; pelvic extension
IIA	Uterus and/or tubes
IIB	Other pelvic tissues
IIC	Malignant ascites cells or peritoneal washings
Stage III	Peritoneal implants; liver; small bowel or omentum
IIIA	Microscopic seeding of peritoneal surfaces
IIIB	<2 cm implants of peritoneal surfaces
IIIC	>2 cm abdominal implants and/or positive retro-peritoneal nodes
Stage IV	Distant metastasis; malignant pleural effusion; liver metastasis

Table 13.2. International Federation of Gynecology and Obstetrics staging of endometrial cancer

Stage I	
Ia	Endometrium
Ib	≤50% myometrium
Ic	>50% myometrium
Stage II	
IIa	Endocervical gland
IIb	Cervical stroma
Stage III	
IIIa	Serosa and/or adnexae, and/or positive peritoneal cytology
IIIb	Vaginal metastasis
IIIc	Pelvic and/or paraaortic nodes
Stage IV	
IVa	Bladder and/or bowel mucosa
IVb	Intra-abdominal and/or inguinal nodes

Table 13.3. International Federation of Gynecology and Obstetrics staging of uterine cervix cancer

Stage 0	In situ, intraepithelial preinvasive
Stage I	Confined to cervix
Ia1	Microscopic invasion of stroma, <3 mm depth and <7 mm width
Ia2	Microscopic invasion of stroma, 3–5 mm depth and <7 mm width
Ib1	Clinical lesion, <4 cm size
Ib2	Clinical lesion, >4 cm size
Stage II	Beyond cervix; upper vagina
IIa	No obvious parametrial involvement
IIb	Parametrial involvement
Stage III	Pelvic wall; lower third of vagina
IIIa	Lower third of vagina; no pelvic wall
IIIb	Pelvic wall; hydronephrosis
Stage IV	Beyond true pelvis
IVa	Bladder or rectum
IVb	Distant organs

Meticulous surgical staging should be performed for early-stage ovarian cancer. According to the FIGO (International Federation of Gynecology and Obstetrics) system (Table 13.1), stage I has a 5-year survival rate of 80–90%; stage II 40–60%; stage III 10–15%; and stage IV less than 5%.

Carcinoma of the uterine endometrium is easily diagnosed, but a well-differentiated carcinoma may be confused with atypical hyperplasia. Most endometrial carcinomas are pure adenocarcinomas, which are usually classified by three grades: grade I, well-differentiated lesions (70%–75%); grade II, moderately differentiated lesions; and grade III, poorly differentiated lesions. Adenosquamous carcinoma is a mixed tumor in which the squamous element is malignant. Uterine papillary serous carcinoma is similar in its clinical behavior to ovarian papillary serous carcinoma and characterized by a high relapse rate, a propensity for transperitoneal seeding, and a poor prognosis [27]. Papillary (villoglandular) endometrioid carcinoma may respond to hormone therapy. Mucinous adenocarcinoma accounts for fewer than 1% of all endometrial carcinomas and is usually associated with a good prognosis. Mesonephroid carcinoma is similar to clear cell carcinoma arising in the ovaries and tends to be deeply invasive. Undifferentiated carcinoma has no glandular, squamous, or sarcomatous differentiation and a poor prognosis. An atypical Papanicolaou smear suggests an adenocarcinoma. Postmenopausal bleeding is the presenting symptom in 90% of women. Tumor spread may be by direct extension to adjacent structures, transtubal passage of exfoliated cells, or lymphatic or hematogenous dissemination [28]. Staging by FIGO has incorporated surgical information (Table 13.2).

Staging is the most important prognostic factor. The 5-year survival rates of stage I and IV diseases are 76.3% and 10.3%, respectively. The risk of pelvic-node metastasis is increased fourfold if the vascular space has been invaded. Estrogen- and progesterone-receptor levels are inversely proportional to tumor grade, stage, and depth of invasion. Tumor grade/stage and invasiveness correlate with the expression of several oncogenes (fms, neu, fos, myb, erb-B, and myc) and the production of growth factors, and TGF-α and EGF receptor [29].

The majority of *uterine cervical cancers* are squamous cell carcinomas which may be either keratinizing or nonkeratinizing. Histologic grading has no significant impact on prognosis. Adenocarcinomas of the uterine cervix account for about 14% of cervical carcinomas and have been increasing over the past few decades. Adenocarcinoma has a worse prognosis than squamous cell carcinoma [30]. Adenosquamous carcinomas are associated with a higher risk of pelvic nodal metastasis than squamous cell carcinomas or adenocarcinomas, and glassy-cell carcinoma is a poorly differentiated form of adenosquamous carcinoma. Verrucous carcinoma is an extremely well-differentiated variant of squamous cell carcinoma. Small cell carcinomas have a very poor prognosis, and the most aggressive tumors are those with neuroendocrine differentiation. Other cervical malignancies include sarcomas, melanomas, lymphomas, germ-cell tumors, and trophoblastic tumors. The development of invasive cervical carcinoma has been viewed as a continuum that begins with mild dysplasia designated as cervical intraepithelial neoplasia (CIN)-1. Moderate dysplasia is designated as CIN-2, and severe dysplasia and carcinoma in situ are grouped together as CIN-3. CIN-2 and CIN-3 lesions are generally associated with aneuploidy and HPV infection, and are grouped together as high-grade CIN. Low-grade squamous intraepithelial lesion (SIL) includes CIN-1 and cellular changes associated with HPV. High-grade SIL combines CIN-2 and CIN-3. Invasive cervical carcinoma (stage I–IV) usually presents as vaginal bleeding or discharge. Patients may have dull pelvic pain and sciatica with involvement of pelvic, para-aortic, mediastinal, and supraclavicular nodes. Hematogenous metastasis to lungs, bones and liver occurs late. The most widely used staging system is the one developed by FIGO (Table 13.3).

The FIGO system uses findings from physical examinations, colposcopy, biopsies, ECG, chest X-ray, intravenous pyelography (IVP), cystoscopy, and proctosigmoidoscopy to determine the clinical stage. A CT scan is used in place of an IVP to evaluate whether obstructive uropathy is present. Clinical staging correlates with tumor burden, as well as with the risk for lymph-node and distant metastases [31]. The 5-year survival rate ranges from 91% in patients with tumors smaller than 2.5 cm^3 to 48% for patients with tumors larger than 50 cm^3 [23]. The presence of periaortic and pelvic lymph-node metastases results in lower survival rates. Tanaka et al. [25] reported a 10% 5-year survival rate for patients with periaortic lymph node metastasis, 49% for those with involved pelvic lymph nodes, and 92% for patients with negative lymph-node involvement. The 5-year-survival rate was 62% for those with one node positive for tumor, 36% for two positive nodes, 20% for three or four positive nodes, and 0% for those with five or more positive nodes. A higher rate of recurrence was seen in patients with an S-phase fraction greater than or equal to 20% [21]. The overexpression of the HER-2/neu and c-myc oncogene has been found to be associated with a poor prognosis, exhibiting both anemia (hemoglobin <12 g/dl) and thrombocytosis (>4,000,000/μl) [26].

Magnetic Resonance Imaging

The role of magnetic resonance imaging (MRI) in evaluating patients with suspected adnexal tumors lies in lesion detection, characterization, staging, and follow-up. The sensitivity of MRI in the detection of adnexal lesions is comparable with CT and ultrasound, ranging from 87% to 100% [32]. In the characterization of adnexal masses, MRI has an accuracy ranging from 83% to 95%, compared with 63% to 88% on ultrasound and 66% to 94% on CT [33]. On MRI, ovarian cancer usually appears as a large heterogeneous solid and cystic lesion which is commonly bilateral. Well-differentiated tumors of low malignant potential appear primarily cystic with intracystic vegetations, while undifferentiated tumors tend to have large amounts of solid tissue, necrosis, and hemorrhage. Solid components of an ovarian cancer usually demonstrate low-to-intermediate signal intensity on T_1-weighted images and high signal intensity on T_2-weighted images. Cystic ovarian cancers containing proteinaceous or hemorrhagic material may manifest high signal intensity on both T_1- and T_2-weighted images. Cystic carcinomas may demonstrate thick walls or septa (>3 mm) and contain vegetations or regions of soft-tissue nodularity. These findings are best shown on T_2-weighted or gadolinium-enhanced T_1-weighted images. Gadolinium is useful for determining wall thickness or the presence and thickness of septations, identifying vegetation or soft-tissue nodules, and depicting tumor necrosis. The likelihood of malignancy increases with the amount of soft tissue present within a lesion [34]. Primary criteria suggesting malignancy include: size greater than 4 cm, solid lesion, wall thickness greater than 3 mm, septa greater than 3 mm, vegetation or nodularity, and presence of necrosis. Ancillary criteria include: involvement of pelvic organs or sidewall; peritoneal, mesenteric or omental disease; ascites; and lymphadenopathy. The findings most predictive of malignancy or multivariant analysis of these criteria are presence of necrosis within a solid lesion, vegetations within a cystic lesion, presence of peritoneal metastases, and ascites [35].

MRI may be superior to CT in the assessment of pelvic involvement by ovarian cancer [36]. Low-signal-intensity tumor implants or standing may be identified on T_1-weighted images with

CHAPTER 13 Gynecologic Cancers   203

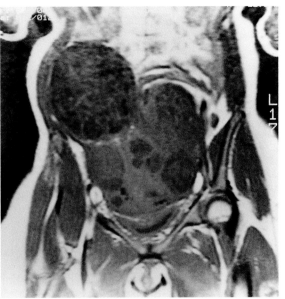

Fig. 13.2. T_1-weighted coronal image of the abdomen and pelvis shows multiple uterine extraserosal and intramural fibroids with heterogeneous intermediate signal intensity, suggesting degeneration

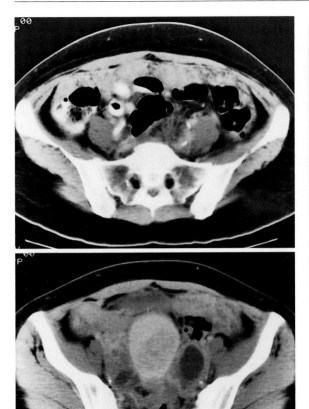

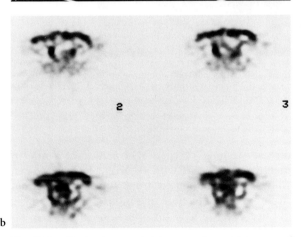

Fig. 13.1. a Contrast-computed-tomography axial images of the pelvis show a left cystic ovarian carcinoma (*lower*) with omental (*upper*) and mesenteric (*lower*) metastases. **b** Selected positron-emission tomography axial images of the pelvis at comparable levels show moderately increased uptake of ^{18}F-fluoro-2-deoxy-D-glucose in the rim of left ovarian cancer (*lower*) and markedly increased activities in the omental and mesenteric metastases (*upper*)

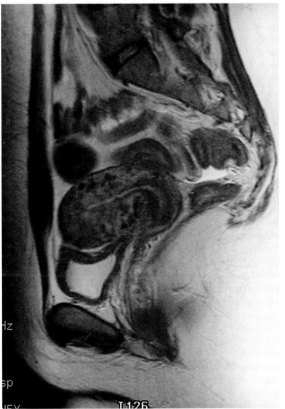

Fig. 13.3. T_2-weighted sagittal image of the pelvis shows an anteroverted uterus with serpiginous low-signal-intensity areas in the myometrium, indicating bilateral uterine vessels in a patient with a hydatidiform mole

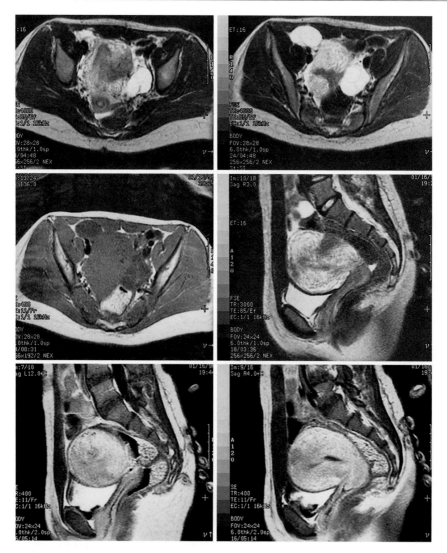

Fig. 13.4. T$_2$- (*top*) and T$_1$- (*middle left*) weighted axial images of the pelvis show cystic lesions in the bilateral ovaries. A choriocarcinoma is seen in the posterior myometrium on a T$_2$-weighted sagittal image of the pelvis (*middle right*). Note also contrast enhancement and dilated uterine vessels on post-gadolinium T$_1$-weighted sagittal images of the pelvis (*bottom*)

corresponding regions of high signal intensity on T$_2$-weighted images. Pelvic implants will enhance after gadolinium injection. The presence of ureteral obstruction, as well as extension of cancer to the pelvic wall or retroperitoneum, may also be seen on MRI. Outside of the pelvis, MRI may be useful in detecting ascites, peritoneal implant, and presence of omental and mesenteric lesions.

Due to limitations in identifying small peritoneal implants and mesenteric nodules, overall staging accuracy by MRI or CT is only moderate compared with surgical staging (Fig. 13.1). However, prediction of tumor resectability is excellent for both MRI and CT [36]. Second-look laparotomy should be limited to patients with minimal disease (lesions <2 cm). MRI may have a role in identifying patients with recurrent lesions >2 cm, who would not benefit from surgical debulking. Accuracy in detection of lesions >2 cm is 82%, but decreases to 33% for lesions <2 cm [37].

MRI shows no specificity for endometrial tumor detection. The signal intensity of small endometrial cancers is often similar to that of normal endometrium [38]. Indirect signs of the endometrial cancer include increased thickness or lobulation of the endometrial cavity, or a heterogeneous but lower-signal-intensity mass on T$_2$-weighted images. Endometrial cancer demonstrates variable contrast enhancement. It is possible to differentiate cancer from necrosis or fluid (hematometria

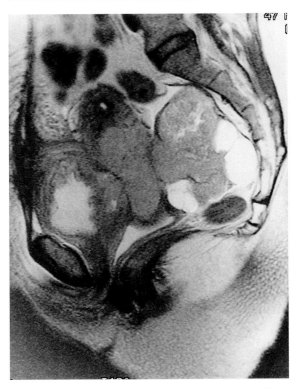

Fig. 13.5. T$_2$-weighted sagittal image of the pelvis shows cervical as well as ovarian cancers with heterogeneous intermediate-to-high signal intensities. Note also invasion of the cervical cancer into the lower uterine segment as well as the upper vagina

or pyometria) on contrast-enhanced images. The most reliable MRI criterion for myocardial invasion is a disruption of the junctional zone. However, this zone may not be consistently noted in postmenopausal women or women taking oral contraceptives. Most recent studies have demonstrated an MRI staging accuracy ranging from 91% to 74%, the latter not utilizing gadolinium or a high-field scanner [39]. Dynamic contrast-enhanced images help in differentiating endometrial cancer from adenomyosis or leiomyoma. Nondegenerating leiomyomas demonstrate a homogeneous intermediate signal intensity on T$_1$- and T$_2$-weighted images, and degenerating nodules show a high signal intensity on T$_2$-weighted images (Fig. 13.2). Accuracy for differentiating stage-I and -II from stage-III and -IV endometrial cancers was found to be 96%, with a sensitivity of 100% and a specificity of 71% [38]. The accuracy in detection of pelvic-node involvement by MRI is similar to that of CT, with both techniques relying on increased nodal size for tumor detection. Neither MRI nor CT can distinguish malignant from hyperplastic nodes. MRI may be useful in the evaluation of therapeutic changes of trophoblastic diseases (Fig. 13.3 and 13.4)

Cervical cancer is identified as an abnormal area of high signal intensity on T$_2$-weighted images (Fig. 13.5). It is isointense with normal cervix, uterus, and vagina on T$_1$-weighted images. Although contrast enhancement allows distinction between viable tumor and necrosis, it has not been shown to increase diagnostic accuracy [40]. For the staging of cervical cancer, MRI had an accuracy of 90%, compared with 65% for CT. MRI was more accurate than CT (94% vs 76%) in assessing parametrial invasion [41]. Tumor staging based on MRI follows FIGO staging criteria. In a cost-effectiveness study of 120 patients with cervi-

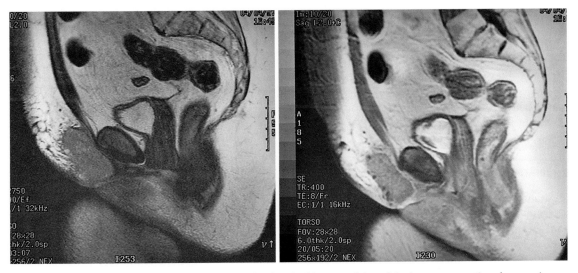

Fig. 13.6. T$_2$- (*left*) and post-gadolinium T$_1$- (*right*) weighted sagittal images of the pelvis show a metastatic vulvar carcinoma with contrast enhancement in the subcutaneous tissue abutting the anterior cortex of the symphysis pubis

cal carcinoma, use of MRI resulted in net-cost savings, especially compared with patients subjected to unnecessary exploratory laparotomy. In patients with cervical cancers measuring 2 cm or greater, pretreatment MRI decreased the number of diagnostic tests and invasive procedures [42]. Cervical carcinoma spreads to parametrial nodes, followed by obturator nodes and then internal and external iliac chains. The MRI accuracy in detecting adenopathy is particularly high when an axial diameter of greater than 1 cm is used as an indicator of lymphadenopathy (Fig. 13.6).

Magnetic Resonance Spectroscopy

There have been very few magnetic resonance spectroscopy (MRS) studies of gynecologic tumors in human patients because of problems related to motion artifacts of gynecologic organs and contamination from surrounding tissues and air. The use of ^{1}H MRS has been reported to document changes arising in the lipid chemistry of biopsies from the human uterine cervix [43]. Proton chemical-shift imaging was further used to determine the spatial location of lipid change in ex vivo human biopsy specimens and provided insight into the chemistry of neoplastic transformation. In vivo and in vitro ^{31}P MRS studies demonstrated the phosphocreatine/adenosine triphosphate (PCr/ATP) ratio as an expression of the energy metabolic state of human uterine myometrium in comparison with striated skeletal muscles [44]. The content of PCr and adenylates in biopsies of uterine smooth muscle and abdominal rectus muscle from seven term-pregnant women were determined in vitro and compared with results obtained in vivo from the uterine and gastrocnemius muscles of eight non-pregnant women. The PCr/ATP ratio in the striated skeletal muscle was about three times higher than that of the myometrium. In the biopsies, both PCr and ATP concentrations were significantly lower in the myometrium than in the rectus muscle, but the difference for PCr was more pronounced, accounting for the significantly lower PCr/ATP ratio in the uterine smooth muscle.

Positron-Emission Tomography

In a study of nine patients evaluated for recurrent ovarian carcinoma and confirmed by second-look laparotomy, positron emission tomography (PET) had a sensitivity of 83%, whereas CT and ultrasound had sensitivities of 67% and 33%, respectively (Fig. 13.7) [45]. In a larger study of 33 patients, PET had a sensitivity for recurrent disease

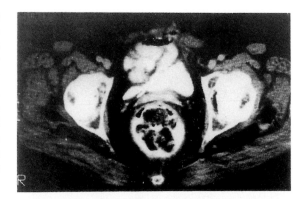

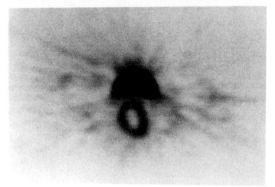

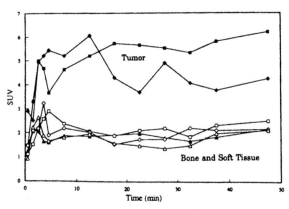

Fig. 13.7. Follow-up contrast-computed-tomography axial image of the pelvis (*top*) shows no definite recurrent ovarian cancer. A comparable positron-emission tomography image (*middle*) shows a focal area of markedly increased uptake of ^{18}F-fluoro-2-deoxy-D-glucose in the pelvis. Note also a ring-shaped lesion in the posterior mid-pelvis. These were found to be metastatic ovarian cancers with standard uptake values of 5.62 and 6.85, respectively (reprinted with permission from [46])

of 93%, whereas CT had an 87% sensitivity for recurrent disease. The specificity of PET was 80% and that of CT was 50% [46]. These authors found a good correlation between PET and histological findings, and concluded that patient management will benefit from PET because PET can identify occult foci that are not apparent on morphological imaging studies (Fig. 13.8). PET may

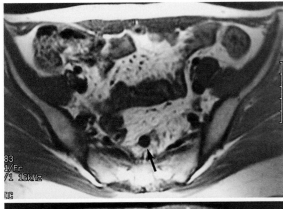

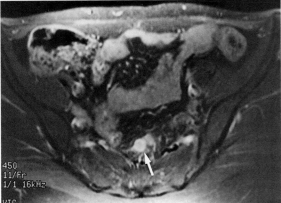

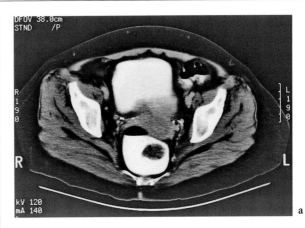

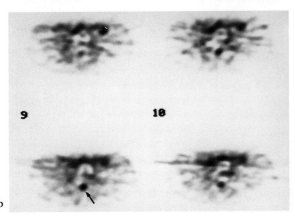

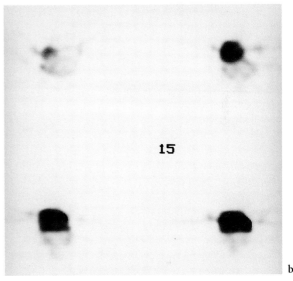

Fig. 13.8. a T$_1$-weighted axial magnetic resonance images of the pelvis before (*upper*) and after injection of gadolinium-diethylenetriaminepentaacetic acid show a contrast-enhanced small nodular metastatic ovarian mesothelioma (*arrows*) in the presacral space. Note also slight contrast enhancement of the rectus abdominis muscle (*lower*). **b** Selected positron-emission tomography axial images show a focal area of markedly increased uptake of ^{18}F-fluoro-2-deoxy-D-glucose, indicating active malignant tumor. Note also increased activity in the area of the rectus abdominis which was subsequently found to be a metastasis

Fig. 13.9. a Axial contrast-computed-tomography image of the pelvis shows an ill-defined contrast-enhanced leiomyosarcoma in the lower anterior uterine myometrium. **b** Selected axial positron-emission tomography images of the pelvis show a markedly increased uptake of ^{18}F-fluoro-2-deoxy-D-glucose in the mid-pelvis, indicating malignant tumor. Bladder activity was drained by applying a Foley catheter

be useful in the differentiation of recurrent gynocologic cancers and post-treatment changes (Figs. 13.9–13.11).

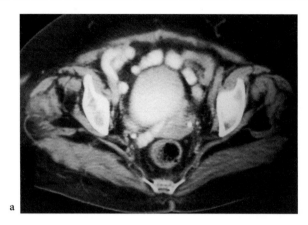
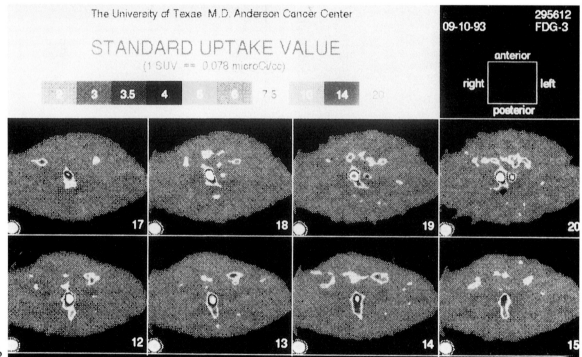

Fig. 13.10. a Axial contrast-computed-tomography image of the pelvis shows a possible recurrent cervical cancer or post-treatment change. b Selected positron-emission tomography axial images of the pelvis show a focal area of markedly increased uptake of ^{18}F-fluoro-2-deoxy-D-glucose with 7.5 standard uptake value, indicating recurrent malignant tumor. Bladder activity was drained using a Foley catheter

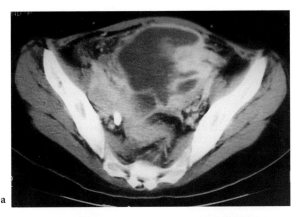

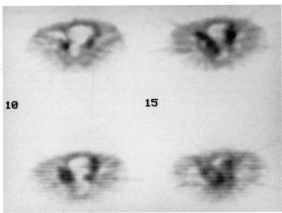

Fig. 13.11. a Contrast-computed-tomography axial image of the pelvis shows diffusely enhanced metastatic vaginal sarcomas in the right pelvis obstructing the right distal ureter and also left anterior mesentery. **b** Selected positron-emission tomography axial images of the pelvis show focal areas of markedly increased uptake of ^{18}F-fluoro-2-deoxy-D-glucose in the right posterior and left anterior pelvic walls, indicating malignant tumors

References

1. Landis SH, Murray T, Bolden S, Wingo PA (1998) Cancer statistics, 1988. CA Cancer J Clin 48:6–29
2. National Center for Health Statistics (1994) Vital statistics of the United States, 1991. Public Health Service, Washington
3. Schieldkraut JM, Thompson WD (1988) Familial ovarian cancer: a population-based case control study. Am J Epidemiol 128:456–466
4. Hawkinson SE, Colditz GA, Hunter DJ (1992) A quantitative assessment of oral contraceptive use and risk of ovarian cancer. Obstet Gynecol 80:708–714
5. Berek JS, Martinez-Maza O, Hamilton T (1993) Molecular and biological factors in the pathogenesis of ovarian cancer. Semin Oncol 4:S3–16
6. Gotlieb WH, Abrams JS, Watson JM (1992) Presence of IL-10 in the ascites of patients with ovarian and other intra-abdominal cancers. Cytokine 4:385–390
7. Berchuck A, Kamel A, Whitaker R (1990) Overexpression of HER-2/neu is associated with poor survival in advanced epithelial ovarian cancer. Cancer Res 50:4087–4091
8. Marks JR, Davidoff AM, Kerns BJ (1991) Overexpression and mutation of p53 in epithelial ovarian cancer. Cancer Res 51:2979–2984
9. Chin KV, Veda K, Pasaan I (1992) Modulation of activity of the promoter of the human MDR1 gene by ras and p53. Science 255:459–462
10. Wong GHW, Goeddel DV (1994) Fas antigen and p53 TNT receptor signal apoptosis through distinct pathways. J Immunol 52:1751–1755
11. Tholander B, Lindgren A, Taube A (1992) Immunohistochemical detection of CA 125 and CEA in ovarian tumors in relation to corresponding preoperative S levels. Int J Gynecol 2:263–270
12. Chambers JT, Merino JM, Kohory EI (1998) Borderline ovarian tumors. Am J Obstet Gynecol 59:1088–1094
13. Dembo AJ, Davy M, Stenwig AE, Berle EJ (1990) Prognostic factors in patients with stage I epithelial ovarian cancer. Obstet Gynecol 75:263–273
14. Potter ME, Hatch KD, Soong SJ (1992) Second look laparotomy and salvage therapy: a research modality only? Gynecol Oncol 44:3–9
15. Morgan MA, Nourmoff JS, King S (1992) A formula for predicting the risk of a positive second look laparotomy in epithelial ovarian cancer: implications for a randomized trial. Obstet Gynecol 80:944–948
16. Kedar RP, Bourne TH (1994) Effects of tamoxifen on uterus and ovaries of postmenopausal women in a randomized breast cancer prevention trial. Lancet 343:1318–1321
17. Rayter Z, Shepperd J, Gazrt JC (1993) Tamoxifen and endometrial lesions. Lancet 343:1124–1127
18. Devesa SS, Silverman DT, Young JL (1987) Cancer incidence and mortality trends among whites in the United States, 1947–84. J Natl Cancer Inst 79:701–770
19. Hoppe-Seyler F, Butz K (1993) Repression of endogenous p53 transactivation function in HeLa cervical carcinoma cells by human papillomavirus type 16 Eg, human indan-2, and mutant p53. J Virol 67:3111–3117
20. Dyson N, Howley P, Münger K (1989) The human papillomavirus 16 E7 oncoprotein is able to bind to the retinoblastoma gene product. Science 243:934–937
21. Strang P, Eklund G, Stendahl B (1987) S-phase rate as a predictor of early recurrence in carcinoma of the uterine cervix. Anticancer Res 7:807–810
22. Bourhis J, Le MG, Barrios M (1990) Prognostic value of c-myc proto-oncogene overexpression in early invasive carcinoma of the cervix. J Clin Oncol 8:1789–1796
23. Burghardt E, Baltzer J, Tulusan AH (1992) Results of surgical treatment of 1028 cervical cancers studied with volumetry. Cancer 70:648–655
24. Coia L, Won M, Lanciano R (1990) The patterns of care outcome study for cancer of the uterine cortex: results of the second national practice survey. Cancer 66:2451–2456
25. Tanaka Y, Sawada S, Murata T (1984) Relationship between lymph node metastases and prognosis in patients irradiated postoperatively for carcinoma of the uterine cervix. Acta Radiol Oncol 23:455–459
26. Hernandez E, Lavine M, Dunton CJ (1992) Poor prognosis associated with thrombocytosis in patients with cervical cancer. Cancer 69:2975–2977
27. Mallipeddi P, Kapp DS (1993) Long-term survival with adjuvant whole abdominopelvic irradiation for uterine papillary serous carcinoma. Cancer 71:3076–3081
28. Berman ML, Berek JS (1990) Uterine corpus. In: Haskel C (ed) Cancer treatment, 3rd edn. Saunders, Philadelphia, pp 338–350
29. Frank AH, Tseng PC (1991) Adjuvant whole abdominal radiation therapy in uterine papillary serous carcinoma. Cancer 68:1516–1519
30. Eifel PJ, Morris M, Oswald J (1990) Adenocarcinoma of the uterine cervix. Cancer 65:2507–2514

31. Fagundes H, Perez CA, Grigsby PW (1992) distant metastases after irradiation alone in carcinoma of the uterine cervix. Int J Radiat Oncol Biol Phys 24:197–204
32. Jain KA, Friedman DL, Pettinger TW, Alagappan R, Jeffrey RB Jr, Sommer FG (1993) Adnexal masses: comparison of specificity of endovaginal US and pelvic MR imaging. Radiology 186:697–704
33. Ghossain MA, Buy JN, Ligneres C (1991) Epithelial tumors of the ovary: comparison of MR and CT findings. Radiology 181:863–870
34. Komatsu T, Konishi I, Mandai M (1996) Adnexal masses: transvaginal US and gadolinium-enhanced MR imaging assessment of intratumoral structure. Radiology 198:109–115
35. Chen M, Hricak H, Sica GT (1995) MR imaging characterization of adnexal masses (abstract). Radiology 197(p):354
36. Forstner R, Hricak H, White S (1995) CT and MRI of ovarian cancer. Abdom Imaging 20:2–8
37. Forstner R, Hricak H, Powell CB, Azizi L, Frankel SB, Stern JL (1995) Ovarian cancer recurrence: value of MRI. Radiology 196:715–720
38. Hricak H, Rubinstein L, Gherman GM, Karstaedt N (1991) MR imaging evaluation of endometrial carcinoma: results of an NCI cooperative study. Radiology 179:829–832
39. Yamashita Y, Mizutani H, Torashima M, Takahashi M, Miyazaki K, Okamura H, Ushijima H et al. (1993) Assessment of myometrial invasion by endometrial carcinoma: transvaginal sonography vs contrast-enhanced MRI. AJR Am J Roentgenol 161:595–599
40. Sironi S, De Cobelli F, Scarfone G, Colombo E, Bolis G, Ferrari A, DelMaschio A (1993) Carcinoma of the cervix: value of pain and gadolinium-enhanced MRI in assessing degree of invasiveness. Radiology 188:797–801
41. Subak LL, Hricak H, Powell CB, Azizi L, Stern JL (1995) Cervical carcinoma: CT and MRI for preoperative staging. Obstet Gynecol 86:43–50
42. Hricak H, Powell CB, Yu KK, Washington E, Subak LL, Stern JL, Cisternas MG, Arenson RL (1996) Invasive cervical carcinoma: role of MRI in pretreatment workup – cost minimization and diagnostic efficacy analysis. Radiology 198:403–409
43. Mountford CE, Mackinnon WB, Russell P, Tutter A, Delikatny EJ (1996) Human cancers detected by proton MRS and chemical shift imaging ex vivo. Anticancer Res 16:1521–1531
44. Steingrimasdottir T, Ericsson A, Franck A, Waldenstrom A, Ulmsten U, Ronquist G (1997) Human uterine smooth muscle exhibits a very low phosphocreatine/ATP ratio as assessed by in vitro and in vivo measurements. Eur J Clin Invest 27:743–749
45. Casey MJ, Gupta NC, Muths CK (1994) Experience with positron emission tomography scans in patients with ovarian cancer. Gynecol Oncol 53:331–338
46. Hubner KF, McDonald TW, Niathammer JG (1993) Assessment of primary and metastatic ovarian cancer by positron emission tomography using 2-[18 F]-deoxyglucose. Gynecol Oncol 51:197–204

Chapter 14

Brain Tumors

F.C.L. Wong and E.E. Kim

Basic Considerations

In 1998, it is estimated that 17,400 new cases of primary brain and nervous-system tumors will occur, with 13,300 deaths [1]. Every year approximately 35,000 adult Americans develop primary or metastatic brain tumors [2]. Central nervous system (CNS) tumors are the most prevalent solid tumors in children under 15 years of age, the second leading cancer-related cause of death (after leukemia) in children and the third leading cancer-related cause of death in adolescents and adults between the ages of 15 years and 35 years [2]. The majority of intracranial tumors occur in patients over the age of 45 years, and recent evidence suggests that the incidence of malignant gliomas among the elderly is increasing [3].

About 16% of patients with brain tumors have a family history of cancer [2], and various genetic disorders can predispose people to brain tumors. Chromosomal abnormalities include an increased number of copies of chromosome 7 or 22, and nonrandom losses associated with chromosomes 9p, 10p, 10q and 17p [4]. Loss of chromosome 17p with or without p53-gene alteration is seen in lower grades of astrocytoma [5], loss of 9p appears to represent an intermediate event that occurs in most higher-grade astrocytomas [6], and loss of a portion of chromosome 10 is a late event seen primarily in glioblastoma multiforme tumors [7]. Patients with multifocal gliomas are more likely than other glioma patients to have germline cell p53 mutations, to have a second malignancy or to have other family members with cancer [8]. Multiple deletions of chromosome 22 have been associated with meningiomas. It has been postulated that such chromosomal losses may result in the deletion of tumor-suppressor genes that normally inhibit tumorigenesis [9]. In addition to chromosomal abnormalities, cytokine and receptor aberrations are also seen in brain tumors. Of cells that produce tumor growth factor, alpha cells are more often demonstrated in high-grade and more aggressive astrocytomas. Likewise, increased levels of epidermal-growth-factor receptors are seen in high-grade astrocytomas [7].

Symptoms of intracranial tumors are produced primarily by the tumor mass itself, the surrounding edema or the infiltration and destruction of normal tissue. The symptoms are headache, nausea and vomiting, behavioral and personality changes, slowing of psychomotor function, visual changes and speech disturbances. Seizures are the presenting symptoms in only about 20% of patients. In most primary spinal-axis tumors, symptoms and signs do not arise from parenchymal invasion, but from spinal-cord and nerve-root compression. Motor weakness is dominant with impairment of function at the affected levels. Radicular spinal syndrome presents as a sharp pain in the distribution of a sensory nerve root. Local paresthesia, impaired sensations of pain and touch, weakness and muscle wasting are common. Intramedullary spinal tumors also produce syringomyelic dysfunction, destroying lower motor neurons and resulting in segmental muscle weakness, wasting and loss of reflexes. Pain and temperature sensations are lost, but the sense of touch is preserved.

Pathology, Grading, Classification and Diagnosis

Gliomas include astrocytomas, oligodendrogliomas, ependymomas, and mixed-type tumors. Astrocytomas are the most common type of malignant brain tumor in adults, accounting for 75–90% of such lesions. Histologically, astrocytomas are categorized as low-grade astrocytoma, mid-grade anaplastic astrocytoma or high-grade glioblastoma multiforme.

Cell density, pleomorphism, anaplasia, nuclear atypia, mitoses, endothelial proliferation and necrosis are used to grade astrocytomas [10]. The presence of necrosis differentiates anaplastic astrocytomas from glioblastoma multiforme [11]. Necrosis was found to be a significant predictor of short survival time [12].

Low-grade gliomas constitute about 10–20% of all adult primary brain tumors. The majority are astrocytomas; approximately 5% are oligodendrogliomas or mixed oligoastrocytomas. They are well differentiated and lack all the cellular features (high cellularity, pleomorphism, mitoses, vascular endothelial proliferation and necrosis) that characterize anaplastic glioma.

Much less common than the astrocytic tumors, oligodendrogliomas have a somewhat even peak incidence in people between the ages of 25 years and 49 years. They tend to infiltrate the cerebral cortex more than do astrocytomas [13]. Clinically, these tumors present in the typical fashion of hemispherical astrocytomas in the frontal or temporal lobe. Ependymomas are tumors arising from cells of ependymal lineage. Sixty percent of intracranial ependymomas are infratentorial, and the fourth ventricle is the most common site. Of the supratentorial ependymomas, 50% are primarily intraventricular. Intraventricular tumors frequently cause increased intracranial pressure and hydrocephalus. As a result, most patients present with headache, nausea, vomiting, papilledema and ataxia. The deletion of tumor-suppressor genes is involved in the development of ependymomas [14].

Medulloblastomas most likely originate from germinative neuroepithelial cells in the roof of the fourth ventricle. Most (50%–60%) medulloblastomas occur in children 1–10 years of age, with a peak between age 5 and age 9. Childhood medulloblastoma typically arises in the cerebellum, mostly in the midline and posterior vermis. In adults, it typically arises in a cerebellar hemisphere. The risk of metastasis within the craniospinal intradural axis is relatively high [15]. Up to 30% of cases will have positive cytology or myelographic evidence of spinal metastasis. Extra-CNS metastases occur in less than 5% of cases, and most metastases are to long bones. The overall disease-free 5-year survival rate for medulloblastoma is approximately 50% [16].

Meningiomas arise from arachnoidal cells in the meninges. The majority of meningiomas are differentiated, with low proliferative capacity and limited invasiveness. Less commonly, meningiomas are more anaplastic, have a higher proliferative capacity and are invasive. On computed tomography (CT) and magnetic resonance imaging (MRI) scans, meningiomas are well-defined lesions that are easily enhanced with the contrast agent [17]. The major tumors occurring in the cerebellopontile angle are acoustic-nerve tumors and meningiomas. Acoustic neuromas or neurilemomas can originate on the VIIIth cranial nerve. Neurilemomas can compress the Vth, VIIth, IXth and Xth cranial nerves. Acoustic schwannomas are more common among people in the fifth decade of life, but can occur earlier when they are associated with familial neurofibromatosis. Auditory and vestibular-branch involvement occurred in 98% of cases, facial weakness with disturbances of taste in 56% and gait abnormality in 41% [18].

Only about 1% of all non-Hodgkin's lymphomas are primary CNS lymphomas. Increased incidence of CNS lymphoma is correlated with the disappearance of intermediate-grade histology, suggesting a shift in the biology of the tumors [19]. Both AIDS-related and non-AIDS-related primary CNS lymphomas are frequently B-cell lymphomas of the histiocytic type. CNS lymphomas most often occur in men. It has been found that 52% of cases were supratentorial, 34% were multiple, 12% were cerebellar, 2% were in the brainstem and less than 0.5% were spinal [20]. The contrast-enhanced CT and MRI appearance of these lesions is sometimes distinctive. Multiple lesions and homogeneous enhancement of signal is suggestive of CNS lymphoma. Brain metastases occur in 25%–35% of all cancer patients, of which approximately 15% will be symptomatic. Eighty percent of brain metastases are supratentorial [21]. Most cerebral metastases originate from lung, melanoma, kidney, colon, soft-tissue sarcoma, breast and non-Hodgkin's lymphoma.

Meningeal carcinomatosis is found in 5%–8% of patients with solid tumors [22]. The most common tumors to metastasize to the leptomeninges are lung, breast cancers, non-Hodgkin's lymphoma, melanoma and genitourinary cancer. Mode of spread is via hematogenous seeding of the arachnoid. Direct examination of the spinal fluid for tumor cells is a common way to make a diagnosis, and MRI with gadolinium (Gd)-diethylenetriaminepentaacetic acid (DTPA) is helpful in the diagnosis.

Magnetic Resonance Imaging

Imaging studies play an important role in the diagnosis and anatomic localization of intracranial tumors and provide information about the morphology and pathology of these lesions. The advent of MRI scanning, with its multiplanar-imaging capabilities, high inherent contrast sensitivity for normal neural tissue and pathologic processes, and availability of Gd-DTPA to characterize intracranial lesions further, has made this the primary imaging modality for assessing suspected brain tumors [23].

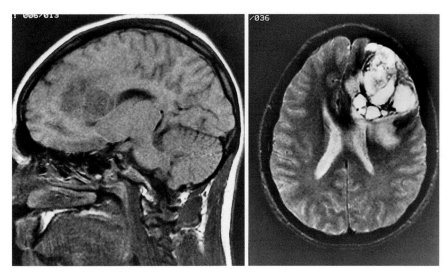

Fig. 14.1. T_1-weighted sagittal image of the head (*left*) shows an ill-defined mass with slightly heterogeneous intermediate signal intensity in the left frontal lobe. The T_2-weighted axial image (*right*) shows a markedly heterogeneous hyperintense mass surrounded by a vasogenic edema. Surgery revealed a glioblastoma multiforme. Note a significant shift of the midline to the right

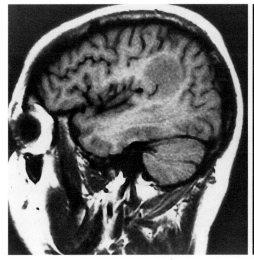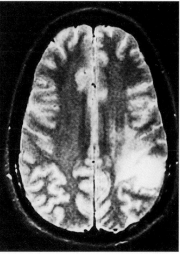

Fig. 14.2. T_1-weighted sagittal image of the head (*left*) shows a rounded mass with intermediate signal intensity in the left parietal lobe. The T_2-weighted axial image (*right*) shows a hyperintense mass surrounded by a vasogenic edema. Surgery revealed an astrocytoma, grade II

Glioblastoma multiforme has a predilection for the white matter of the cerebral hemispheres, especially the frontal lobes, and frequently infiltrates extensively into adjacent lobes and deep structures. Invasion of the cortex, leptomeninges, and dura also occurs. The tumor is typically heterogeneous with focal areas of necrosis and hemorrhage centrally, and often one or more cysts. There is usually a rim of viable tumor and extensive perifocal edema. The tumor on MRI [24] is usually large and often heterogeneous in intensity, producing hypointensity on T_1-weighted images and hyperintensity on T_2-weighted images (Figs. 14.1–14.3). Focal areas of acute hemorrhage or hemosiderin deposition are often best seen on gradient-echo (GE) images, but may produce areas of marked hypointensity on T_2-weighted images (or, less commonly, hyperintensity on T_1-weighted images). There are vasogenic edema and microscopic tumor infiltration of white-matter tracts. These tumors usually demonstrate moderate heterogeneous contrast enhancement, but irregular thick-rim or nodular enhancement is also seen (Fig. 14.4). In tumors clinically in remission, the white-matter changes seen on T_2-weighted images are much more extensive than the volume of any residual tumor. In recurrent tumors, the abnormal signal intensity on T_2-weighted images has been correlated with tumor extent [25]. Areas of increased signal intensity on T_2-weighted

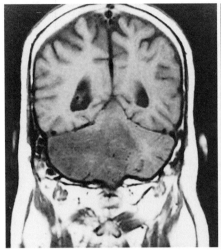
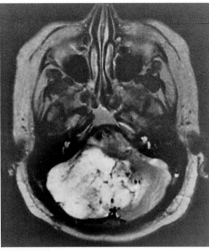

Fig. 14.3. T_1-weighted coronal image of the head (*left*) shows a large mass with slightly heterogeneous intermediate signal intensity in the right cerebellum extending into the left side. The T_2-weighted axial image (*right*) shows a heterogeneous high signal intensity. Surgery revealed an astrocytoma, grade III

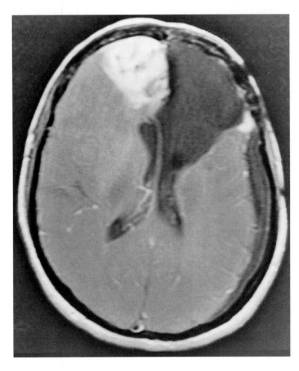

Fig. 14.4. Post-gadolinium-diethylenetriaminepentaacetic-acid injection, T_1-weighted axial image of the head shows a large post-surgical cavity in the left frontal lobe. There is a large area of heterogeneous contrast enhancement in the right frontal lobe. There is also a small focal enhanced lesion in the left frontal lobe adjacent to the cavity. Biopsy revealed recurrent glioblastoma

images that demonstrate increased metabolic activity on positron-emission-tomography (PET) scans are likely to represent tumor. Lesions that are hypometabolic usually represent edema, gliosis or radiation necrosis.

On MRI, low-grade diffuse fibrillary astrocytomas typically have well-defined margins and little associated edema or mass effect. They are usually superficial in location, and involvement of gray matter may be identified as thickening of the cortical mantle. They are fairly homogeneous, isointense to hypointense on T_1-weighted images and mildly hyperintense on T_2-weighted images, with no necrosis or hemorrhage. Contrast-enhancement patterns are variable (Figs. 14.5 and 14.6) [24]. Low-grade gliomas may present as discrete focal masses with smooth margins. Atypical (cystic) meningiomas may mimic low-grade gliomas on MRI. Gliomas may also mimic vasogenic edema or encephalomalacia when they infiltrate white-matter tracts. Anaplastic astrocytomas are often heterogeneous with areas of necrosis and cystic formation. There is usually vasogenic edema of adjacent white matter, and more intense irregular contrast enhancement. MRI, with its high sensitivity for parenchymal lesions, detects more multifocal gliomas with the same signal characteristics as solitary tumors of similar grade. Gliomatosis cerebri is an extreme form of diffuse glioma characterized by diffuse glial overgrowth [26]. CT of gliomatosis cerebri may reveal normal, demonstrate ventricular asymmetry or symmetric slit-like ventricles. Nonenhancing hypodensities in the white matter are also seen. MRI may show areas of diffuse enlargement or thickening, especially of midline structures.

Oligodendrogliomas are usually heterogeneous in signal intensity, but predominantly isointense to gray matter on T_1-weighted images and hyperintense on T_2-weighted images. The heterogeneity reflects cystic change, blood products and tumoral calcification. GE pulse sequences are more reliable than spin-echo scans in detecting calcification and hemorrhage. MRI with sagittal and coronal images demonstrates the route of spread of in-

Fig. 14.5. T$_1$-weighted sagittal images before (*left*) and after (*right*) injection of gadolinium-diethylenetriaminepentaacetic acid shows a contrast-enhanced glioma in the brain stem

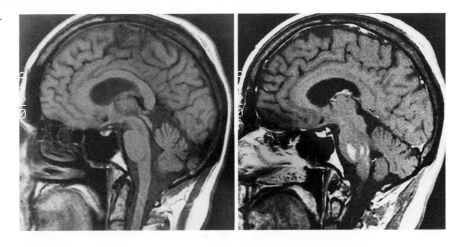

Fig. 14.6. T$_1$-weighted sagittal images before (*left*) and after (*right*) injection of gadolinium-diethylenetriaminepentaacetic acid show a craniopharyngioma with rim enhancement in the suprasellar area

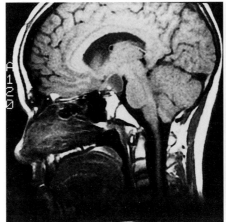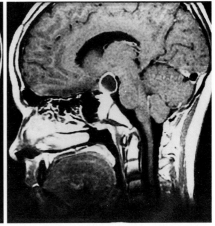

traventricular ependymomas and subependymomas well. On T$_1$-weighted images, the solid components of supratentorial ependymomas are hypointense to isointense and are hyperintense on T$_2$-weighted images. On MRI, choroid plexus papillomas are usually homogeneous and slightly hypointense to normal white matter on T$_1$-weighted images and slightly hyperintense on T$_2$-weighted images. These tumors are generally hyperdense on CT. Meningiomas tend to be nearly isotense to gray matter on all pulse sequences on MRI; 30–40% are mildly hypointense in T$_1$-weighted images and mildly hyperintense on T$_2$-weighted images (Fig. 14.7a). The presence of a dural tail, shown as homogeneously enhancing dural thickening, is highly suggestive. As with CT, enhancement of meningiomas is usually homogeneous and intense (Fig. 14.7b).

Lesions of primary CNS lymphoma tend to be hypointense to gray matter on T$_1$-weighted images and hyperintense on T$_2$-weighted images. There is a variable zone of abnormal high signal intensity on T$_2$-weighted images surrounding the lymphomatous mass, consisting of edema and infiltrating tumor cells. There is usually intense and homogeneous enhancement of the lesions on T$_1$-weighted images [27]. Epidural metastases tend to be hypointense to brain on T$_1$-weighted images and hyperintense on T$_2$-weighted images. They usually demonstrate homogeneous enhancement. T$_2$-weighted images may demonstrate sulcal effacement, and postcontrast scans reveal marked nodular or sheetlike leptomeningeal enhancement. The blood-brain barrier does not exist for metastatic lesions because they elaborate their own vascular supply [28]. Contrast-enhanced MRI is the most sensitive method for assessing the cerebral metastasis (Fig. 14.8)[29]. On MRI, metastases are usually hypointense to isointense on T$_1$-weighted images. On T$_2$-weighted images, the solid components of metastases are usually isointense to gray matter (Fig. 14.9). Hypointensity may be encountered in hemorrhagic or calcified lesions and sometimes in melanoma (Fig. 14.10). Vasogenic edema appears as extensive areas of increased signal intensity on T$_2$-weighted images. The pattern of en-

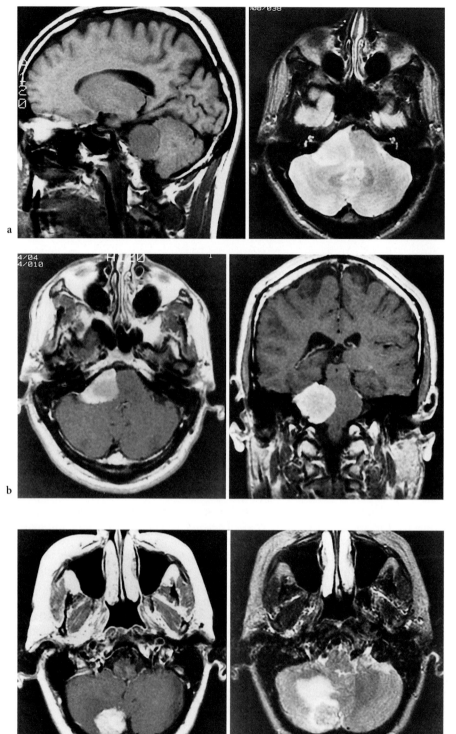

Fig. 14.7. a Proven meningioma in the right cerebellopontine angle shows a hypointensity on T_1-weighted sagittal image (*left*) and a hyperintensity on T_2-weighted axial image (*right*). **b** Post-gadolinium T_1-weighted axial (*left*) and coronal (*right*) images of the head show a fairly intense contrast enhancement in the meningioma

Fig. 14.8. Post-gadolinium injection T_1-weighted axial image of the head (*left*) shows a contrast-enhanced metastatic breast cancer in the right cerebellum. The T_2-weighted axial image (*right*) shows an extensive hyperintense vasogenic edema anterior to the metastasis

hancement on MRI may vary from homogeneous to rim enhancing. Rim enhancement may be thick walled, nodular and irregular.

The advent of rapid techniques greatly improved MR tissue sensitivity and specificity without sacrificing its high spatial resolution, allowing us to measure alterations in tissue perfusion and diffusion as well as other functional parameters. Functional MR images can provide information about tissue hemodynamics, water mobility and

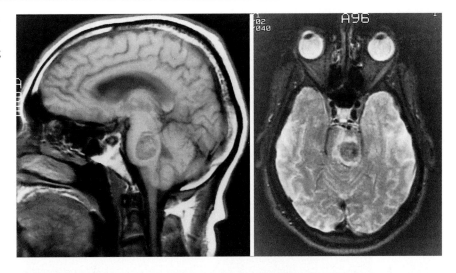

Fig. 14.9. T_1-weighted sagittal (*left*) and T_2-weighted axial (*right*) images of the head show a metastatic lung cancer in the pons

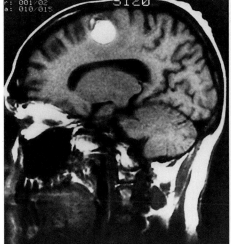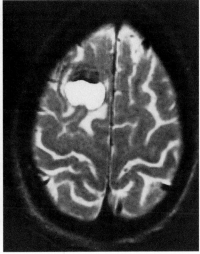

Fig. 14.10. T_1-weighted sagittal (*left*) and T_2-weighted axial (*right*) images of the head show a metastatic melanoma in the right frontal lobe. Paramagnetic melanin or hemorrhage in the lesion is responsible for the hyperintensity on T_1-weighted image

diffusion for characterization of pathophysiologic brain conditions. A zone of nonfunctioning, but still viable tissue, surrounding the infarct (penumbra zone) may recover its function if blood flow can be restored [30]. Cell death may cause the demand for oxygen to fall, the oxygen tension to rise and biochemical cascade. Whatever the mechanism may be, reperfusion does not re-establish normal perfusion or blood volume, nor does it involve the normal number of perfused capillaries. In an acute reperfusion stage, blood flow and volume increase [31]. It appears that the greater the extent to which cell death has occurred, the more excessive the reperfusion. During reperfusion, the supply of oxygen often exceeds its demand, and postischemic increases in flow above normal levels may actually lead to increased tissue damage in the form of hemorrhage and edema. Moreover, the release of oxygen free radicals may increase during reperfusion and directly harm the tissue. The reactive hyperemia (increased flow and blood volume) following ischemia is of no immediate relation to cell viability or functional integrity. Diffusion-weighted MR images may be useful for the classification of malignant brain tumors. Microvascular perfusion, cell size and distribution of water in the extravascular space may have an impact on the measured apparent diffusion coefficient (ADC) [32]. Diffusion-weighted imaging may prove informative in differentiating epidermoid tumors from extra-axial cysts [33].

Recent concepts in tumor biology point to the importance of tumor vascularity (angiogenesis) as critical in the regulation of tumor growth and malignant potential [34]. Expression of angiogenic growth-factor genes in astrocytomas may contribute to their growth and progression. Measurement of tissue microvascular blood volume appears to

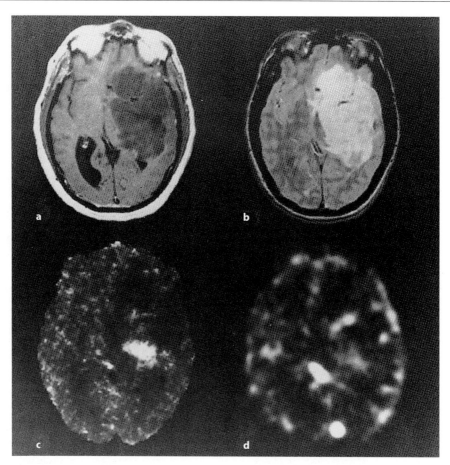

Fig. 14.11 a–d. T$_1$-weighted postcontrast (**a**), proton density (**b**), magnetic-resonance-imaging cerebral blood-volume (MRI CBV) (**c**) and positron-emission-tomography-carbon monoxide (PET-CO) (**d**) axial images of the head show the ability of MRI CBV mapping to depict areas of high microvascularity in the tumor not seen in the postcontrast or T$_2$-weighted images. The MRI CBV map is particularly sensitive to capillary blood volume and relatively insensitive to larger vessels in the brain, which are prominent in the PET CO study (reprinted with permission from [35])

be sensitive to the phenotypic expression of angiogenesis, particularly increased microvascular density. In comparing MRI cerebral blood-volume maps with PET using carbon monoxide, the MRI maps were particularly sensitive for microvasculature and relatively insensitive for larger vessels in the brain (Figs. 14.11 and 14.12) [35]. It is not possible to make a differential diagnosis between high-grade and low-grade gliomas based on the measured ADC, due to overlapping diffusion values. The edema surrounding tumors has a higher diffusion coefficient than the surrounding normal brain tissue, while the necrotic areas of gliomas have a higher diffusion coefficient compared with the active tumor area. Low-grade gliomas are typically more homogeneous on MRI. MRI cerebral blood-volume mapping may be useful when evaluating radiation necrosis, showing diminished cerebral blood volume. It may also be useful in guiding optimal sites for stereotactic biopsies.

Magnetic Resonance Spectroscopy

MR spectroscopy (MRS) can noninvasively measure numerous biochemicals and pH. Various pulse sequences have been used for single-voxed techniques, but the most commonly used technique is image-selected in vivo spectroscopy (ISIS) [36]. ISIS is the preferred ^{31}P pulse sequence because many metabolites have relatively short T$_2$-relaxation time constants. The minimum spatial resolution or volume of interest is determined by the signal-to-noise ratio (S/N) and is about 50 ml. T$_2$ relaxation time constants of ^{1}H-bearing metabolites are relatively long. Echo-localized sequences are advantageous compared with the ISIS technique. The commonly used spin-echo technique is called point resolved spectroscopy (PRESS) or proton imaging of metabolites (PRIME) [37, 38]. Water suppression is typically performed using a water-eliminated Fourier transform (WEFT) or chemi-

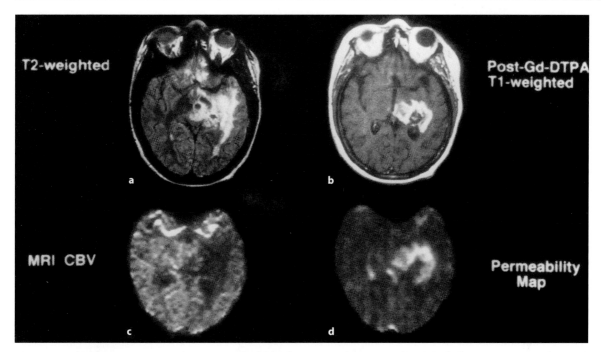

Fig. 14.12 a–d. Magnetic-resonance-imaging cerebral-blood-volume axial map shows a focal area of decreased blood volume in the left temporal white matter at a site of radiation necrosis verified by biopsy. The blood-brain barrier permeability map shows the leaky area, corresponding well with the gadolinium-enhanced area (reprinted with permission from [35])

cal-shift-selective (CHESS) sequence [39]. The CHESS technique applies one or more frequency or chemical-shift-selective 90° pulses to the water resonance. The advantage of stimulated-echo acquisition mode (STEAM) over PRESS is that it is technically much easier to acquire spectra with short Tes (~20 ms). The limitation of STEAM is that it suffers from a 2-S/N loss. The minimum spatial resolution or volume of interest (VOI) is determined by S/N and is about 1 ml [40].

MRS imaging combines the advantages of MRI and MRS in that spectral information is obtained from multiple volume elements within a designated field of view (FOV) (Fig. 14.13) [39]. Much pathology in the brain is multifocal, and tumors are not metabolically or anatomically homogeneous.

^{31}P MRS can provide information concerning tissue energetics, phospholipid metabolism and intracellular pH. An acute change in the phosphocreatine (PCr)/inorganic phosphate (Pi) ratio is a sensitive measure of ischemia. Adenosine triphosphate (ATP) is necessary for all life processes that require energy, such as membrane potentials, muscle contraction and macromolecule synthesis. Phosphomonoesters (PME) and phosphodiesters (PDE) represent precursors to membrane synthesis and breakdown products, respectively. Changes in PME and PDE may be useful markers of cell proliferation. The pH can be determined by the chemical shift between Pi and PCr resonances. ^{1}H MRS can provide information concerning neuronal density, membrane constituents, amino acid metabolism and glycolysis. N-acetyl aspartate (NAA) is a neuronal marker and is absent in glial cells.

The most common features of tumor spectra are decreased PDE, PDE/ATP ratio and decreased pH. The large variation in spectral pattern may be the result of partial volume effects, since large VOIs must be used to maintain S/N. ^{1}H MRS has been more reliable, and tumor spectra are easily discerned from normal tissue by decreased NAA and increased choline (Cho) (Figs. 14.13 and 14.14) [41]. Increased inositols, alanine (Ala), lactate (Lac) and lipids (Lip) and decreased creatine (Cr) have been also reported [42]. Tumor cell death following treatments was characterized by increasing Pi and decreasing PME, PDE and high-energy phosphates [43]. Pi is the terminal product of high-energy phosphate reactions, and Lac represents deficit metabolism but not necessarily cell death. Lac is the product of active glycolysis when pyruvate cannot enter the citric acid (TCA) cycle. Lac is a specific marker of mitochondrial damage or relative hypoxia and not overt cell death. Late brain injury after radiation therapy is thought to arise from endothelial damage which results in reduced regional blood flow to the treated areas. Early radiation damage can be detected by ^{1}H

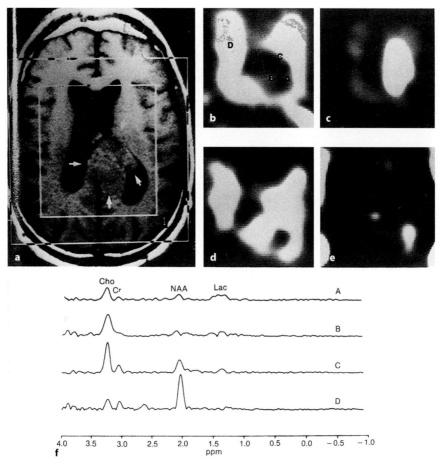

Fig. 14.13a–f. Scout axial T$_1$-weighted image (**a**) of the head in a patient with grade-III oligodendroglioma shows the tumor extension (*arrows*) from midline through the corpus callosum. The inner box represents the volume of interest in the corresponding volume-selective spectroscopic measurement, and the outer box indicates the field of view of the phase-encoding spectroscopic measurement. Metabolite maps of *N*-acetyl aspartate (**b**), choline (**c**), creatine (**d**), and lactate (**e**) were reconstructed from the spectroscopic data set. a–d in **b** are the locations from which the selected spectra in **f** were obtained (reprinted with permission from [38])

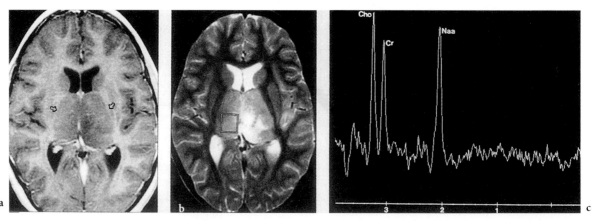

Fig. 14.14a–c. Post-gadolinium T$_1$-weighted axial image of the head (**a**) shows relatively iso-to-hypointense low-grade glioma in the bilateral thalami with minimal contrast enhancement. Axial T$_2$-weighted image (**b**) shows increased signal intensity in the thalami with the voxel positioned within abnormal right thalamus. **c** Single-voxel proton brain exam (PROBE/SV) using point-resolved ^{1}H magnetic resonance spectroscopy shows mildly decreased *N*-acetylaspartate (NAA) level compared with the levels of choline (Cho) and creatine (Cr) (reprinted with permission from [40])

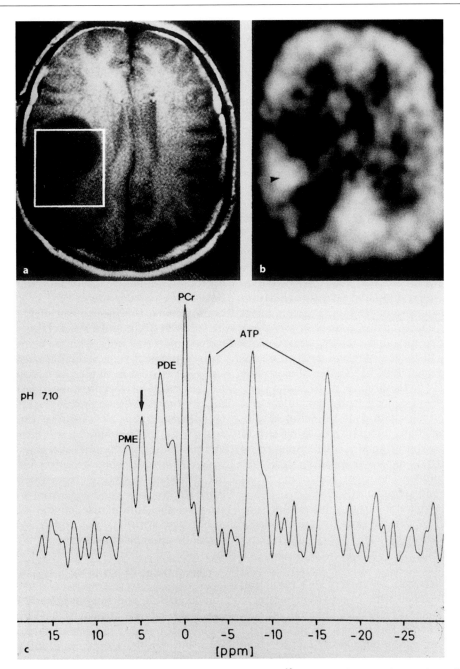

Fig. 14.15 a–c. Post-gadolinium injection T_1-weighted axial magnetic resonance image of the head (**a**) shows a volume of interest in the right temporal lobe with no focal contrast enhancement. Axial positron-emission tomography image at the comparable level (**b**) shows a slightly increased uptake of ^{18}F-fluoro-2-deoxy-D-glucose (*arrowhead*) in the glioblastoma. ^{31}P spectrum (**c**) shows reduction and possible splitting of phosphodiesters (PDE), and also some decrease of phosphocreatine (PCr) signals. The tumor pH was 7.1 (reprinted with permission from [45])

MRS which may be useful for managing supportive therapies to prevent progression to fatal injury. Highly depressed levels of NAA, Cho, and Cr with an intense, broad proton peak between 0 ppm and 2 ppm were consistent with tissue necrosis. ^{31}P MRS also showed depressed levels of all metabolites in the treated tumor region (Fig. 14.15). ^{31}P MRS of the infectious lesions showed a marked loss of phosphorus signal. The Lac/Cho ratio was also significantly elevated in patients with infection, while the NAA/Cho ratio was significantly depressed in patients with tumors. Multivoxel spectroscopy technique can define the extent of the tumorous tissues and characterize the peritumorous regions in biochemical terms, which may be useful for treatment planning [44]. MR spectroscopic imaging maps generally show that the tumor area has high Cho, low NAA, relatively normal Cr and increased Lac. Ischemic tumor tissue can be seen on the Lac image. Metastases and glioblastomas had much higher Lac levels. The abnormalities shown by MRS imaging extended beyond the tumor as defined by MRI [45].

Positron Emission Tomography

Basic Considerations

In the study of patients with brain tumors, anatomic changes that are clinically significant occur starting at sizes of millimeters (mm), and the pathologic processes occurs at sub-millimolar concentration. In fact, genetic aberrations and early subcellular injuries occur at sub-picomolar ranges. Before imaging studies become available, the above events are usually identified on autopsy or by surgical biopsy, followed by histochemistry and detailed microscopic examination. Imaging studies analyze the chemical signals of the brain and the tumors and display these signals, along with their differences, in spatial coordinates with good resolution. Evaluation of human brain tumors by imaging techniques therefore requires good spatial resolution of the anatomic details as well as sensitive signals reflecting the pathologic processes occurring at organic, cellular and subcellular levels.

Traditional structural imaging modalities such as CT and MRI remain the primary study tools of human brain cancer because of their superior resolution, currently at sub-millimeter levels. The spatial resolution of CT and MRI are an order of magnitude better than the current PET resolution of 5–8 mm. Together with contrast-enhancement techniques, CT or MRI provides anatomic as well as gross physiologic aberrations, such as tumor mass, edema and rupture of blood-brain barriers. These anatomic and gross pathologic changes occur at the molar and millimolar ranges. The use of CT and MRI are limited by their current abilities to detect cellular or molecular alterations at concentrations below millimolar levels. However, current PET technologies detect molecular changes from molar to sub-picomolar ranges and are the only imaging modalities to fill the large void left by CT or MRI, i.e., the cellular and subcellular events at the millimolar to picomolar levels.

The study of human brain tumors using PET started in the 1970s. Gross pathology at the vascular level, such as perfusion abnormalities, were reported with ^{15}O-water PET [46]. Breakdown of blood-brain barriers were reported by ^{68}Ga-PET [47]. Differential vascular responses between vessels in tumor versus brain were reported under adenosine pharmacologic stimulation using ^{15}O-water PET [48]. Vascular response to physiologic stimulation in patients with brain tumors in order to identify motor or sensory representation in brain parenchyma has been used as a clinical tool for presurgical planning [49]. Down to the cellular and subcellular levels, the study of tumor regional perfusion, oxygen consumption and glucose utilization have been in the literature since the late 1970s [50]. In the 1980s, increased ^{18}F-fluoro-2-deoxy-D-glucose (FDG) uptake in gliomas was correlated with tumor grades [51]. Because of its uptake by the normal cerebral cortex, ^{18}F-FDG has remained the main tracer to study the brains of patients with and without tumors. Despite the popular use of FDG in PET studies of brain tumors, the mechanism of FDG uptake remains to be fully understood. Likely explanations include increased hexose kinase activities [52], increased uptake by surrounding macrophages [53] and increased levels of glucose transporters [54].

The search for specific tumor markers in imaging continues, with increasing emphasis on tumor-specific molecules such as essential amino acids (e.g., L-methionine) [55], nucleotides (thymidine) [56], dopamine D2 receptors [57] and peripheral benzodiazepine receptors [58]. Because of the stringent technical requirements, most of these studies were conducted from a research perspective; the clinical use of this expensive PET technology, which is not widely available, often demands different considerations.

Clinical Utility of PET in Brain Tumors

Tumor grading and staging remains an important task of the clinical oncologist. There are earlier reports on correlation of glioma grades with ^{18}F-FDG PET. However, the acceptance of this notion varies. Often PET is not used to grade human brain tumor.

Because of limited availability of the short-lived tracers, which require a nearby cyclotron and rapid synthesis as well as quality assurance, clinical PET is available only to large academic medical centers. Furthermore, because of the inferior spatial resolution, PET is best positioned to study the brain tumor patients for whom CT and MRI offer little help. In fact, owing to improved early diagnosis and treatment, brain tumor patients have improved survival rates and, ironically, they have proved difficult for CT or MRI to evaluate. Since either the tumor or the treatment or both have altered the architecture of normal brain pa-

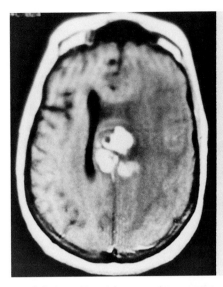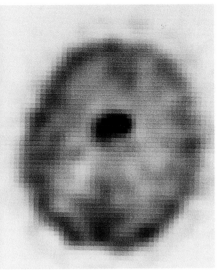

Fig. 14.16. Post-gadolinium T_1-axial magnetic resonance image of the head (*left*) shows a contrast-enhanced lesion in the corpus callosum suggesting glioblastoma or radiation necrosis. Axial positron-emission tomography image (*right*) at the comparable level shows a markedly increased uptake of ^{18}F-fluoro-2-deoxy-D-glucose, indicating active malignant tumor

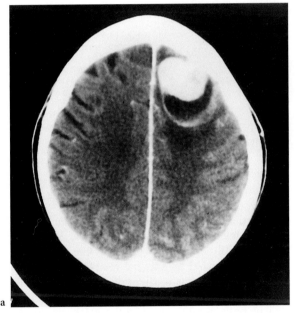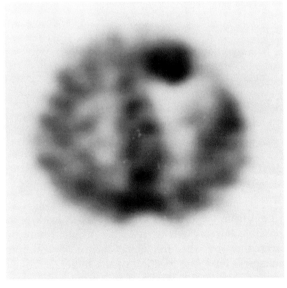

Fig. 14.17. a Contrast computed tomography axial image of the head shows a metastatic ovarian sarcoma with enhanced solid and nonenhanced cystic components in the left frontal lobe. **b** Axial positron-emission tomography image at the comparable level shows a markedly increased uptake of ^{18}F-fluoro-2-deoxy-D-glucose in the solid portion of the lesion, indicating active malignant lesion

renchyma, grossly abnormal CT/MRI signals such as contrast enhancement often remain, regardless of whether there is recurrent tumor. PET remains most useful in the differentiation of recurrent brain tumor from post-treatment necrosis.

The most frequently used tracer in clinical PET is ^{18}F-FDG. When used to study patients with brain tumors, it posts a technical challenge. The tumor is expected to have higher uptake (and hence contrast) than the surrounding tissue without tumor (Fig. 14.16–14.18). However, the gray matter in normal human cerebral cortex already has higher FDG uptake than the white matter. The contrast of the signal from the tumor versus the

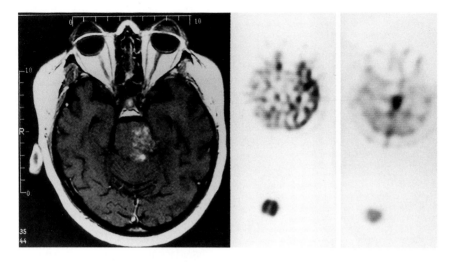

Fig. 14.18. Post-gadolinium injection axial image of the head (*left*) shows a contrast-enhanced lesion in the left side of pons. Axial positron-emission tomography images at the comparable level show no significant uptake of ^{18}F-fluoro-2-deoxy-D-glucose (*middle*), but marked uptake of ^{11}C-methionine (*right*). Biopsy revealed an astrocytoma, grade II

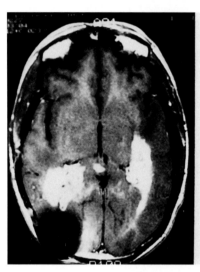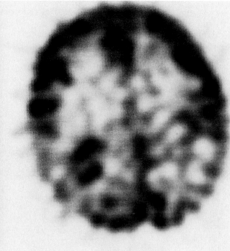

Fig. 14.19. Post-gadolinium T_1-axial image of the head (*left*) shows a focal enhanced lesion anterior to the surgical cavity in the right inferior parietal lobe. Axial positron-emission-tomography image (*right*) at the comparable level shows a moderately increased uptake of ^{18}F, indicating active recurrent anaplastic astrocytoma

signal from the brain is thus decreased, leading to possible lowered sensitivity. This problem may be overcome by the following technically simple schemes. First, the location of the hypermetabolic tumor helps to identify tumors in the hypometabolic white matter. Second, comparison with prior studies may find a lesion with increasing uptake. Third, coregistration with anatomic imaging, such as MRI, will reveal the exact locations of the lesions. Finally, presentation of the images in standard uptake value (SUV) or other semi-quantitative parameters will help to assess the contrast of the signals.

To be clinically useful, the results of the PET study should have direct impact on the treatment plans. Most PET studies of brain tumors are concerned with primary brain tumor, i.e., gliomas, because the findings may direct the subsequent treatment plans, such as continuing chemotherapy, further surgery or observation. Other tumors, such as meningiomas and metastases, have only been scantily reported because the treatment plans are directed by surgery for meningioma. In the case of metastases, therapy is directed by the treatment of the primary tumor. Furthermore, PET of both meningiomas and metastases are reported to have variable uptake of FDG. Therefore, the usefulness of FDG-PET in the routine clinical evaluation of brain tumors other than gliomas remains to be established. Although glioma refers to a group of brain tumors of varying grade, and there is an apparent trend of higher uptake with higher grade, there are very few studies further delineating the FDG uptake of the various gliomas.

There is a unique place for PET in the differentiation of recurrent tumor versus post-treatment necrosis because MRI of these post-treatment pa-

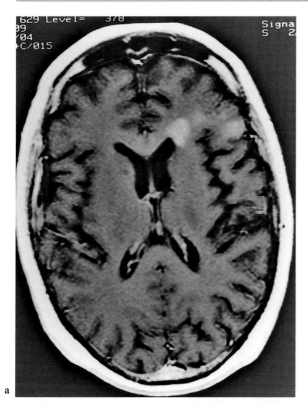

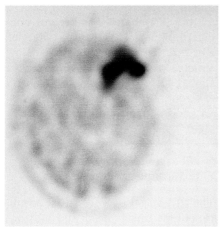 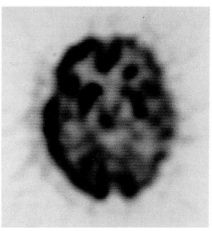

Fig. 14.20. a Post-gadolinium injection T_1-weighted axial image of the head shows patchy areas of contrast enhancement in the medial and lateral aspects of left frontal lobe. **b** Positron-emission-tomography axial images at the comparable level show a markedly increased uptake of ^{11}C-methionine in the enhanced lesions of left frontal lobe and a moderately increased uptake of ^{18}F-fluoro-2-deoxy-D-glucose only in the medial enhanced lesion, a recurrent glioblastoma verified by biopsy. The lateral lesion showed a gliosis

tients often reveals persistent contrast enhancement. However, necrotic tissues often have little FDG uptake, while tumors exhibit marked uptake (Figs. 14.19 and 14.20). It has been found that immediately after radiation treatment, FDG uptake by brain and tumor may slightly increase, only to return to normal and then subnormal in a few weeks [59]. Furthermore, surgery and systemic steroid did not produce any significant FDG-uptake change during the next few days (Fig. 14.21). Since the chronic effects of radiation treatment on the normal brain are depressed perfusion and metabolism, the post-treatment effects are expected to enhance the tumor contrast on FDG-PET scans. This will add to the ability to detect tumors in the brain, which has a known high uptake of FDG. There is an argument that there are many micrometastases in a patient with primary glioma and, therefore, distinction of tumor versus no tumor may not be very important because tumors are already spread throughout the entire brain, including the post-treatment necrotic tissues. One recent study has shown that the FDG uptake in brain tumor tissue correlates with prognosis and survival [60]. Therefore, FDG uptake in the evaluation of post-treatment necrosis versus residual

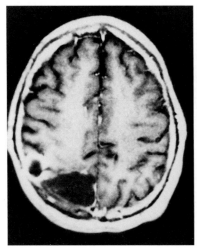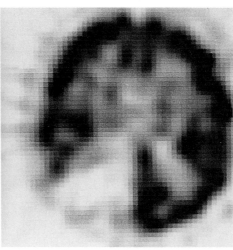

Fig. 14.21. Post-gadolinium axial T$_1$-weighted magnetic-resonance image of the head (*left*) shows a post-surgical cavity in the right posterior parietal lobe. An axial positron-emission-tomography image (*right*) at the comparable level shows a markedly decreased uptake of ^{18}F-fluoro-2-deoxy-D-glucose in the right parietal lobe

tumor is indeed important for the clinical management of brain-tumor patients.

Although ^{11}C-methionine PET is mostly restricted to research studies, it is most promising as an alternative to ^{18}F-FDG-PET, because there is minimal background activity in the brain and, therefore, the lesions stand out with good contrast (Fig. 14.2). This technology is, however, limited by the requirement of very short synthesis time because of the short half-life of ^{11}C (20 min). Occasionally, post-treatment necrosis also exhibits high uptake of the tracer.

Practical Considerations in Clinical Use of PET to Evaluate Brain-Tumor Patients

The patient's mental status and mood may be affected by the tumor and, therefore, the patient may not understand or comply with instructions. The patient's ambulatory status as well as bowel and bladder control may require special attention. Usually, a PET-scan session may not last more than an hour. On special occasions, repeated studies, e.g., with different positron tracers, may require large intervals between scans on the same day to allow for decay of the tracer from the earlier scan.

In order to avoid excessive patient motion or to provide external coregistration with CT/MRI, the patient may be fitted with a thermoplastic mask with openings for the eyes, nose and mouth. Again, close monitoring of these brain-tumor patients is necessary for a safe and successful scanning session.

In order to provide PET images useful to the clinicians, the images should be available shortly after acquisition and presented in formats readily understood by the clinicians. With such time and logistic constraints, some of the optimal theoretical requirements, such as attenuation correction and blood sampling, may need compromises. There is a current trend to present the PET images with a SUV color-coded format along with a color scale so that the SUV value is readily discerned from the images [61].

Since a sustainable clinical PET operation requires a steady and positive cash flow, payment for the PET studies has become one of the major determinants of its success. Meticulous planning and accurate accounting, as well as pre-scan assurance of payment is crucial. Currently, in the United States, some of the PET studies are actually reimbursable. Therefore, success also depends on good documentation and compliance with regulatory requirements.

PET as a Research Tool to Study Human Brain Tumors

The advantages of PET include absolute quantification of the tracers inside the body or the head on a pixel-to-pixel basis. With FDG PET, it is possible to calculate the tracer or metabolite at micromolar concentrations for the region of interest. With other tracers, such as ^{11}C-*N*-methylspiperone (NMSP) for D2 receptors in pituitary adenomas, it is even possible to quantify molecular events at picomolar levels. This level of precision in research requires meticulous attention to protocol details. Furthermore, it is necessary to calibrate the tracer activities measured on the image to the tracer activities measured in the blood. For tracers that undergo metabolism during the scan duration, metabolites should also be accurately accounted. Therefore, quantification of tracers in human brain tumors may require rigorous procedures, such as arterial catheterization, accurate blood collection up to seconds, readily accessible analytical tools such as high-performance liquid chromatography and labor-intense computer iterations.

Perfusion PET studies of brain tumors typically involve ^{15}O-water, which has a high extraction coefficient by the brain and tumor tissues. However, because of the wide regional variation of perfusion within the gliomas, the perfusion pattern itself is not of great research interest. However, the advantage of ^{15}O-water PET became apparent after repeated studies comparing baseline study and studies under pharmacologic or physiologic stimulation [46]. The 2-min half-life of ^{15}O allows multiple, rapid, successive testing while the patient is still in the scanner. However, when exact quantification or repeated scanning is not required, perfusion studies are mostly accomplished by the less expensive and more available SPECT with ^{99m}Tc-labeled hexamethylpropyleneamine oxime or ethyl cysteinate dimer as tracers.

For the identification of pathology at subcellular levels, ^{18}F-FDG remains the main thrust in the study of human-brain tumors. Exact quantification requires arterial blood sampling to obtain the input function and invariably leads to patient discomfort. Alternatives include monitoring carotid or ventricular activities to estimate the input function. The uptake of FDG by brain or tumor is also affected by the insulin and glucose levels. Therefore, the glucose and postprandial status in patients should be controlled. In fact, the uptake of FDG by the brain has been found to be too large in variation because of technical factors routinely encountered in a clinical setting [62]. Enhanced-FDG contrast in brain gliomas has also been reported by suppression of the baseline high cortical uptake under barbiturate coma [63].

Some amino acid-transporter levels are markedly elevated in tumors. The contrast of tumor to background in ^{11}C-methionine PET is higher than in FDG PET because of the low uptake by normal brain parenchyma. The uptake of ^{11}C-methionine in tumor and brain tissues is suppressible by oral ingestion of L-phenylalanine. However, high uptake of ^{11}C-methionine has also been reported with radiation necrosis, which is less suppressible by oral L-phenylalanine, therefore, providing a basis for distinction from tumors [64]. Recently, ^{123}I-labeled iodomethyltyrosine, a SPECT tracer, has been shown to exhibit similar biologic characteristics, and may prove to be a less expensive and more widely available alternative to ^{11}C-methionine [64].

Tumor tissues require large amounts of nucleotides for replication of DNA, while nontumor tissues do not normally divide and do not concentrate nucleotides. ^{11}C-labeled thymidine PET has been reported to show high tumor uptake of the tracer [56]. However, ^{11}C-thymidine undergoes rapid hepatic metabolism and the ^{11}C label is typically cleaved from the molecule to join the general circulation, adding to a rising background activity over a few minutes. The cleavage rate depends to some degree whether the ^{11}C label is in the 2 position or the 5 position. Nevertheless, multiple-compartment kinetic modeling and measurement of metabolites are required for quantification. Because of thymidine metabolism, iododeoxyuridine (IUDR) is another compound used to detect tumors. When labeled with ^{124}I, IUDR-PET has demonstrated elevated uptake in human gliomas in a pattern not identical to FDG or thallium SPECT [66]. However, it is also subject to rapid hepatic clearance with a serum half-life of 1.6 min.

Elevated dopamine D2 receptor has been reported in pituitary adenomas using ^{11}C-NMSP. A nonspecific increase in peripheral benzodiazepine receptor has also been reported using ^{11}C-PK14105. However, the elevation of these receptors is not specific to the tumors and is observed in other cerebral pathologies such as schizophrenia and multiple sclerosis.

In summary, PET tracers have proved to be able to detect pathologic processes of brain tumors at the cellular and subcellular levels. This technology has largely remained a research tool. To be a useful clinical tool, PET has to continue to improve to provide speedy and accurate services and be user friendly for clinicians.

References

1. Landis SH, Murray T, Bolden S, Wingo PA (1998) Cancer statistics, 1998. CA Cancer J Clin 48:6–29
2. Mahaley MS Jr, Mettlin C, Natarajan N (1989) National survey of patterns of care for brain-tumor patients. J Neurosurg 71:826–836
3. Grieg NH, Ries LG, Yancik R (1990) Increasing annual incidence of primary malignant brain tumors in the elderly. J Natl Cancer Inst 82:1621–1624
4. Pershouse MA, Stubble field E, Hadi A (1993) Analysis of the functional role of chromosome 10 loss in human glioblastomas. Cancer Res 53:5043–5050
5. Lang FF, Miller DC, Koslow M (1994) Pathways leading to glioblastoma multiforme: a molecular analysis of genetic alterations in 65 histocytic tumors. J Neurosurg 81:427–436
6. Bigner SH, Mark J, Burger PC (1988) Specific chromosomal abnormalities in malignant human gliomas. Cancer Res 48:405–409
7. Wong AJ, Zoltick PW, Moscatello DK (1994) The molecular biology and molecular genetics of astrocytic neoplasms. Semin Oncol 21:126–138

8. Kyritsis AP, Bondy ML, Xiao MI (1994) Germline p53 gene mutations in subsets of glioma patients. J Natl Cancer Inst 86:344–349
9. Dumanski JP, Rouleau GA, Nordenskjold M (1990) Molecular genetic analysis of chromosome 22 in 81 cases of meningioma. Cancer Res 50:5863–5868
10. Daumas-Dupont C, Scheithauer B, O'Fallon J (1988) Grading of astrocytomas, a simple and reproducible method. Cancer 62:2152–2157
11. Bruner JM (1994) Neuropathology of malignant gliomas. Semin Oncol 21:126–138
12. Nelson JS, Tsukada Y, Schoenfeld D (1983) Necrosis as a prognostic criterion in malignant supratentorial astrocytic gliomas. Cancer 52:550–555
13. de la Monte SM (1989) Uniform lineage of oligodendroglioma. Am J Pathol 135:529–540
14. Sawyer JR, Sammartino G, Husain M (1994) Chromosome aberrations in four ependymomas. Cancer Gent Cytogenet 74:132–138
15. Deutsch M (1984) The impact of myelography on the treatment results for medulloblastoma. Int J Radiat Oncol Biol Phys 8:2023–2028
16. Carrie C, Lasset C, Blay JY (1993) Medulloblastoma in adults. Surgical and prognostic factors. Radiother Oncol 29:301–307
17. Murtagh R, Linden C (1994) Neuroimaging of intracranial meningioma. Neurosurg Clin North Am 5:217–233
18. Jackler RK, Pitts LH (1990) Acoustic neuroma. Neurosurg Clin N Am 1:199–204
19. Miller DC, Hochberg FH, Harris NL (1994) Pathology with clinical correlations of primary central nervous system non-Hodgkin's lymphoma. Cancer 74:1383–1397
20. Murray K, Kun L, Cox J (1986) Primary malignant lymphoma of the central nervous system. J Neurosurg 65:600–606
21. Delathe JY, Krol G, Thaler HT (1988) Distribution of brain metastases. Arch Neurol 45:741–744
22. Patchell RA, Posner JB (1985) Neurologic complications of systemetic cancer. Neurol Clin 3:729–750
23. Brant-Zawadzki M, Badami P, Mills CM (1984) Primary intracranial brain imaging. A comparison of magnetic resonance and CT. Radiology 150:435–440
24. Dean BL, Drayer BP, Bird CR (1990) Gliomas: classification with MR imaging. Radiology 174:411–415
25. Johnson PC, Hunt SJ, Drayer BP (1989) Human cerebral gliomas: correlation of postmortem MR imaging and neuropathologic findings. Radiology 170:211–217
26. Spagnoli MV, Grossman RI, Packer RJ (1987) Magnetic resonance imaging of gliomatosis cerebri. Neuroradiology 29:15–18
27. Roman-Goldstein SM, Goldman DL, Howieson J (1992) MR of primary CNS lymphoma in immunologically normal patients. AJNR Am J Neuroradiol 13:1207–1213
28. Healy ME, Hesselink JR, Press GA (1987) Increased detection of intracranial metastases with intravenous Gd-DTPA. Radiology 165:619–624
29. Yuh WT, Engelken JD, Muhonen MR (1992) Experience with high dose gadolinium MR imaging in the evaluation of brain metastases. AJNR Am J Neuroradiol 13:335–345
30. Hakim AM (1987) The cerebral ischemic penumbra. Can J Neurol Sci 14:557–559
31. Crumrine RC, LaManna JC (1991) Regional cerebral metabolites, blood flow, plasma volume and mean transit time in total cerebral ischemia in the rat. J Cereb Blood Flow Metab 11:272–282
32. LeBihan D, Turner R Moonen CTW, Pekar J (1991) Imaging of diffusion and microcirculation with gradient sensitization: design, strategy and significance. J Magn Reson Imaging 1:7–28
33. Tsuruda J, Chew W, Moseley M, Norma D (1991) Diffusion-weighted MRI of extraaxial tumors. Magn Reson Med 19:316–320
34. Weidner N, Semple JP, Welch WR, Folkman J (1991) Tumor angiogenesis and metastasis – correlation in invasive breast carcinoma. N Engl J Med 324:1–8
35. Rosen BR, Aronen HJ, Cohen MS, Belliveau JW, Hamberg LM, Kwong KK, Fordham JA (1993) Diffusion and perfusion fast scanning in brain tumors. Neuroimaging Clin N Am 3:631–648
36. Ordidge RJ, Connelly A, Lohman JAB (1986) Image-selected in vivo spectroscopy (ISIS). A new technique for spatially selective NMR spectroscopy. J Magn Reson 66:283–294
37. Bottomley PA (1987) Spatial localization in NMR spectroscopy. Ann N Y Acad Sci 505:33–348
38. Luyten P, Marien AJH, Heindel W (1990) Metabolic imaging of patients with intracranial tumors. H-1 MR spectroscopic imaging and PET. Radiology 176:791–799
39. Frahm J, Bruhn H, Gyngell ML (1989) Localized high-resolution proton NMR spectroscopy using stimulated echoes: initial applications to human brain in vivo. Magn Reson Med 9:79–93
40. Tien RD, Lai PH, Smith JS, Lazeyras F (1996) Single-voxel proton brain spectroscopy exam (PROBE/SV) in patients with primary brain tumors. AJR Am J Roentgenol 167:201–209
41. Alger JR, Frank JA, Bizzi A (1990) Metabolism of human gliomas: assessment with H-1 MR spectroscopy and F-18 fluorodeoxyglucose PET. Radiology 177:633–641
42. Frahm J, Bruhn H, Hanicke W, Merboldt KD, Mursch K, Markakis E (1991) Localized proton NMR spectroscopy of brain tumors using short echo time STEAM sequences. J Comput Assist Tomogr 15:915–922
43. Mattiello J, Evelhoch JL, Brown E (1990) Effect of photodynamic therapy on RIF-1 tumor metabolism and blood flow examined ^{31}P and ^{1}H NMR spectroscopy. NMR Biomed 3:64–70
44. Segebarth CM, Baleriaux DF, Luyten PR (1990) Detection of metabolic heterogeneity of human intracranial tumors in vivo by ^{1}H NMR spectroscopic imaging. Magn Reson Med 13:62–76
45. Heiss WD, Heindel W, Herholz HK, Rudolf J, Bunke J, Jeske J, Friedman G (1990) PET of F-18-deoxyglucose and image-guided P-31 MRS in brain tumors. J Nucl Med 31:302–310
46. Ito M, Lammertsma AA, Wise RSJ, Bernardi S, Frackowiak RSJ, Heather JD, McKenzie CG, Thomas DGT, Jones T (1982) Measurement of regional cerebral blood flow and oxygen utilization in patients with cerebral tumors using ^{15}O and positron emission tomography: analytical techniques and preliminary results. Neuroradiology 23:63–74
47. Yamamoto YL, Thompson CJ, Meyer E, Robertson SJ, Feindel W (1977) Dynamic positron emission tomography for study of cerebral hemodynamics in a cross section of the head using positron-emitting ^{68}Ga-EDTA and ^{77}Kr. J Comp Assist Tomogr 1:43
48. Baba T, Fukui M, Takeshita I, Ichiya Y, Kuwabara Y, Hasuo K (1990) Selective enhancement of intratumoral blood flow in malignant gliomas using intra-arterial adenosine triphosphate. J Neurosurg 72:907–911
49. Nariai T, Senda M, Ishii K, Maehara T, Wakabayashi S, Toyama H, Ishiwata K, Hirakawa K (1997) Three-dimensional imaging of cortical structure, function and glioma for tumor resection. J Nucl Med 38:1563–1568
50. Rhodes CG, Wise RJS, Gibbs JM, Frackowiak RSJ, Hatazawa J, Palmer AJ, Thomas DGT, Jones T (1983) In vivo disturbance of the oxidative metabolism of glucose in human cerebral gliomas. Ann Neurol 14:614–626
51. Di Chiro G, De La Paz RL, Brooks RA, Sokoloff L, Kornblith PL, Smith BH, Patronas NJ, Kufta CV, Kessler RM, Johnston GS, Manning RG, Wolf AP (1982) Glucose utilization of cerebral gliomas measured by ^{18}F-fluorodeoxyglucose and PET. Neurology 32:1323–1329

52. Weber G (1977) Enzymology of cancer cells I. N Engl J Med 296:486–492
53. Kubota R, Kubota K, Yamada S, Tada M, Ido T, Tamahashi (1994) Active and passive mechanisms of [Fluorine-18] fluorodeoxyglucose uptake by proliferating and prenecrotic cancer cells in vivo: a microautoradiographic study. J Nucl Med 35:1067–1075
54. Fulham MJ, Melisi JW, Nishimiya J, Dwyer AJ, Di Chiro G (1994) Neuroimaging of juvenile pilocytic astrocytomas: an enigma. Radiology 189:221–225
55. Derlon J-M, Bourdet C, Bustany P, Chatel M, Theron J, Darcel F, Syrota A (1989) [^{11}C] L-methionine uptake in gliomas. Neurosurgery 25:720–728
56. Conti PS, Hilton J, Wong DF, Alauddin MM, Dannal RF, Ravert HT, Wilson AA, Anderson JH (1994) High performance liquid chromatography of carbon-11-labeled compounds. J Nucl Med 21:1045–1051
57. Yung BCK, Wand GS, Blevins L, Dannals RF, Ravert HT, Chan B, Wong DF (1993) In vivo assessment of dopamine receptor density in pituitary macroadenoma and correlation with in vitro assay (abstract). J Nucl Med 34:133p
58. Pappata S, Cornu P, Samson Y, Prenant C, Benavides J, Scatton B, Crouzel C, Hauw JJ, Syrota A (1991) PET study of carbon-11-PK-11195 binding to peripheral type benzodiazepine sites in glioblastoma: a case report. J Nucl Med 32:1608–1610
59. Lichtor J, Dohrmann GJ (1987) Oxidative metabolism and glycolysis in benign brain tumors. J Neurosurg 67:336–340
60. Valk PE, Budinger TF, Levin VA, Silver P, Gutin PH, Doyle WK (1988) PET of malignant cerebral tumors after interstitial brachytherapy. J Neurosurg 69:830–838
61. Holzer T, Heerholz K, Jeske J, Heiss WD (1993) J Comput Assist Tomogr 17:681–687
62. Camargo EE, Szabo Z, Links JM, Sostre S, Dannals RF, Wagner HN (1992) The influence of biological and technical factors on the variability of global and regional brain metabolism of 2-[^{18}F]fluoro-2-deoxy-d-glucose. J Cereb Blood Flow Metab 12:281–290
63. Blacklock JB, Oldfield EH, Di Chiro G, Tran D, Theodore W, Wright DC, Larson SM (1987) Effect of barbiturate coma on glucose utilization in normal brain versus gliomas. J Neurosurg 67:71–75
64. O'Tuama LA, Phillips PC, Strauss LC, Carson BC, Uno Y, Smith QR, Dannals RF, Wilson AA, Ravert HT, Loats S et al. (1990) Two-phase [11 C]L-methionine PET in childhood brain tumors. Pediatr Neurol 6:163–170
65. Weber W, Bartenstein P, Gross MW, Kinzel D, Daschner H, Feldmann HJ, Reidel G, Ziegler SI, Lumenta C, Molls M, Schwaiger M (1997) Fluorine-18-FDG PET and iodine-123-IMT SPECT in the evaluation of brain tumors. J Nucl Med 38:802–808
66. Tjuvajev JG, Macapinlac HA, Daghighian F, Scott AM, Ginos JZ, Finn RD, Kothari P, Desai R, Zhang J, Beattie B et al. (1994) Imaging of brain tumor proliferative activity with iodine-131-iododeoxyuridine. J Nucl Med 35:1407–1417

Head and Neck Tumors

F.C.L. Wong and E.E. Kim

Basic Considerations

In the United States, head and neck cancers account for 3.0% (41,400) of all new cancers and 2.2% (12,300) of cancer deaths [1]. The disease is more common in many developing countries. The incidence of head and neck cancer increases with age; most patients are older than 50 years. The male-to-female ratio is approximately 3:1, and the African-American population has experienced a significant increase [2]. The greatest risk factor is tobacco use. It has been shown that heavy smokers have a 5- to 25-fold higher risk of head and neck cancer than nonsmokers. The use of smokeless tobacco is strongly associated with the formation of premalignant oral lesions (hyperkeratosis, epithelial dysplasia), at rates ranging from 16% to 60% [3]. Dietary factors seem to play a role in the risk of oral and pharyngeal cancers. Epidemiologic studies have shown an increased risk of cancer in individuals whose diets lack sufficient quantities of nutrients. Mutagen sensitivity has been shown to be a strong independent risk factor for the development of head and neck cancer and seems to have a multiplicative interaction with smoking. Epstein-Barr virus (EBV) is associated with nasopharyngeal carcinoma (NPC). EBV genome has been found in NPC tissue. Most patients with NPC show evidence of an elevated serum titer of immunoglobulin G (IgG) and IgA antibodies against viral capsid antigen [4]. The association of NPC and EBV is particularly strong in patients with endemic undifferentiated carcinoma [5]. Human papilloma virus, especially types 16 and 18, and herpes simplex virus type I have been detected in the sera and tumor tissues of patients with head and neck cancer [6].

The multiple independent tumor cells may arise and progress in the same patient in a process known as field cancerization. Metachronous second primary tumors develop at a constant rate of 4–7% [7]. Tumorigenesis in the aerodigestive tract is a multistep process via genetic damage caused by continuous exposure to carcinogens. Specific genetic alterations include the activation of oncogenes, the inactivation or mutation of tumor-suppressor genes, and the amplification of growth factors and their receptors. Multiple allelic abnormalities (3p, 9p, 11q, 13q and 17p) have been documented, and they appear to have a prognostic value [8]. The cyclin D1 gene, also known as *PRAD*-1, *bcl*-1 or *CCND*-1, is located on chromosome 11q13 and amplified in 30–50% of patients with head and neck cancers. Overexpression and amplification of cyclin D1 has also been associated with more advanced disease, more rapid and frequent recurrence of disease and shortened survival [9]. Mutations and overexpression of the tumor-suppressor gene *p53*, located on the short arm of chromosome 17, occur in 40–60% of cancer patients and have been associated with a poor prognosis [10]. Tumors with *p53* mutations recurred at a median time of 6 months, compared with 17.4 months for tumors without mutations [11]. Thirty-eight percent of the patients with *p53*-positive margins relapsed, compared with none of the 12 patients found, by polymerase chain reaction, to have all tumor margins free of *p53* mutations [12]. Mutation of *p53* has been associated with tobacco and alcohol use; *p53* mutation was found in 58% of cigarette smokers who also used alcohol. Among patients who smoked but did not drink alcohol, 33% had mutations, whereas only 17% of the patients who neither smoked nor drank alcohol showed mutations of the *p53* gene [13].

Epidermal growth factor receptor (EGFR) is a cellulose oncogene likely to play a role in head and neck tumorigenesis. Its genetic amplification and overexpression have been demonstrated in pre-invasive and invasive lesions [14]. Anti-EGFR monoclonal antibodies upregulate EGFR and may prove useful in enhancing chemotherapeutic efficacy. Proliferating cell nuclear antigen (PCNA) is a nuclear protein whose expression, associated with DNA synthesis, increased 4- to 10-fold as tissue progressed from adjacent normal epithelium to squamous cell carcinoma [15]. Similarly, a high expression of transforming growth factor alpha was also documented to be a strong mitogenic factor, capable of inducing epithelial proliferation.

More than two-thirds of patients with head and neck cancer present with stage-III or -IV disease. For patients with early-stage (I or II) disease, surgery or radiotherapy is used with curative intent. In patients with stage-III disease and most patients with stage-IV disease, surgery followed by radiation therapy is considered standard care. Despite optimal local therapy, more than 50% of patients with stage-III and -IV disease will develop local or regional recurrence, and nearly 30% will develop distant metastases. Chemotherapy is under intense study in locally advanced disease, with promising results.

Pathology, Diagnosis and Staging

Cancers of the head and neck include a great variety of tumors, specifically those involving the upper aerodigestive tract. Head and neck cancers originate in the area under the base of the skull to just below the larynx in a cephalocaudal orientation and by the nasal cavity and vermilion border of the lips, anteriorly, to the pharynx, posteriorly. Greater than 90% of head and neck cancers are squamous carcinomas. There are three histopathologic subtypes of NPC: type 1 – differentiated squamous cell carcinoma; type 2 – nonkeratinizing squamous cell carcinoma; and type 3 – undifferentiated or lymphoepithelioma [16]. About 50–75% of NPCs in the United States are type 1 or 2, whereas in Asian and African areas, type-3 NPC predominates.

Most patients will present with symptoms and signs of locally advanced disease that vary according to the subsite in the head and neck. Sinusitis, unilateral nasal airway obstruction and epistaxis may be early symptoms of cancer of the nasal cavity and paranasal sinus. Persistent hoarseness demands visualization of the larynx. Otitis media that remains unresponsive to antibiotics may indicate a nasopharyngeal tumor. Chronic dysphagia or odynophagia may be the presenting symptom of oropharyngeal or hypopharyngeal cancer. Supraglottic laryngeal tumors rarely present early symptoms. The location of adenopathy provides clues to the specific subsite of head and neck primary tumors. Subdigastric adenopathy suggests primary cancer of the oral tongue or oropharynx, and posterior cervical adenopathy is a frequent result of regional spread of a nasopharyngeal tumor. Leukoplakia and high risk erythroplakia are the common premalignant lesions in the head and neck. Up to 40% of cases of dysplastic oral leukoplakia transform into invasive carcinoma. EBV DNA is found in nasopharyngeal carcinoma, and identification of EBV DNA in the lymph node may suggest a tumor of nasopharyngeal origin [17].

Patients who present with a suspicious neck mass should undergo a flexible fiberoptic nasopharyngoscopy or indirect laryngoscopy. A panendoscopy is the definitive diagnostic and staging procedure. Multiple biopsies of any visualized abnormalities or blind biopsies of random areas are performed to define the extent of the disease. If no primary site is found, fine-needle aspiration of the lymph node is performed to establish the diagnosis.

Staging criteria for head and neck cancers are based on the tumor-node-metastasis (TNM) system, and primary (T) tumor staging is complex, varying with each primary subsite (Table 15.1).

Prognosis of head and neck cancers is influenced by many factors, including tumor grade, size, site, vascularity, lymphatic drainage, host immune response, age, gender, national status and performance status. Differentiation grade has not been consistently accurate in reflecting the biologic aggressiveness of squamous cancer [18]. Better-differentiated tumors that produce more keratin are thought to be less likely to metastasize. Enlarged, hyperchromatic nuclei are associated with less-differentiated tumors. Enlarged nuclear size and staining presumably reflects chromosomal abnormalities and increased DNA content. Aneu-

Table 15.1. Staging for head and neck cancer

TNM	Clinical
TX: Cannot be assessed	0: Tis, N0, M0
T0: No primary tumor	I: T_1, N0, M0
Tis: In situ	II: T_2, N0, M0
T_1: <2 cm	III: T3, N0, M0
T_2: 2–4 cm	T_1, N1, M0
T_3: >4 cm	IV: T4, N0–1, M0
T4: Invades adjacent structures (bone, deep muscle, sinus, skin)	Any T, N2–3, M0
NX: Cannot be assessed	Any T and N, M1
N0: No node metastasis	
N1: Single ipsilateral node (≥3 cm)	
N2: a. Single ipsilateral node (3–6 cm) b. Multiple ipsilateral nodes (<6 cm) c. Bilateral or contralateral nodes (<6 cm)	
N3: Node >6 cm	
MX: Cannot be assessed	
M0: No distant metastasis	
M1: Distant metastasis	

ploidy in 50–70% squamous cancers has been associated with poor prognosis [19]. Features reflecting aggressive cancer include lymphatic invasion, perineural invasion, lymph-node metastases and penetration of tumor through the capsule of involved lymph nodes. Extracapsular spread has been associated with high rates of distant metastasis.

Magnetic Resonance Imaging

Two to five days after laryngoscopy with anesthesia, magnetic resonance imaging (MRI) should be performed using a Helmholtz surface coil to produce images ranging from the oral cavity to the caudal thyroid border (Figs. 15.1 and 15.2). MRI with high soft-tissue contrast and multiplanar scans is a highly sensitive and specific imaging technique for laryngeal and hypopharyngeal tumor staging [20]. Due to different T_1 and T_2 relaxation times, fatty, cystic and muscular tissues can be easily differentiated. However, tumor-spread delineation in mucosal areas is more difficult to define, and MRI overestimates the actual tumor extension in some cases of surrounding inflammatory tissue [21]. Excellent T_2-weighted images allow the best anatomical visualization of tumors as well as cartilage (Fig. 15.3). Accurate plain images, contrast-enhanced images, and a subtraction technique of equal T_1-weighted images before and after gadolinium-diethylene-triaminepentaacetic-acid (Gd-DTPA) application allow good – or at least sufficient – assessment of cartilage invasion for separating tumors from neighboring tissues like cartilage. Gd-DTPA-enhanced MRI showed a sensitivity of 86%, compared with 66% for computed tomography (CT) and 69% for sonography. MR, CT and sonography appear equal in specificity, showing 94–96% [22]. MR or CT adds valuable staging information to laryngoscopy by excluding deep tumor extension and the presence of lymphadenopathy. However, some MR and CT findings are nonspecific; a thickened cord may be due to tumor, fibrosis, edema, inflammation or hemorrhage.

Piriform sinus tumors behave more aggressively than endolaryngeal lesions and comprise 10–20% of laryngeal cancers. They are usually squamous cell carcinomas of inferior hypopharyngeal origin and frequently invade the thyroid

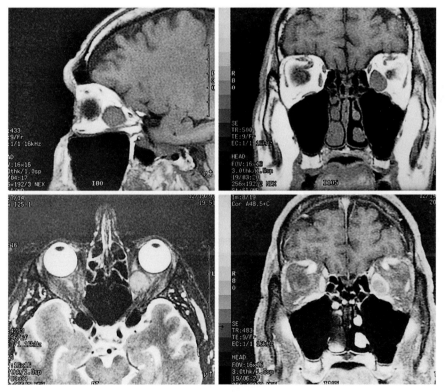

Fig. 15.1. T_1-weighted sagittal (*upper left*) and coronal (*upper right*) images of the head show a metastatic pancreatic islet cell tumor in the medial rectus muscle of the left eye, with an intermediate signal intensity. The T_2-weighted axial image (*lower left*) shows a high signal intensity in the mass. There is slight contrast enhancement on the post-gadolinium T_1-weighted coronal image (*lower right*). Note the excellent anatomy of paranasal sinuses

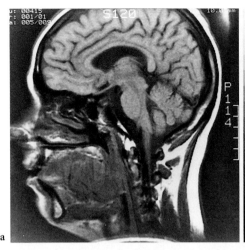
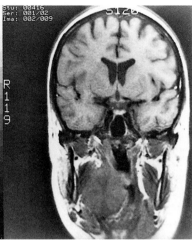

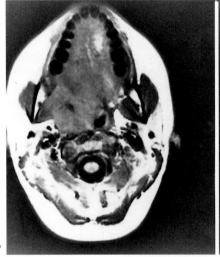
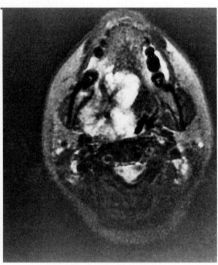

Fig. 15.2. a T_1-weighted sagittal (*left*) and coronal (*right*) images of the head show an ill-defined squamous cell carcinoma in the right tongue with slightly heterogeneous signal intensity, partially obstructing oropharyngeal cavity. **b** Axial images of the mouth show a right tongue cancer partially obstructing the oropharyngeal cavity and involving the right parapharyngeal space as well as the right mandible, with heterogeneous intermediate signal intensity on T_1-weighted image (*left*) and high signal intensity on the T_2-weighted image (*right*)

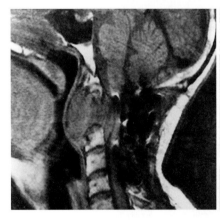
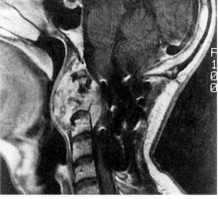

Fig. 15.3. Sagittal images of the neck show a recurrent expansile chordoma involving C2 and C3 vertebral bodies with heterogeneous intermediate signal intensity on the T_1-weighted image (*left*) and high signal intensity on the T_2-weighted image (*right*). Note multiple surgical clip artifacts in the soft tissue posterior to the tumor

cartilage at its posterolateral margins. Supraglottic tumors arising anywhere from the false vocal cords to the epiglottis comprise 20–35% of laryngeal cancers and tend to spread to lymph nodes high in the neck. They often present as more advanced tumors than glottic tumors. Anterior supraglottic tumors have a better prognosis than those of the posterolateral supraglottis. Advanced piriform sinus carcinomas often resemble lateral supraglottic (marginal) tumors. Glottic tumors

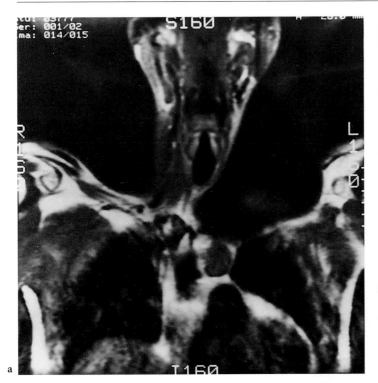 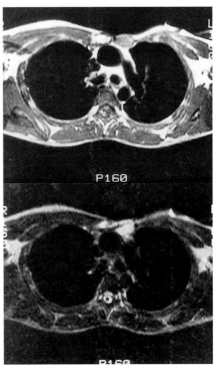

Fig. 15.4. a T-1 weighted coronal image of the neck shows a parathyroid adenoma in the superior mediastinum with intermediate signal intensity above the knob of the aortic arch. **b** Axial images of the upper chest show a diffuse contrast enhancement of the tumor on the post-gadolinium T_1-weighted image (*upper*) and markedly increased signal intensity on the T_2-weighted image (*lower*)

arising from the true vocal cords comprise 50–70% of laryngeal cancers and are usually well-differentiated, slow-growing lesions. About 75% of them arise from the anterior half of the true cord. On scans below the true cords, any soft tissue between the cricoid cartilage and the airway is abnormal and may represent subglottic carcinoma or extension. In a simple goiter with nuclear scan showing a diffuse trace uptake, MRI shows diffuse homogeneous signals in an enlarged thyroid. In Graves' disease, a uniformly high signal intensity is demonstrated on T_2-weighted images. Thyroid adenomas may appear brighter than normal thyroid tissue on T_1-weighted images, possibly related to hemorrhagic degeneration. Thyroid carcinomas show T_1 and T_2 prolongation, and MR tissue characterization is useful in distinguishing post-treatment fibrosis with short T_2 relaxation time from recurrent cancer. Parathyroid adenomas tend to have longer T_2 relaxation times than thyroid adenomas (Fig. 15.4). Discrimination between adenomas and hyperplasia is not possible via MRI. Posterior thyroid adenomas and lymph nodes are the most common cause of false-positive MRI findings. A definite proof of pathological lymph nodes exists at a size of 5–8 mm in MR and in CT. Metastatic nodes, at times, show a contrast enhancement in the rim, with a centrally decreased signal or density. MR has an advantage over CT in the differentiation of lymphadenopathy with various slice-orientation and gradient-echo techniques revealing vessels. MR angiography allows excellent depiction of the carotid vessels and is indicated to evaluate vascular displacement or compression by tumor growth and tumor perfusion.

Magnetic Resonance Spectroscopy

Early experience with in vivo MR spectroscopy (MRS) has shown its potential for obtaining biochemical information, thus enhancing the diagnostic sensitivity of MRI studies [23]. In vivo proton MRS using a 1.5-T scanner was performed in patients with squamous cell carcinoma and also in healthy volunteers. In vitro, correlated proton MRS using an 11-T scanner was also performed in tissue specimens of squamous cell carcinoma of the head and neck, in normal tissue, in metastatic cervical lymph nodes, and in a squamous-cell-carcinoma cell line. The mean in vitro proton MRS choline (Cho)/creatine (Cr) ratio was significantly higher in tumor than in normal tissue. The difference between the mean ratios appeared to increase with increasing echo time. All in vivo tumor Cho/Cr ratios were greater than the calculated mean in vitro tumor ratio, whereas six of the seven volunteers had no detectable Cho or Cr resonance. The data also revealed that a variety of amino acids have a significantly greater likelihood of being detected in tumor than in normal tissues [24].

Positron Emission Tomography in Head and Neck Tumors

Head and neck tumors, either primary or metastatic, have been studied with positron emission tomography (PET) using ^{18}F-fluoro-2-deoxy-D-glucose (FDG) for viability, ^{11}C-methionine for amino acid transport, ^{11}C-thymidine for proliferation, and ^{18}F-fluoromisonidazole (FMISO) for hypoxia. The apparent advantages of these agents are that the background tracer uptake is usually low and they provide higher specificity. The use of ^{18}F-FDG is the most common because FDG is relatively easy to obtain from cyclotron facilities and there are well-established, quick synthetic procedures.

^{18}F-Fluoro-2-Deoxy-D-Glucose PET

The issue of heterogeneous tumor uptake continues to affect the interpretation of FDG-PET, because FDG uptake has been correlated with cyto-

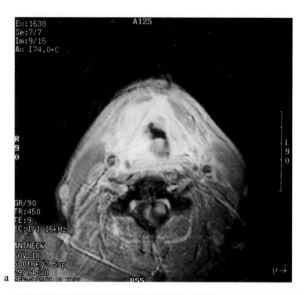

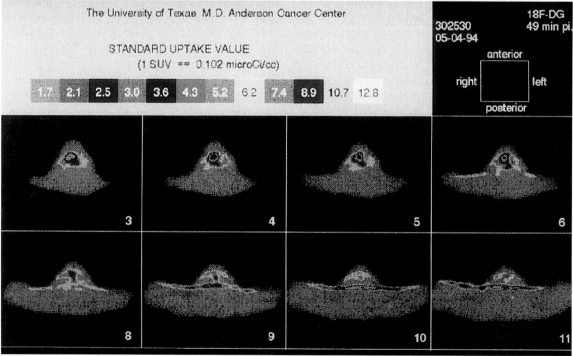

Fig. 15.5. a Post-gadolinium T_1-axial magnetic resonance image of the upper neck shows a diffuse contrast enhancement in the right supraglottic, glottic and paraglottic areas, probably due to irradiation. **b** Selected axial positron-emission-tomography images of the upper neck show an increased uptake of ^{18}F-fluoro-2-deoxy-D-glucose with a 5.2 standard uptake value (*image #3*), indicating recurrent laryngeal cancer which was subsequently proven

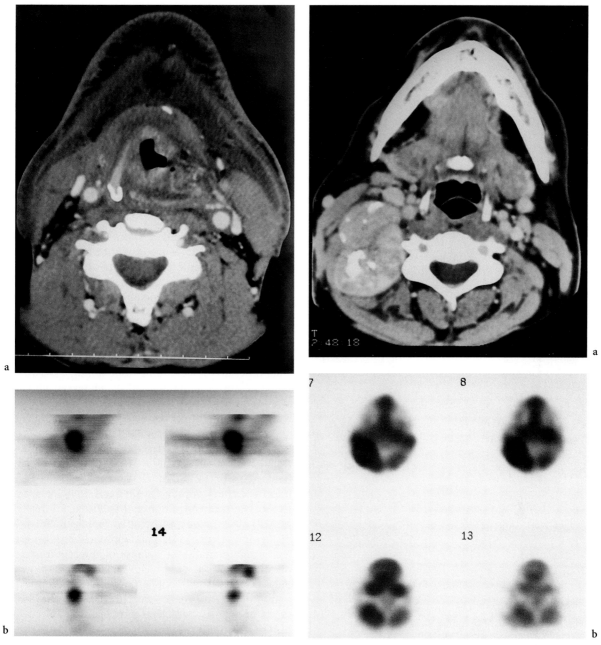

Fig. 15.6. a Axial contrast-enhanced computed tomography image of the upper neck shows an irregular enhanced tissue density in the left supraglottic area, possibly related to prior surgery and irradiation. **b** Selected coronal positron-emission-tomography images of the upper neck show a marked increased uptake of ^{18}F-fluoro-2-deoxy-D-glucose, indicating recurrent squamous cell carcinoma which was subsequently found

Fig. 15.7. a Axial contrast-enhanced computed tomography image of the mouth shows a calcified synovial sarcoma in the right neck, abutting the cervical spine. **b** Selected axial positron-emission-tomography images of the mouth show a markedly increased uptake of ^{18}F-fluoro-2-deoxy-D-glucose (*images #7 and #8*), indicating active malignant tumor in the right posterior neck

metric proliferation indexes to various degrees, but not with the perfusion rate of the tumor [25].

In a recent meta analysis of published studies between 1993 and 1994, the sensitivity of FDG-PET for the detection of primary tumors was 96% (Figs. 15.5–15.8). For the detection of lymph-node metastasis, the sensitivity and specificity are 88% and 93%, respectively (Fig. 15.9). For the differentiation of recurrent tumor from post-treatment changes, they are 94% and 82%, respectively [26].

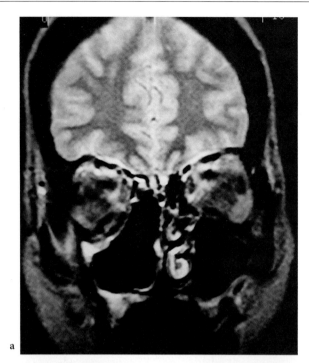

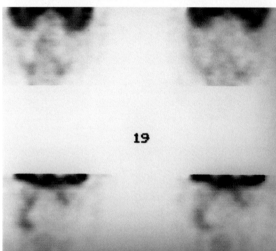

Fig. 15.8. a T_2-weighted coronal image of the face shows a markedly increased signal intensity along the lateral and inferior walls of the right maxillary sinus, probably related to postsurgical changes and/or recurrent sarcoma. **b** Selected coronal positron-emission-tomography images of the face show a minimally increased uptake of ^{18}F-fluoro-2-deoxy-D-glucose in the lateral wall of the right maxillary sinus (*lower*). No recurrent sarcoma was found

The accuracy of FDG-PET is better than either CT or MRI in all of the above applications. Prospective studies of FDG-PET of primary head and neck tumor found a sensitivity and specificity of 67% and 100%, respectively, while CT or MRI was accurate in 54% (7/13) of patients [27].

A study of 13 patients with unknown primary head and neck tumors found that four of five tumors were detected and the remaining eight tumors were correctly excluded [28]. In patients with untreated lymphomas, a higher uptake (differential uptake ratio, or DUR) of FDG was correlated with a worse survival rate [29]. These are similar to the conclusions of another study of the evaluation of benign versus malignant lesions, using a DUR of 4.0 to distinguish the lesions [30]. For the more difficult case of differentiating recurrent laryngeal tumor from post-treatment changes when clinical observations and conventional imaging (CT/MRI) did not provide a clearcut distinction, FDG-PET was found to have a sensitivity of 67% and a specificity of 57% [31] (Fig. 15.6 and 8). More quantitative evaluation will require multiple blood sampling and the calculation of parameters such as regional metabolic rates. In fact, regional metabolic rates do indeed detect recurrent head and neck tumors better than semiquantitative measures such as standard uptake values (SUVs), an index analogous to DUR [32]. When SUV is used to follow the course of chemotherapy of head and neck tumor. FDG-PET demonstrates a general trend of decreased uptake after treatment and may be a good indicator to correlate with clinical response [33].

A more recent development is the coregistration algorithms that correlate anatomic and functional images. In a study of 30 preoperative patients, coregistration of CT or MRI to FDG-PET improved the accuracy to 97% and 100%, respectively. The results are better than either CT (69%) or MRI (80%) alone and altered management in 7 of the 30 patients [34]. This approach is, however, technically demanding because of the requirement of manipulation of images of different types. Furthermore, the flexible contours of the neck may not permit exact registration of the two types of images, which are typically acquired at different times or different days. This latter impediment may require the use of thermoplastic molding for the head and neck, which in turn may cause discomfort to those patients who have ailments in this region.

^{11}C-Methionine PET and ^{11}C-Thymidine PET

Owing to the short half-life of ^{11}C, clinical studies require close proximity to the imaging facilities and expeditious synthesis. Therefore, these types of PET are only carried out in specialized academic centers.

^{11}C-methionine uptake by tumors is presumed to be mediated by neutral amino acid transpor-

Fig. 15.9. a Axial contrast-enhanced computed tomography image of the upper neck shows a large necrotic and hemorrhagic metastatic squamous cell cancer of the left tonsil in the left jugular lymphatic chain. **b** Selected axial positron-emission-tomography images show moderately increased uptake of ^{18}F-fluoro-2-deoxy-D-glucose in the periphery of necrotic active tumors in the left jugular (*images #9–12*) and cervical (*images #16–19*) lymphatic chains

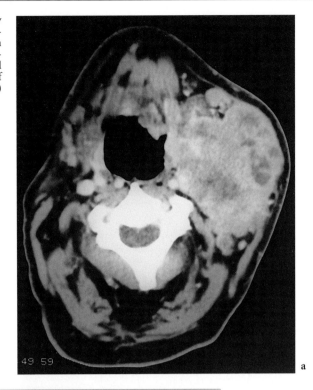

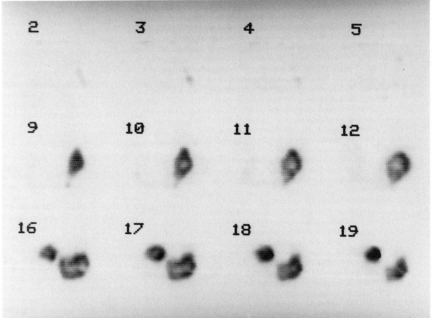

ters. For tumors larger 1.0 cm, ^{11}C-methionine PET detected 91% of malignant head and neck lesions. No correlation was found between the histologic tumor grade and ^{11}C uptake in 30 patients with squamous tumors [35]. The results are comparable with those of FDG in patients who underwent both ^{11}C-methionine PET and FDG PET [36]. Probably through splanchnic shunting and competition at the level of neutral amino acid-transporter mechanisms, tumor uptake of ^{11}C-methionine is subject to significant suppression from food in a nonfasting patient [37]. When used to follow the response of head and neck tumor to radiotherapy, ^{11}C-methionine PET shows markedly lower range of SUV (1.9) in those patients with histologic response, while those with no histologic response had statistically significantly higher SUVs (4.1) [38].

^{11}C-thymidine uptake by tumors has been correlated with the degree of malignancy and the proliferation indexes, as well as the number of cells in the S-phase of the cell cycle. Depending on the 2 position or 5 position of the ^{11}C label, ^{11}C-thymidine undergoes different degrees of rapid metabolism, presumably by the liver, leading to ^{11}C labels released into the general circulation, thus decreasing the signal-to-noise ratio in the tumor. It has been demonstrated that, in 13 patients, during the 10–30 min of PET imaging, the uptake of ^{11}C-thymidine in head and neck tumors remained stable and the kinetic differences were small [39]. However, in another group of nine patients with squamous cell head and neck carcinomas, variations from blood pool ^{11}C activities between –14% and +40% were noted [40]. Because of rapid hepatic clearance of ^{11}C-thymidine, exact measurement of tumor uptake will require individual correction for tumor blood volume and

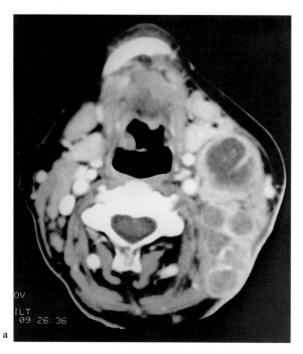

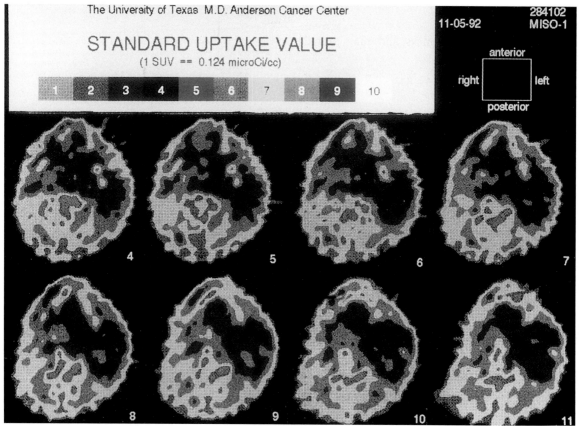

Fig. 15.10. a Axial contrast-enhanced computed tomography image of the upper neck shows a large necrotic squamous cell carcinoma in the left jugular and cervical lymphatic chains. b Selected axial positron-emission tomography images of the upper neck show a markedly increased uptake of ^{18}F-fluoromisonidazole in the left neck, indicating a hypoxic tumor mass

pose another technical requirement to measure the blood volume.

^{18}F-Fluoromisonidazole PET

Originally developed as a radiation enhancer, FMISO has been labeled with ^{18}F, and the resulting PET images were suggested to correlate with hypoxic states of head and neck tumors as well as lung cancers, [41], gliomas [42], strokes and myocardial infarctions.

The uptake site of FMISO is presumed to be a reductase that is found in metabolically active tumors (Fig. 15.10). The promise of FMISO in oncology is that it may provide an in vivo noninvasive indication of hypoxic states of the tumor and direct radiotherapy plans. However, FMISO-PET suffers from three weaknesses. First, the uptake of FMISO is slow and reaches a plateau at 2 h with relatively low uptake. Second, the correlation with in vivo measurement of oxygen tension is still to be conclusively demonstrated, although the human dosimetry has been recently published [43]. Finally, the synthesis is not standardized and the quality assurance procedures not established. Because of these issues, FMISO-PET has remained a research tool available to only a few centers.

Besides PET, other scintigraphic modalities such as ^{111}In-octreotide and ^{99m}Tc-sestamibi single-photon-emission computed tomography (SPECT) have made advances and may provide complementary information and less expensive alternatives to PET in the study of human head and neck tumors

References

1. Landis SH, Murray T, Bolden S, Wingo PA (1998) Cancer statistics, 1998. CA Cancer J Clin 48:6–30
2. Spitz MR (1994) Epidemiology and risk factors for head and neck cancer. Semin Oncol 21:281–288
3. Wray A, McGuire WF (1993) Smokeless tobacco usage associated with oral carcinoma, incidence and treatment outcome. Arch Otolaryngol Head Neck Surg 119:929–933
4. Hadar T, Rahima M, Kahan E (1986) Significance of specific Epstein-Barr virus IgA and elevated IgG antibodies to vital capsid antigens in nasopharyngeal carcinoma patients. J Med Virol 20:329–339
5. Liebowitz D (1994) Nasopharyngeal carcinoma: the Epstein-Barr virus association. Semin Oncol 21:376–381
6. Watts SL, Brewer EE, Fry TL (1991) Human papilloma virus DNA types in squamous cell carcinoma of the head and neck. Oral Surg Oral Med Oral Pathol 71:701–707
7. Cooper S, Pajak TF, Rubin P (1989) Second malignancies in patients who have head and neck cancer: incidence, effect on survival and implications based on the RTOG experience. Int J Radiat Oncol Biol Phys 17:449–456
8. Nawroz H, van der Riet P, Hruban RH (1994) Allelotype of head and neck squamous cell carcinoma. Cancer Res 54:1152–1155
9. Michalides R, van Veelen N, Hart A (1995) Overexpression of cyclin D1 correlates with recurrence in a group of forty-seven operable squamous cell carcinomas of head and neck. Cancer Res 55:975–978
10. Brachman DG (1994) Molecular biology of head and neck cancer. Semin Oncol 21:320–329
11. Brachman DG, Grover DE, Voken E (1992) Occurrence of p53 gene deletions and human papilloma virus infection in human head and neck cancer. Cancer Res 62:4832–4836
12. Brennan JA, Mao L, Hauban RH (1995) Molecular assessment of histopathologic staging. N Engl J Med 332:429–443
13. Brennan JA, Boyle JO, Koch WM (1995) Association between cigarette smoking and mutation of the p53 gene in squamous-cell carcinoma of the head and neck. N Engl J Med 332:712–717
14. Kwok TT, Sotherland RM (1989) Enhancement of sensitivity of human squamous carcinoma cells to radiation by epidermal growth factor receptor. J Natl Cancer Inst 81:1020–1024
15. Shin DM, Voravud N, Ro JY (1993) Sequential increases in proliferation of cell nuclear antigen expression in head & neck tumorigenesis: a potential biomarker. J Natl Cancer Inst 85:971–978
16. Perez CA (1992) Carcinoma of the nasopharynx. In: Brady LW, Peser C (eds) Principles and practice of radiation oncology, 2nd edn. Lippincott, Philadelphia, pp 617–644
17. Feinmesser R, Miyasaki I, Cheung R (1992) Diagnosis of nasopharyngeal carcinoma by DNA amplification of tissue obtained by fine-needle aspiration. N Engl J Med 326:17–21
18. Crissman JD, Liu WY, Gluckman J, Cummins G (1984) Prognostic value of histopathologic parameters in squamous cell carcinoma of the oropharynx. Cancer 54:2995–2999
19. Kokal WA, Gardine RL, Sheibani K, Zak IW, Beatly JD, Rihimaki DU, Wagman LD, Terz JJ (1988) Tumor DNA content as a prognostic indication in squamous cell carcinoma of the head and neck region. Am J Surg 156:276–280
20. Castelijns JA, Kaiser MC, Valk J, Gerritsen GJ, van Hattum AH, Show GB (1987) Magnetic resonance imaging of the laryngeal cancer. J Comput Assist Tomogr 11:134–140
21. Glazer HS, Niemeyer JH, Balfe DM, Hayden RE, Emami B, Devineni VR, Levitt RG, Aronberg DJ, Ward MP, Lee JK et al. (1987) Neck neoplasms: MR imaging Part II. Posttreatment evaluation. Radiology 160:349–354
22. Vogl TJ, Steger W, Balzer J, Dresel S, Grevers G (1991) MRI of the neck, larynx and hypopharynx. In: Hasso AN, Stark DD (eds) Spine and body MRI. Am Roentgen Ray Soc, Boston, pp 99–110
23. Mafee MF, Barany M, Gotsis ED, Dobben GD, Puklin J, Chow JM, Wenig BL (1989) Potential use of in vivo proton spectroscopy for head and neck lesions. Radiol Clin North Am 27:243–254
24. Mukherji SK, Schiro S, Castillo M, Kwock L, Muller KE, Blackstock W (1997) Proton MR spectroscopy of squamous cell carcinoma of the extracranial head and neck: in vitro and in vivo studies. AJNR Am J Neuroradiol 18:1057–1072
25. Haberkorn U, Strauss LG, Reisser C, Haag D, Dimitrakopoulou A, Ziegler S, Oberdorfer F, Rudat V, van Kaick G (1991) Glucose uptake, perfusion, and cell proliferation in head and neck tumors: relation of positron emission tomography to flow cytometry. J Nucl Med 32:1548–1555

26. Conti PS, Lilien DL, Hawley K, Keppler J, Grafton ST, Bading JR (1996) PET and F-18 FDG in oncology: a clinical update. Nucl Med Biol 23:717–735
27. Wong WL, Chevretton EB, McGurk M, Hussain K, Davis J, Beaney R, Baddeley H, Tierney P, Maisey M (1997) A prospective study of PET-FDG imaging for the assessment of head and neck squamous cell carcinoma. Clin Otolaryngol 22:209–214
28. Braams JW, Pruim J, Kole AC, Nikkels PG, Vaalburg W, Vermey A, Roodenburg JR (1997) Detection of unknown primary head and neck tumors by positron emission tomography. Int J Oral Maxillofac Surg 26:112–115
29. Okada J, Oonishi H, Yoshikawa K, Itami J, Uno K, Imaseki K, Arimizu N (1994) FDG-PET for predicting the prognosis of malignant lymphoma. Ann Nucl Med 8:187–191
30. Sakamoto H, Nakai Y, Ohashi Y, Okamura T, Ochi H (1997) Eur Arch Otorhinolaryngol Suppl 1:S123–126
31. Austin JR, Wong FC, Kim EE (1995) Positron emission tomography in the detection of residual laryngeal carcinoma. Otolaryngol Head Neck Surg 113:404–407
32. Lapela M, Grenman R, Kurki T, Joensuu H, Leskinen S, Lindholm P, Haaparaanta M, Ruotsalainen U, Minn H (1995) Head and neck cancer: detection of recurrence with PET and 2-[F-18] fluoro-2-deoxy-D-glucose. Radiology 197:205–211
33. Reisser C, Haberkorn U, Dimitrakopoulou-Strauss A, Seifer E, Strauss LG (1995) Chemotherapeutic management of head and neck malignancies with positron emission tomography. Arch Otolaryngol Head Neck Surg 121:272–276
34. Wong WL, Hussain K, Chevretton E, Hawkes DJ, Baddeley H, Maisey M, McGurk M (1996) Validation and clinical application of computer-combined computed tomography and positron emission tomography with 2-[18F]fluoro-22-deoxy-D-glucose head and neck images. Am J Surg 172:628–632
35. Leskinen-Kallio S, Lindholm P, Lapela M, Joenssuu H, Nordman E (1994) Imaging of head and neck tumors with positron emission tomography and [11C] methionine in imaging of malignant tumors of the head and neck region. Int J Radiat Oncol Biol Phys 30:1195–1199
36. Inoue T, Kim EE, Wong FC, Yang DJ, Bass P, Wong WH, Korkmaz M, Tansey W, Hick K, Podoloff, DA (1996) Comparison of fluorine-18-fluorodeoxyglucose and carbon-11-methonine PET in detection of malignant tumors. J Nucl Med 37:1472–1476
37. Lindholm P, Leskinen-Kallio S, Kirvela O, Nagren K, Lehikoinen P, Pulkki K, Peltola O, Ruotsalainen U, Teras M, Joensuu H (1994) Head and neck cancer: effect of food ingestion on uptake of C-11 methionine. Radiology 190:863–868
38. Lindholm P, Leskinen-Kallio S, Grenman R, Lehikoinen P, Nagren K, Teras M, Ruotsalainen U, Joensuu H (1995) Evaluation of response to radiotherapy in head and neck cancer by positron emission tomography and [11C] methionine. Int J Radiat Oncol Biol Phys 32:787–794
39. Goethals P, van Eijkeren M, Lodewyck W, Dams R (1995) Measurement of [methyl-carbon-11]thymidine and its metabolites in head and neck tumors. J Nucl Med 36:880–882
40. van Eijkeren ME, Thierens H, Seuntjens J, Goethals P, Lemahieu I, Strijckmans K (1996) Kinetics of [methyl-11C] thymidine in patients with squamous cell carcinoma of the head and neck. Acta Oncol 35:737–741
41. Rasey JS, Koh WJ, Evans ML, Peterson LM, Lewellen TK, Graham MM, Krohn KA (1996) Quantifying regional hypoxia in human tumors with positron emission tomography of [18F] fluoromisonidazole: a pretherapy study of 37 patients. Int J Radiat Oncol Biol Phys 36:417–428
42. Valk PE, Mathis CA, Prados MD, Gilbert JC, Budinger TF (1992) Hypoxia in human gliomas: demonstration by PET with fluorine-18-fluoromisonidazole. J Nucl Med 33:2133–2137
43. Graham MM, Peterson LM, Link JM, Evans ML, Rasey JS, Koh WJ, Caldwell JH, Krohn KA (1997) Fluorine-18-fluoromisonidazole radiation dosimetry in imaging studies. J Nucl Med 38:1631–1636

Musculoskeletal Tumors

T. INOUE, J. AOKI, and E. E. KIM

Basic Considerations

Sarcomas are a heterogeneous group of tumors originating from mesenchymal tissues. According to American Cancer Society estimates, approximately 9,400 new cases will be diagnosed in 1998, including 7,000 cases of soft-tissue sarcomas and 2,400 cases of bone tumors [1]. Soft-tissue sarcomas are extremely rare tumors, represent 0.7% of adult malignancies [1], occur more frequently in children and are indicated as 6.5% of all cancers in children younger than 15 years of age. Soft-tissue sarcomas are the fifth leading cause of cancer death in this age group, and 4,300 deaths are expected to occur from this disease in the United States in 1998 [1]. Bone sarcomas account for 0.2% of all primary cancers in adults and approximately 5% of childhood malignancies; 1,400 deaths will be caused by bone sarcomas in the United States in 1998 [1].

Soft-Tissue Sarcomas

The majority of soft-tissue sarcomas are of mesodermal origin, but some sarcomas are derived from the ectoderm. Some histological subtypes share some epithelial features [2]. Recent advances in molecular biology indicate that genetic mutations in mesenchymal stem cells may be responsible for the development of sarcomas. Alteration in the retinoblastoma (*Rb*) and *p53* genes have been found in a variety of soft-tissue sarcomas [3]. Mutations of *p53* have been associated with high histological grade and poor prognosis [4]. Specific cytogenetic alterations have been associated with some sarcomas. About 50% of alveolar rhabdomyosarcomas show a t(2;13) translocation and t(11;22) is present in 90% of patients with extraskeletal Ewing's sarcomas (ESs) [5]. Myxoid liposarcomas have been found to have a t(12;16) translocation, clear cell sarcoma a t(12;22) translocation, extraskeletal myxoid chrondrosarcoma a t(9;22) translocation and synovial sarcoma a t(x;18) translocation [6]. Genetic alterations of the *Rb* gene have been identified in cases of osteosarcoma [7], and loss of heterozygosity and DNA alterations of the *Rb* gene in sporadic osteosarcomas indicate a poor prognosis [8]. Expression of the MIC2 gene has been reported in ES and peripheral primitive neuroectodermal tumors (pPNETs) [9]. A chromosomal translocation t(11;22) (q24;q12) is a characteristic abnormality of ES, but it has also been reported in pPNET [10].

Most soft-tissue sarcomas (60%) develop in the extremities; other sites include the trunk (31%), as well as the head and neck region (9%). The majority of soft-tissue sarcomas in children are identified as rhabdomyosarcomas, arising in 20% of cases in the extremities, 37% of head and neck cases and in 25% of genitourinary cases [11].

Bone Sarcomas

Osteosarcoma is a high-grade, malignant, spindle cell tumor of the bone characterized by the production of osteoid by the malignant spindle-cell stromas. It is the most common primary malignant bone tumor and affects males more than females (male-to-female ratio 1.5:1). There is a bimodal age distribution; the first peak occurs during childhood and adolescence and the second peak occurs during the sixth decade of life. During childhood and adolescence, 80–90% of osteosarcomas occur in a lower limb, indicating that osteosarcoma is associated with rapid growth of weight-bearing long bones [12]. Fifty percent of all osteosarcomas occur in the knee-joint area; the proximal humerus is the next most common site, with 25% of the cases. The axial skeleton is rarely involved [12]. In patients older than 40 years, the most frequent sites of osteosarcoma become the skull, pelvis and mandible. Patients with Paget's disease have a tenfold risk of developing bone cancer. Other conditions associated with an increased risk for osteosarcoma have been noted with hereditary multiple exostoses, enchondromatosis, polyostotic fibrous dysplasia and osteogenesis imperfecta [13].

Ionizing radiation is the only environmental agent known to cause bone tumors [14]. Chondrosarcoma of bone is the second most common primary malignant spindle-cell tumor of the bone, characterized by cartilaginous neoplastic tissue without direct osteoid formation. Chondrosarcomas usually present in patients older than 40 years of age. The most common sites are the pelvis (30%), femur (20%) and shoulder girdle (15%) [15].

ES is a rare tumor that usually occurs in bone and presents most frequently during the second decade of life; it is an unusual occurrence before 5 years or after 30 years of age. In patients up to 13 years old, it occurs with equal frequency in females and males; after age 13 years, it is more common in males. ES is believed to be of neuroectodermal origin [16]. ES can affect any bone, although it most commonly presents in the femur and pelvis. The axial skeleton is often involved. In long bone, ES usually localizes in the diaphysis, with frequent extension through the bone cortex into the soft tissues. Malignant fibrous histiocytoma (MFH) of bone is a high-grade tumor in bone as well as in soft tissues. It usually occurs during adulthood and commonly involves the metaphyseal ends of long bones, especially those of the knee joint.

Most soft-tissue sarcomas are treated according to their grade, size and location. Tumors treated via wide en bloc excision have a local recurrence rate of 20–30% for low-grade lesions and as high as 50% for high-grade lesions. Pre- and post-operative radiotherapy has been used in conjunction with surgery to improve local control of the tumor. Adjuvant chemotherapy is considered standard therapy for rhabdomysarcomas and extraskeletal ES [17]. Local recurrence should be treated with aggressive surgical resection or with preoperative chemotherapy followed by local therapy. Limb-salvage surgery is preferred for a significant number of patients with osteosarcoma or MFH of bone. Because radiotherapy can establish good local control of ES, the role of surgery in ES treatment has historically been limited to diagnostic biopsy and primary control of an expendable bone. The beneficial role of adjuvant chemotherapy is now proven and has significantly improved the disease-free survival rate at 2–3 years [18].

Diagnosis, Pathology and Staging

Diagnosis

The most common manifestations of soft-tissue sarcomas are swelling and pain. Patients with pelvic sarcomas might present with leg swelling that simulates iliofemoral thrombosis, or with pain in the distribution of the femoral or sciatic nerve. Hypoglycemia is rare and usually associated with large retroperitoneal sarcomas. The most common presenting symptom of osteosarcoma is pain with a slightly tender, firm, palpable soft-tissue mass fixed to the underlying bone. Fewer than 1% of patients with osteosarcoma will have a pathologic fracture.

Chondrosarcomas usually reach a significant size before symptoms such as a palpable mass with pain or pressure are noted. ES presents as a rapidly enlarging mass causing poorly localized pain. Metastases are present at the time of initial diagnosis in 15–50% of ES cases. The lungs are the most common sites of metastasis, followed by bone and bone marrow. Metastases to the central nervous system occur in fewer than 1% of patients.

Radiologic evaluation should include a chest X-ray and a computed tomography (CT) scan of the lungs as well as a CT scan or, preferably, a magnetic-resonance-imaging (MRI) scan of the primary tumor-bearing area. A bone scan should be obtained for bone tumors or soft-tissue sarcoma to determine whether there is periosteal invasion or reaction.

Pathology

The biopsy of soft-tissue sarcoma, and bone-marrow biopsy, as well as aspirate studies for ES, are important for obtaining morphological details necessary for electron microscopy, DNA flow cytometry, cytogenetics, immunohistochemistry and molecular biological studies.

There are approximately 70 different histological types of soft-tissue sarcomas. Most sarcomas are classified according to the normal cell type they mimic. In children, the most common sarcoma is rhabdomyosarcoma which represents 5–8% of all childhood cancers. Rhabdomyosarcoma has four subtypes: embryonal, botryoid, alveolar and pleomorphic. Immunohistochemistry is helpful in the differential diagnosis. The embryonal subtype is the most frequent and constitutes 75% of all rhabdomysarcomas. The differential diagnosis of the particular type includes small cell tumors, such as lymphoma, oat cell carcinoma of lung, mesenchymal chondrosarcoma, and ES. Botryoid subtype has a polypoid or grape-like appearance and is found in the urogenital tract of infants and children. The alveolar subtype occurs in patients who are 10–25 years older and occurs more frequently in the extremities; it has a poorer prognosis than the embryonal type. Pleomorphic subtype is the least common and occurs in adults, more often in the extremities; it should be differentiated from other pleomorphic lymphomas, melanomas and carcinomas.

In adolescents and young adults, the most common soft-tissue tumors are synovial sarcoma, clear cell sarcoma and primitive neuroectodermal tumors. Synovial sarcoma usually occurs near the large joints of the lower extremities in patients 15–40 years of age and has a slightly higher incidence of lymph-node metastasis [18]. Synovial sarcomas frequently calcify, which is rare for soft-tissue tumors. Calcification may also occur in extraskeletal osteosarcoma and mesenchymal chondrosarcoma. In adults, the most common soft-tissue sarcoma is MFH, which accounts for 10–20% of all soft-tissue sarcomas. MFH usually occurs in the thigh and retroperitoneum of adults 40–80 years of age, and generally refers to a high-grade sarcoma, with the exception of myxoid MFH, which usually has an intermediate grade [19].

Liposarcomas are the second most common adult sarcoma and usually occur in the deep soft tissue of the extremities and retroperitoneum. They occur slightly more frequently in men than in women and can vary in behavior, ranging from low-grade, well-differentiated to high-grade pleomorphic liposarcoma [20]. Leiomyosarcomas commonly arise from smooth muscle in the retroperitoneum, but can occur anywhere in the body. Neurofibrosarcomas originate from the neural sheath and are frequently associated with Recklinghausen's disease, in which patients have a 15% risk of developing neurofibrosarcomas. Angiosarcomas include hemangiosarcomas and lymphangiosarcomas, which arise from blood vessels and lymphatic vessels, respectively. They are rare and almost always high-grade tumors, and the 5-year survival rate is only 12% [21].

Alveolar soft-tissue sarcomas have no benign counterpart and evolve slowly. Most patients develop brain metastases that progress gradually over 5–15 years before death occurs.

Staging

Soft-tissue sarcomas are classified according to their grade, which represents the most important

Table 16.1. TNM classification of soft tissue sarcoma

T=	Primary Tumor
T1	Tumor smaller than 5 cm
T2	Tumor 5 cm or larger
G=	Histological grade
G1:	Low
G2:	Moderate
G3:	High
N=	Regional lymph node
N0:	No node metastasis
N1:	Node metastasis
M=	Metastasis
M0:	No distant metastasis
M1:	Distant metastasis
Stage I	IA: G1, T1, N0, M0 IB: G1, T2, N0, M0
Stage II	IIA: G2, T1, N0, M0 IIB: G2, T2, N0, M0
Stage III	IIIA: G3, T1, N0, M0 IIIB: G3, T2, N0, M0
Stage IV	IVA: G1–3, T1–2, N1, IVB: G1–3, T1–2, M0 N0–1, M1

Table 16.2. Surgical staging of bone sarcomas

Stage	Grade	Site
I A	Low (G1)	Intracompartmental (T1)
I B	Low (G2)	Extracompartmental (T2)
II A	High (G2)	Intracompartmental (T1)
II B	High (G2)	Extracompartmental (T2)
III	Any G	Any T
		Regional or distant metastases

prognostic factor [22]. Grade I describes well-differentiated disease and, at the other extreme, grade III refers to poorly-differentiated disease. Necrosis has been shown to be the best parameter for predicting prognosis [23]. The next important prognostic factors are the size and location of the tumor. Sarcomas located in extremities generally have a better prognosis than those not in extremities. The staging system of the American Joint Committee on Cancer depends largely on grade and tumor-node-metastasis (TNM) classification (Table 16.1). The lungs are the most frequent sites of metastasis (33%), followed by bone (23%) and the liver (15%).

A surgical staging system proposed by the Musculoskeletal Tumor Society in 1980 is used for bone sarcomas [24] (Table 16.2).

Bone tumors metastasize almost exclusively through hematogeneous spread, with pulmonary metastases usually occurring first, followed by bony involvement. Lymphatic involvement occurs rarely and is considered a poor prognostic sign.

There are different types of osteosarcoma. The classic osteosarcoma may present a lesion that can range from nearly normal to extremely dense radiographically or even involve complete destruction of the bone. About 14% of osteosarcomas are purely lytic and cannot be distinguished from telangiectatic osteosarcomas, giant cell tumors, aneurysmal bone cysts or MFH of bone. About 75% of all osteosarcomas belong to the conventional type, which includes osteoblastic, chrondroblastic and fibroblastic subtypes.

Parosteal and periosteal osteosarcomas are the most common variants of osteosarcoma. Parosteal sarcoma accounts for 4% of all osteosarcomas and usually occurs in older people, with a slightly higher incidence in women [25]. The distal femur is involved in 75% of cases and arises from the cortex of bone. It presents as a mass and grows slowly with late metastasis, and overall survival rates range between 75% and 85% [25]. Dedifferentiated and parosteal osteosarcoma and high-grade surface osteosarcoma have a much poorer prognosis. Periosteal osteosarcoma originates in the cortex, usually of the tibial shaft, and is pathologically a high-grade chondroblastic osteosarcoma. A small radiolucent lesion, bone spicules and Codman's triangle are characteristic on a plain radiography.

Chondrosarcomas are pathologically classified as grade I to grade III (high grade), which has the worst prognosis, with a risk of metastasis of 75% [26]. There are five types of chondrosarcoma: central, peripheral, mesenchymal, dedifferentiated and clear cell [27]. The most common variants are central and peripheral chondrosarcomas. Clear-cell chondrosarcoma is the rarest type, grows slowly and locally recurs with some malignant potential; it is often confused with chondroblastoma. Mesenchymal chondrosarcoma is a rare, aggressive tumor that affects younger patients; it shows a predilection for flat bones. Malignant fibrous histiocytoma (MFH) of bone presents an osteolytic lesion in the metaphysis with cortical disruption and minimal cortical or periosteal reaction.

There is no uniformly accepted staging system for ES, but a TNM system seems appropriate. Lymph-node involvement is rare, and the presence of a gross extraosseous extension, metastatic disease and less-than-optimal response to preoperative chemotherapy are poor prognostic factors.

Magnetic Resonance Imaging

Benign Lesions

Benign lesions account for the majority of soft-tissue masses, with 50–100 times higher incidence than malignant lesions [28]. Lesions that morphologically look benign do not always turn out to be benign. The signal characteristics of both benign and malignant tumors overlap frequently. MR examination should include at least T_1- and T_2-weighted images in at least two orthogonal planes, always including the axial plane.

Lesions with T_1-Shortening (High Signal)

■ **Lipomatous Tumors.** Benign lipomatous tumors are fat-containing tumors which generally have a characteristic signal pattern. Benign lipomas are encapsulated mature fat masses and are, by far, the most common mesenchymal tumor. They show characteristic high T_1 signal, intermediate T_2 signal, and loss of signal on fat-suppression techniques. They may contain lobulations and fibrous septa. They can be simple, multiple, superficial or deep-seated [29]. There are histological variants of lipoma, such as angiolipoma and spindle-cell lipoma. Heterotrophic lipomas are adipose-tissue masses in association with other tissues and include intramuscular lipoma, tendon sheath lipoma, fibrolipomatous hamartoma, macrodystrophia lipomatosa and lumbosacral lipoma. Lipomatosis syndrome is a benign symmetric lipomatosis (Madelung's disease) in middle-aged men associated with chronic alcoholism. Hibernoma is a benign tumor of brown fat.

■ **Subacute Soft-Tissue Hemorrhage.** Soft-tissue trauma may lead to intramuscular hemorrhage, hematoma, inflammation, subcutaneous fat necrosis and myositis ossificans. Intramuscular hemorrhage and inflammation show a feathery/infiltrative appearance of signal intensity. Hematomas can mimic hemorrhagic tumors (Fig. 16.1) [30], tend to be well marginated and are usually confined to one compartment with homogeneous signal intensity. Most subacute (weeks to months) hematomas demonstrate increased T_1 and T_2 signal owing to extracellular methemoglobin, and more chronic hematomas shows a rim of low signal due to hemosiderin deposition.

■ **Hemangioma.** Hemangioma is common and represents 7% of all benign tumors and the most common soft-tissue tumor in infancy and childhood [31]. It is divided pathologically into capillary, venous, cavernous and arteriovenous types. The MRI representation is characteristic, with scattered serpentine signal-void structures, representing high-flowing vascular channels (Fig. 16.1) [32]. There is an increase in signal intensity of hemangiomas on T_2-weighted images. Most hemangiomas are extremely bright on gradient-echo sequences, and hemosiderin and phleboliths are demonstrated as signal void foci.

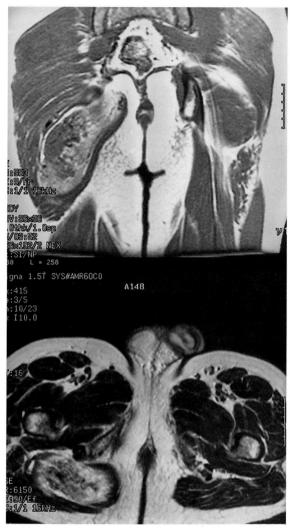

Fig. 16.1. T$_1$-weighed coronal (*upper*) and T$_2$-weighted axial (*lower*) images of the pelvis show a mass with heterogeneous high signal intensity in the right gluteus maximus muscle in a patient with a history of trauma. Surgery found a hemangioma with subacute hematoma

Lesions with T$_2$-Shortening (Low Signal)

T$_2$-shortening is due to the paramagnetic effect of tumor content, such as hemosiderin, hypocellularity or low water, high collagen, fibrotic scar, mineralized tissue, foreign body, air and fast-flowing vessels.

■ **Fibromatosis.** Aggressive fibromatosis is characterized by proliferation of fibrous tissue and local aggressive behavior with recurrence following resection. MRI findings are often variable and infiltrative, suggesting a malignancy [33]. T$_2$-shortening is attributed to low cellularity and abundant collagen.

■ **Nodular Fasciitis.** Nodular fasciitis is relatively common and composed of active proliferating fibroblasts with a rich intervening myxoid matrix. It is an infiltrative process in subcutaneous tissue and most commonly seen in young adults. On MRI, it is well-defined and homogeneous and exhibits decreased signal intensity on all pulse sequences.

■ **Elastofibroma Dorsi.** Elastofibroma dorsi is a rare slow-growing pseudotumor, and presents as a mass in the subscapular lateral chest wall. It appears isointense to muscle, reflecting a fibrous tissue with interspersed fat entrapped.

■ **Morton's Neuroma.** Morton's neuromas is a benign fibrotic lesion and consists of perineural fibrosis and degeneration of the interdigital nerve, predominantly in females. On MRI, the tumor shows low signal intensity on both T$_1$- and T$_2$-weighted images, and good contrast enhancement.

■ **Pigmented Villonodular Synovitis and Giant Cell Tumor of Tendon Sheath.** Pigmented villonodular synovitis (PVNS) is a benign soft-tissue lesion characterized by synovial proliferation and hemosiderin deposition. The knees are most frequently involved (80%), followed by the hip. MRI shows a reflection of heterogeneous composition (lipid, hemosiderin, fluid, cellular element and fibrous stroma) [34]. The synovial sac is distended with discrete masses of low signal intensity on T$_1$- and T$_2$ images. The differential diagnosis includes juvenile rheumatoid arthritis, amyloidosis, calcified synovial osteochondromatosis and hemophilic arthropathy. PVNS, when extra-articular, is referred to as a giant cell tumor of the tendon sheath. It is a benign growth of histiocyte-like cells associated with giant cells, foam cells and hemosiderin-laden cells. It typically occurs in small joints and is the second most common tumor of the hand after ganglion [35]. The tumor has a homogeneous low signal on T$_1$- and T$_2$-weighted images due to abundant collagenous stroma.

■ **Cystic Lesions.** Features of simple cysts include round or oval shape, thin wall and lack of enhancement. Proteinaceous or hemorrhagic fluid shows high or intermediate signal on T$_1$-weighted images. Popliteal (Baker's) cysts are common, and the synovium-lined cysts occur by extension of knee-joint fluid into the gastrocnemius-semimembranous bursa medially. Ganglia are locular benign cystic lesions containing mucous fluid and lined with a pseudosynovial capsule composed of spindle cells and collagen materials. On MRI, ganglia appear as a septated, ovoid cystic mass in proximity to the anterior cruciate ligament of the knee. Bursitis and trauma can result in fluid collection.

■ **Myxoma.** Myxoid tissues are in fibromatosis, chondroid tumor and myxoid liposarcoma, and show low signal on T_1- and T_2-weighted images. Intramuscular myxoma is a benign mesenchymal tumor in the lower extremity, and shows low T_1 signal, markedly increased T_2 signal, and gadolinium-diethylenetriaminepentaacetic-acid (Gd-DTPA) enhancement [36].

Lesions with Characteristic Shape, Course and Location

■ **Peripheral Nerve Sheath Tumor.** Peripheral nerve sheath tumors (PNSTs) are neurofibroma, schwannoma and their malignant counterparts. Neurofibromas arise either sporadically or in association with neurofibromatosis, which is characterized by multiple tumors or plexiform-type neurofibroma, and is also associated with an increased risk for sarcomatous degeneration. Malignant lesions tend to be larger. Schwannomas are the most common type, invariably solitary and arise in trunks of large nerves. They are slow growing along the long axis of a host nerve. The target pattern on MRI refers to a central decreased signal with a peripheral hyperintense rim on T_2-weighted images. This appearance has been seen in both neurofibromas and schwannomas due to peripheral myxomatous tissue and central fibrocartilaginous tissue [37]. However, this feature has not been identified in malignant nerve-sheath tumors.

■ **Normal Muscles Mimicking Tumor.** Anomalous or accessory muscles occur more frequently in the upper extremities. Normal muscle that has herniated through normal fascial planes can present as a palpable mass [38].

■ **Glomus Tumor.** Glomus tumor is a rare, benign, painful hamartomatous growth of the neuromyoarterial system and most commonly occurs in the distal finger in a subungual location. It appears as a well-defined lesion with T_1 and T_2 prolongation on MRI [39].

Others

■ **Cat-Scratch Disease.** Cat-scratch disease is a cause of unilateral lymphadenitis in young patients, presenting as a mass around the joint. MRI shows a mass with T_2 shortening. A focus of decreased signal is seen in the center of the soft-tissue mass, corresponding to the foreign body.

■ **Myositis Ossificans.** Myositis ossificans is a benign, ossifying, soft-tissue lesion in the skeletal

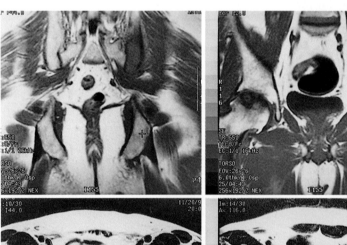
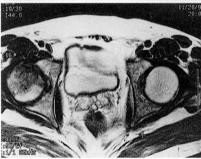
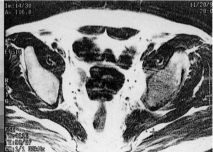

Fig. 16.2. T_1-weighted coronal (*upper*) and axial (*lower*) images of the pelvis show metastatic lung cancer lesions in the left iliac ala (*upper left*) and left acetabulum (*upper right*) with heterogeneous intermediate signal intensities. Note also aseptic necrosis in the right femoral head (*upper right* and *lower left*)

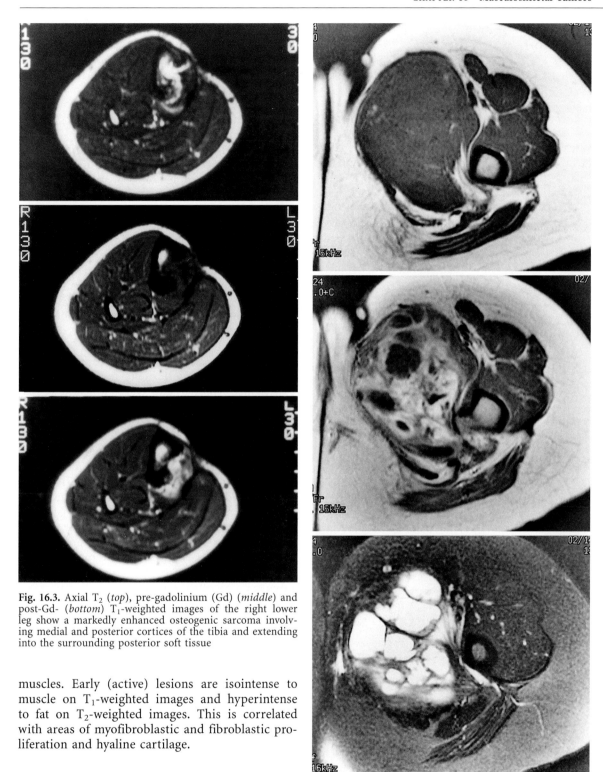

Fig. 16.3. Axial T_2 (*top*), pre-gadolinium (Gd) (*middle*) and post-Gd- (*bottom*) T_1-weighted images of the right lower leg show a markedly enhanced osteogenic sarcoma involving medial and posterior cortices of the tibia and extending into the surrounding posterior soft tissue

muscles. Early (active) lesions are isointense to muscle on T_1-weighted images and hyperintense to fat on T_2-weighted images. This is correlated with areas of myofibroblastic and fibroblastic proliferation and hyaline cartilage.

Malignant Lesions

MRI has largely replaced CT for initial evaluation of malignant soft-tissue tumors, but calcifications that may suggest specific diagnoses are not apparent on MR images. It also has the potential inabil-

Fig. 16.4. Pre- (*top*) and post- (*middle*) gadolinium-diethylenetriaminepentaacetic-acid T_1-weighted images of left thigh show a markedly heterogeneous contrast enhancement of the synovial sarcoma in the medial-anterior compartment. Note cystic components with uniform high signal intensity in the lesion on T_2-weighted image (*bottom*)

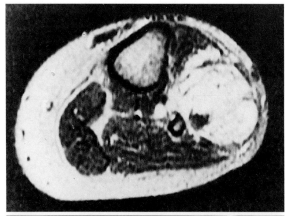
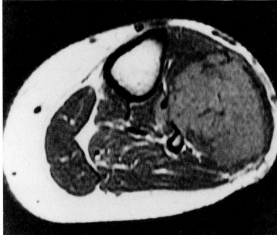
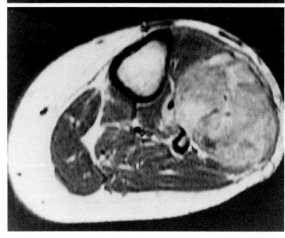

Fig. 16.5. T_2- (*top*), pre- (*middle*) and post- (*bottom*) gadolinium-diethylenetriaminepentaacetic-acid T_1-weighted images of the proximal left lower leg show a malignant fibrous histiocytoma (MFH) mass in the anterior compartment with heterogeneous signal intensities and contrast enhancement. Note also involvement of the anterior cortex of the left fibula by MFH

ity to detect a soft-tissue abscess, which may appear to be a tumor. The primary goals of MRI are to define the margins of the lesion, assess its rela-tionship to major vessels and organs and to determine whether the lesion invades adjacent bones or joints. T_1-weighted images are useful for displaying possible involvement of bone marrow and cortical bone (Fig. 16.2). T_2-weighted images provide excellent contrast between tumor and adjacent tissues. Short inversion-time recovery (STIR) shows improved conspicuity of primary tumors, enlarged lymph nodes and marrow metastases. Contrast enhancement helps define the vascularized as opposed to necrotic portions of tumor (Fig. 16.3). Active tumor, peritumoral edema and reactive granulation tissue show a strong enhancement on static T_1-weighted images. Dynamic Gd-DTPA-enhanced imaging measures the rate of enhancement, and calculating the slopes of time-intensity curves can help in differentiating malignant disease from less rapidly enhancing necrotic contents and adjacent edema [40]. It is also a method of evaluating response to chemotherapy, because slopes of responsive tumors become less steep [41].

Most tumors display intermediate signal on T_1-weighted images, intermediate to high signal on T_2-weighted images and variable contrast enhancement (Fig. 16.4). Low T_2-weighted signal of soft-tissue lesions suggests tumor hypocellularity and abundant collagen content. MR imaging cannot reliably distinguish between benign and malignant soft-tissue tumors. Benign tumors tend to be well-marginated with homogeneous signal intensities and do not encase neurovascular structures or invade bone. Malignant lesions generally demonstrate irregular margins, are larger and are more likely to outgrow their blood supply, with resultant necrosis. They show heterogeneous T_2-weighted signal intensity and often encase neurovascular structures and involve adjacent bone (Fig. 16.5).

MFH is the most frequently diagnosed soft-tissue sarcoma in late adulthood in white males, and most frequently occurs in the lower extremities. MR features of MFH are nonspecific, with ill-defined, heterogeneous and commonly hemorrhagic signal intensities (Fig. 16.6). Lipomatous or well-differentiated liposarcomas have a high fat content and may resemble benign lipomas. Most liposarcomas show inhomogeneous high signal intensity on T_2-weighted images. Myxoid types resemble benign myxoma on MRI, and tumors with fibroblastic or spindle cells show thick low-intensity bands (Fig. 16.7). Pleomorphic types may be confused with rhabdomyosarcoma. Alveolar rhabdomyosarcomas are common in the extremities and trunk. Embryonal rhabdomyosarcoma is the most common subtype, while pleomorphic rhabdomy-

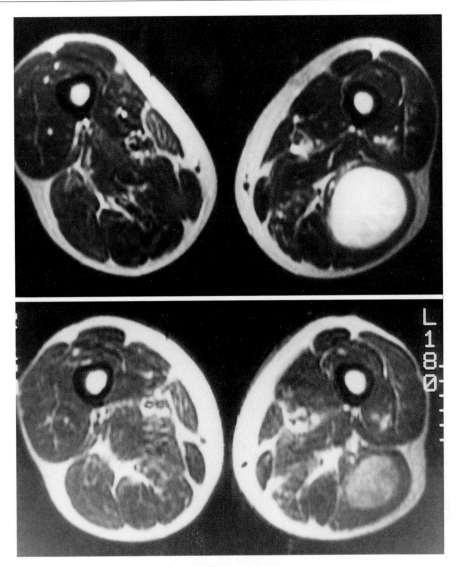

Fig. 16.6. T_1-weighted axial images of bilateral thighs, prior to (*upper*) and after (*lower*) chemotherapy, show significant changes of hemorrhagic malignant fibrous histiocytoma in the posterior compartment of left thigh, with decreased size and increased heterogeneity

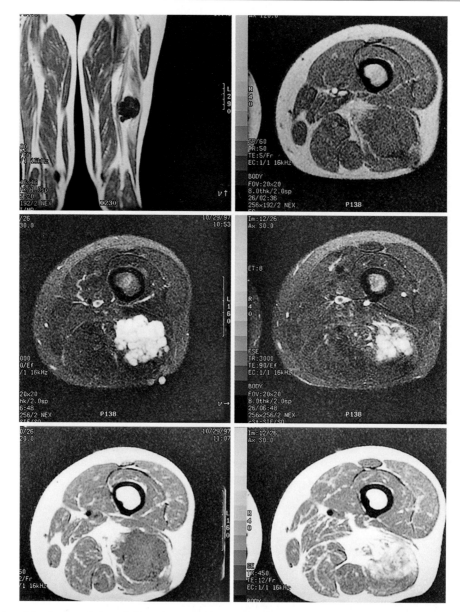

Fig. 16.7. T_1-weighted coronal (*top left*) and T_2-weighted axial (*middle*) images of the left thigh show a lobulated or septated myxoid liposarcoma in the posterior compartment. Pre- (*bottom left*) and post- (*bottom right*) gadolinium-diethylenetriaminepentaacetic-acid T_1-weighted axial images show a heterogeneous contrast enhancement. The gradient-echo axial image (*top right*) shows patent femoral vessels

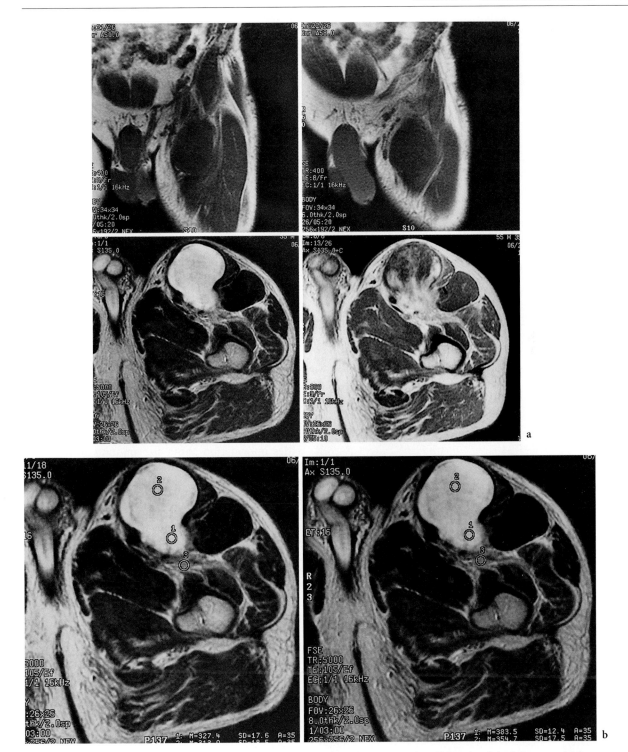

Fig. 16.8. a T_1-weighted coronal (*upper*), T_2-weighted axial (*lower left*) and post-gadolinium T_1-weighted axial (*lower right*) images of the left upper thigh show a malignant fibrous histiocytoma after chemotherapy with fairly uniform high signal intensity on the T_2-weighted image (*lower left*) but markedly heterogeneous contrast enhancement (*lower right*). **b** T_2-weighted axial images of the left upper thigh at the same level using multisliced (*left*) and single-sliced (*right*) fast spin-echo (FSE) pulse sequences show three small areas of interest outlined by circles to generate magnetic transfer ratios (MTRs). Higher MTR suggests a malignant tumor

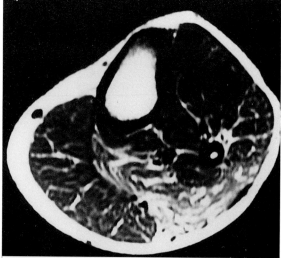
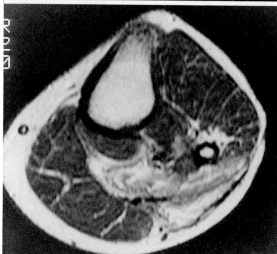
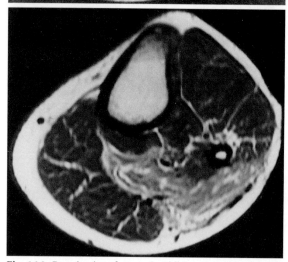

Fig. 16.9. Pre- (*top*) and post- (*middle*) gadolinium T_1- and T_2-weighted (*bottom*) axial images of the left lower leg show a diffuse high signal intensity with feathery appearance in atrophic soleus and lateral head of gastrocnemius muscles following wide local resection for unclassified sarcoma. No recurrent tumor was found

sarcoma is the least common subtype. Metastases to the lung, lymph nodes, mediastinum, brain, liver and bone often occur. MRI findings of rhabdomyosarcoma are nonspecific and usually indistinguishable from those of other soft-tissue sarcomas. After surgery and chemotherapy, a complex image with high T_2-weighted signal due to granulation tissue, fluid collection and radiation effects may obscure a recurrent tumor (Figs. 16.8 and 16.9). Successful results show a decrease in tumor size with low signal on T_2-weighted images. Unlike scar tissue, most recurrent sarcomas display intermediate to high signal on T_2-weighted images.

Magnetic Resonance Spectroscopy

Basic Considerations

MR spectroscopy (MRS) is unique in its ability to provide information about the metabolism of cancers in a noninvasive manner. ^{1}H MRS has been successfully used to study brain disorders. In the brain, ^{1}H MRS gives information about the amounts of choline and choline-containing metabolites, creatine and phosphocreatine (PCr), N-acetyl-aspartate, inositols, some amino acids, lactate and abnormally mobile lipids. ^{13}C MRS provides information about the amounts of the same metabolites observed in ^{1}H MRS as well as ethanolamine-containing metabolites, glycolytic intermediates and other amino acids [42]. ^{31}P MRS provides information about the amounts of phospholipid metabolites and energy metabolites as well as a means to measure intracellular pH. Studies in experimental cancer cell lines and transplanted tumors in animals suggest that the nature and concentrations of phospholipid metabolites observed in ^{31}P MRS are related to cell proliferation and tumor growth, tumor cell death and treatment sensitivity and resistance (Fig. 16.10) [43]. Almost all of the 67 evaluable spectra from soft-tissue sarcomas had relatively strong signal intensities in the phosphomonoester (PME) and phosphodiester (PDE) regions and an alkaline intracellular pH of about 7.25 (Fig. 16.11) [44].

Contamination with phospholipid metabolite signals from adjacent tissues is especially a problem for cancers occurring within organs such as the liver and brain, which contain large amounts of PMEs and PDEs. PME could emerge as a diagnostic discriminant between malignant and benign musculoskeletal lesions, but poor resolution of overlapping signals has made it impossible to distinguish individual components within the

Fig. 16.10a–c. Magnetic-resonance-imaging-guided ^{31}P magnetic resonance spectroscopy in a patient with an undifferentiated soft-tissue sarcoma in the left lumbar paraspinal region. The 8×8 array of 3×3×3 cm chemical-shift-imaging (CSI) voxels overlie the axial T$_2$-weighted image (**a**). The highlighted region indicates the CSI voxels that contain the ^{1}H-decoupled, nuclear-Overhauser-effect (NOE)-enhanced ^{31}P spectra (**b**). **c** The spectrum with the square borders was accurately localized to sarcoma tissue by voxel-shifting the data sets and shows strong phosphomonoester and nucleoside triphosphate signals (reprinted with permission from [43])

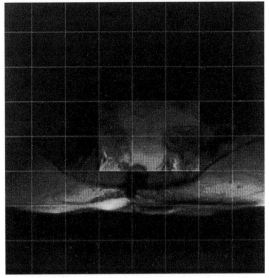

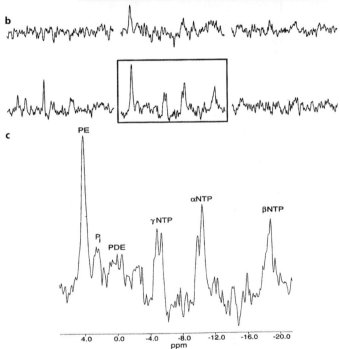

PME regions. Broadening of ^{31}P signals may be eliminated by radiofrequency irradiation of protons during acquisition of the ^{31}P signal using ^{1}H-decoupling. In addition, irradiation of protons between acquisitions can increase the ^{31}P signal by nuclear Overhauser effect (NOE) enhancement.

Diagnosis of Musculoskeletal Tumor

The ^{31}P MR spectrum of muscle has a large signal from PCr and little or no signal from PMEs and PDEs, the opposite of what was found in sarcomas. The difference between sarcomas and muscle is magnified by expressing the metabolite signals as ratios of one another. Almost no overlap was found between the PME/PCr and PDE/PCr ratio found in malignant bone tumors and those found in muscle [45]. The ratio of PME signal intensity to that of the nucleoside triphosphates (NTP) was also significantly different in benign and malignant lesions, with a sensitivity of 1.00 and a specificity of 0.93 [46]. Of all the potential markers of biological or clinical aggressiveness of a soft-tissue sarcoma, histological

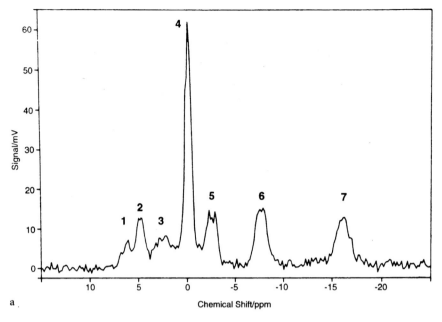

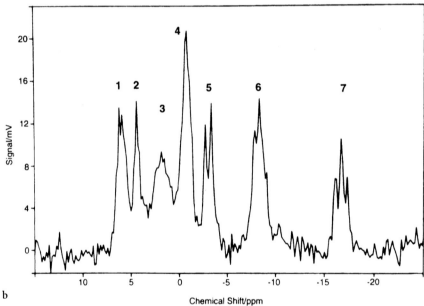

Fig. 16.11. a ^{31}P magnetic resonance spectra obtained from a hemangioma using surface coils primarily show signals from the surrounding muscle (inorganic phosphate: 2, phosphocreatine(PCr): 4, adenosine triphosphate: 5–7). **b** The spectrum from a spindle cell sarcoma shows prominent phosphomonoester (1) and phosphodiester (3) peaks and a relatively low PCr (4) signal (reprinted with permission from [44])

grade remains the most reliable, and it would be interesting biologically to explore the ability of MRS to provide metabolic markers that correlate with histological grade.

The spectra from soft-tissue sarcomas have several features (Figs. 16.10 and 16.11): high signal intensities in the PME region; broad signal within the PDE region due to membrane phospholipids; slightly alkaline pH (mean 7.4); and prominent NTP signals. An alkaline pH contradicted expectations that cancer cells should be acidic because of production of lactate from glycolysis.

Monitoring Treatment Response

Measurable complete responses to chemotherapy occur in only about 10% of recurrent or metastatic soft-tissue sarcomas, and obvious lack of response occurs in about 45% [47]. Because the metabolic changes associated with cell death ought to be apparent in MR spectra, MRS might be useful in determining the actual response of sarcomas with stable or slightly smaller size. Significantly higher PME/PDE ratios were found in sarcomas that responded to chemotherapy than in those that did not [48]. It has also been found that the mean pH (7.30) of sarcomas that responded to treatment was significantly higher than the mean pH (7.16) of those that did not [49]. There was also a suggestion that all tumors with a pretreatment pH of 7.3 or higher or a mean water proton T_2 of 100 msec or longer will respond to treatment. It has been indicated that a decrease in PME-signal intensity soon after initiation of treatment often occurred in cancers that ultimately responded to treatment [45]. An increased PME/NTP ratio following the first hyperthermia treatment correlated with eventual response as measured by the fraction of necrosis [50]. The correlation between a more alkaline pH prior to treatment and response to radiation plus hyperthermia was seen in the same study.

Positron Emission Tomography

Nuclear-medicine techniques offer potentially unique information with regard to the biochemical and pathophysiological characteristics of the malignant soft-tissue tumors, including musculoskeletal tumors. In particular, positron-emission tomography (PET) oncology is now a rapidly developing area in this field. In this chapter, recent papers describing PET oncology used with patients suffering from soft-tissue sarcoma, including musculoskeletal tumors, will be reviewed and a few illustrative cases of ^{18}F-2-deoxy-2-fluoro-D-glucose (FDG) PET conducted at our institute will be shown.

Blood-Flow Imaging

Most malignant soft-tissue sarcomas and malignant bone tumors seem to be hypervascular due to neovascularisation, which sets them apart from benign lesions and normal tissue. In general, the perfusion pattern showing increased peripheral perfusion with decreased flow to the central area of the tumor lesion is seen in aggressive malignant tumors. A blood-flow image can be obtained using PET with ^{15}O-water and ^{13}N-ammonia. In a patient with high-grade sarcoma consistent with MFH of the thigh, ^{13}N-ammonia and ^{15}O-water PET revealed increased blood flow along the periphery of the tumor, with diminished flow in the central area [51]. MFH, rhabdomyosarcoma, ES, osteosarcoma and chondrosarcoma all seem to be highly hypervascular. A "doughnut pattern of perfusion" is more typical of malignancies than the pattern of diffuse hyperperfusion in the tumor [52].

Metabolic Imaging

With respect to tumor metabolism, malignant tumors are characterized by a heightened proliferative activity consistent with a wide range of metabolic consequences. Alteration of cell membrane potentials, increased protein or nucleic-acid synthesis, acceleration with increased glycolysis and alteration in glucose-transporter-protein expression are associated with the malignant tumors. FDG is a metabolic tracer most widely used in the field of clinical PET oncology; it is an analogue of glucose, which is transported into cells by a range of transporters. However, physiological FDG uptake is present in the skeletal muscle and enhanced by exercise [53]. Since the physiological muscle uptake hampers the visual interpretation of tumor FDG uptake (Fig. 16.12), patient fasting for at least 4 h, inhibition of muscle exercise before study and transportation by wheelchair of a patient with a lower-extremity lesion are performed in preparation for the FDG-PET scan, in order to reduce the background radioactivity of the surrounding lesion. Enhanced glucose metabolic activity causes the intense FDG uptake in malignant tumors including soft-tissue and bone sarcomas. Intratumoral FDG distribution may be related to the population of viable tumor cells. Also, heterogeneity of proliferative activity and viable cells are often observed on the FDG-PET images. FDG-PET can be effective in informing us about the most representative area of the tumor. The obtained data is important, since the clinical behavior, patient's prognosis and the most appropriate patient management are usually determined by the highest grade of tumor histology within the lesion [54]. This FDG-PET may also provide useful information about the suitable biopsy site [55]. Some illustrative cases of FDG-PET application in patients with musculoskeletal tumors are shown in Figs. 16.13–16.17.

As an amino acid compound, ^{11}C-methionine (CMET) may reflect protein synthesis in the tumor and correlate with tumor proliferative activity [55]. However, its clinical use is limited because of the short half-life of ^{11}C. ^{18}F-fluoromisonidazole (FMISO) is a unique compound in that it accumulates and remains in hypoxic cells. Malignant tumor usually has some hypoxic cell components resistant to radiation therapy. PET scans with FMISO may provide useful information in selecting the most appropriate form of adjuvant therapy for soft-tissue sarcomas [56].

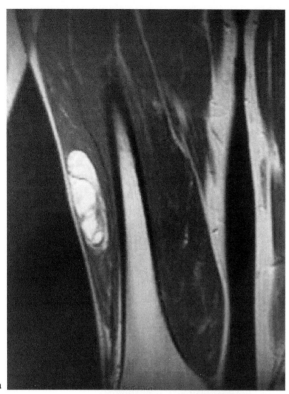

Fig 16.12a,b. Case 1: a 46-year-old male with an intramuscular lipoma. The patient noticed the soft-tissue mass of the right thigh 6 months earlier. Tumor had been gradually growing, and the patient complained of pain in the right leg when he walked. **a** Coronal T_1-weighted spin-echo magnetic resonance image. A mass with some compartments and a clear boundary is shown. Increased signal intensity within the lesion is observed. **b** Contiguous coronal sections of fluoro-2-deoxy-D-glucose positron-emission tomography (FDG-PET) images. Since the patient ran to the examination room, physiological intense uptake of the muscle is shown and hampers the visual interpretation of tumor FDG uptake. A fasting of at least 4 h, inhibition of muscle exercise before study and transportation by a wheelchair for a patient with a lower-extremity lesion are usually performed as preparation for FDG-PET scans to reduce the background radioactivity surrounding the lesion. The standard uptake value of the corresponding area was relatively low (1.0), and lipoma was proven by histopathological examination of the surgical specimen

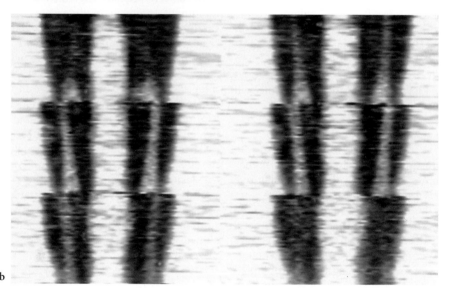

Fig 16.13a–d. Case 2: a 52-year-old female with lipoma of the right neck. The patient noticed the soft large mass (10×8 cm) without clinical symptoms. **a** Computed tomography of the neck. The low-density lesion of the right neck is recognized and a round mass in the right thyroid gland is also observed. **b** Coronal T_1-weighted spin-echo magnetic resonance image. A huge mass with increased signal intensity which extends from the right neck to the supraclavicular region is shown. **c** Contiguous transverse sections of fluoro-2-deoxy-D-glucose positron-emission tomography (FDG-PET). **d** Coronal section of FDG-PET. FDG-PET revealed no uptake of the lesion in the neck [standard uptake value (SUV)=0.5] (*arrow*) and intense uptake of the thyroid mass (SUV=5.4) (*arrow head*). Benign lipoma was proven by examining a surgical specimen of the neck lesion; the thyroid mass with high FDG uptake was also benign adenoma

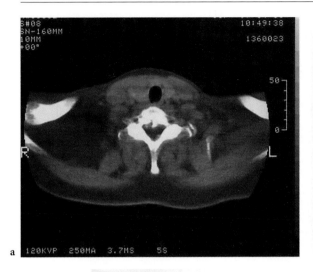
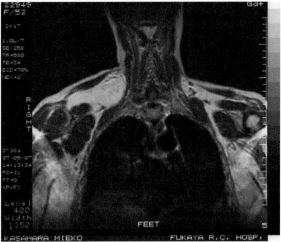
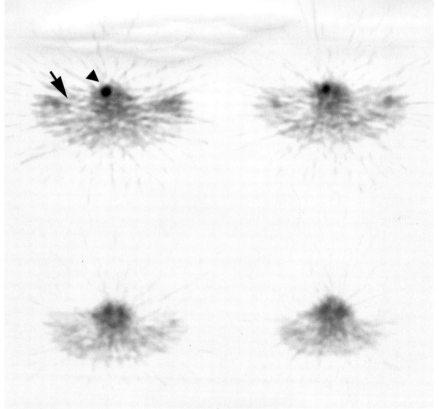
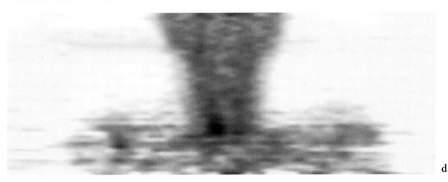

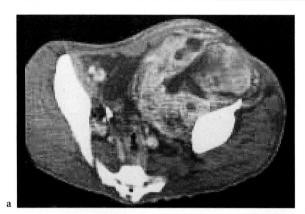

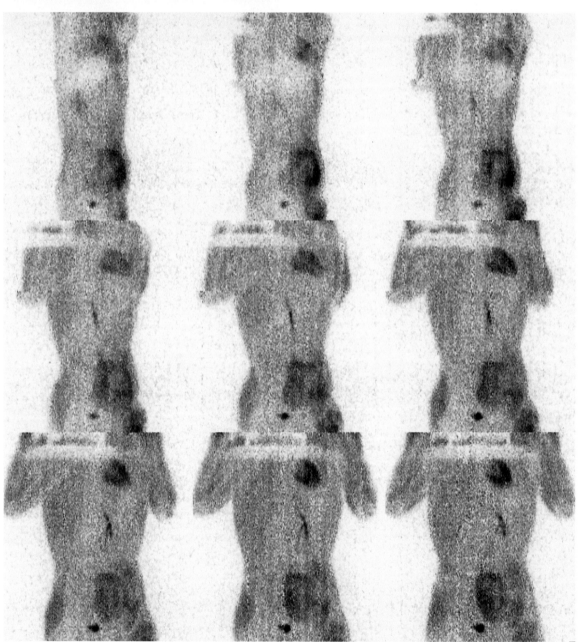

Fig 16.14a–c. Case 3: a 35-year-old male with malignant schwannoma. **a** A huge pelvic mass with heterogeneous densities is seen on a diagnostic contrast-enhanced computed tomography scan. **b** Planar images of whole body fluoro-2-deoxy-D-glucose positron-emission tomography (FDG-PET) from right lateral view (*upper left*) to anterior view (*bottom right*). **c** Transverse sections of FDG-PET images from upper thigh (*upper left*) to the pelvis. PET scans (**b** and **c**) show the irregular intense FDG uptake in the huge soft-tissue tumor, which implies the malignancy of this tumor (**c** see p. 261)

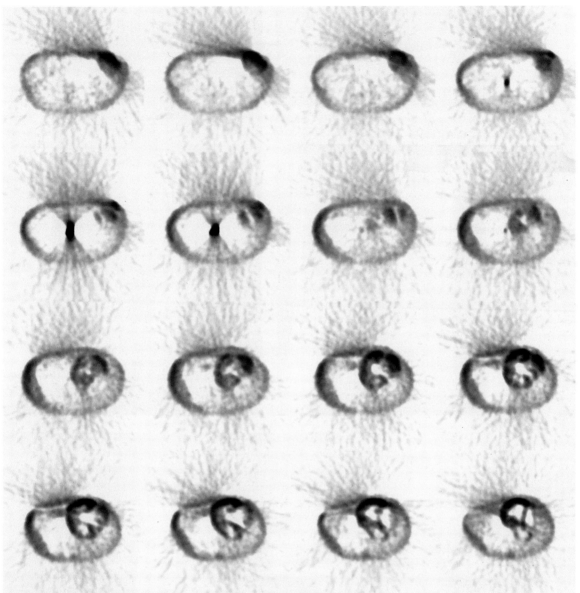

Fig. 16.14c

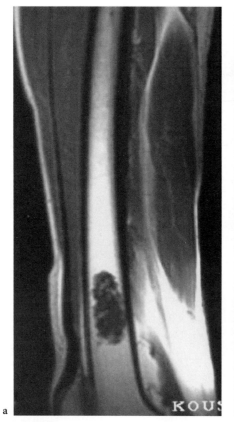 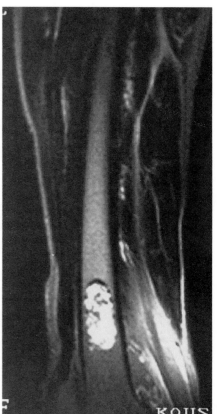
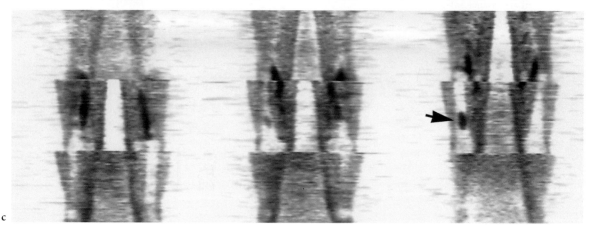

Fig. 16.15a–c. Case 4: a 37-year-old male with enchondroma of the right femur. The patient complained spontaneous pain of the right leg. **a** Coronal T_1-weighted spin-echo magnetic resonance (SE-MR) image of the right thigh. **b** Coronal T_2-weighted SE-MR image of the right thigh. The T_1-weighted MR image demonstrated the right femoral bone mass to be of nodular low signal intensity (**a**) and the T_2-weighted MR image revealed the corresponding lesion with high signal intensity (**b**). **c** Nine contiguous coronal sections of fluoro-2-deoxy-D-glucose positron-emission-tomography images. FDG-PET scan showed visible tracer uptake within the lesion (*arrow*), but the standard uptake value was low (1.1). Bone tumor was removed surgically and benign enchondroma was proven by histopathological examination of the surgical specimen

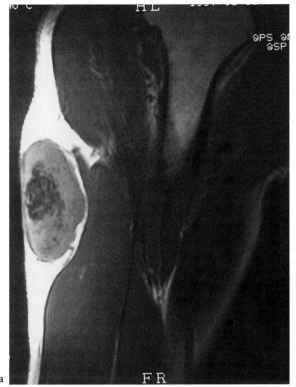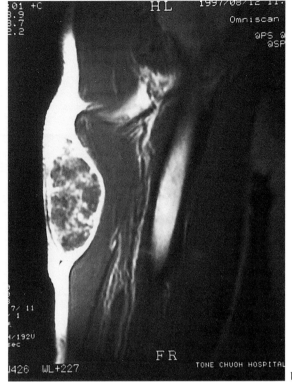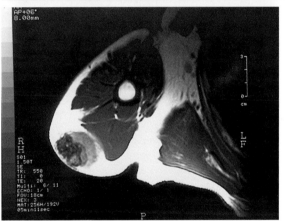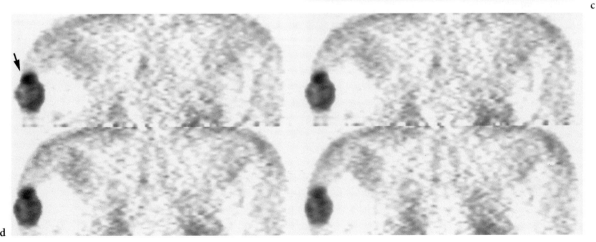

Fig 16.16 a–e. Case 5: a 54-year-old male with a soft-tissue mass of the right upper arm. **a** Coronal T_1-weighted spin-echo magnetic-resonance (SE-MR) image of the right upper arm. **b** Contrast-enhanced T_1-weighted SE-MR image. **c** Transverse section of the right upper arm of the T_1-weighted SE-MR image. MR scan revealed a mass in the fat tissue of the right upper arm, and mixed signal intensity with irregular contrast-enhancement was observed in the lesion. **d** Coronal sections of fluoro-2-deoxy-D-glucose positron-emission-tomography (FDG-PET) image. FDG-PET scan showed intense FDG uptake in the lesion (*arrow*) (standard uptake value=2.5).

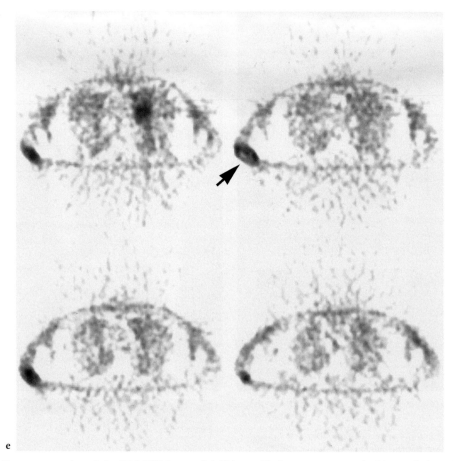

Fig. 16.16e Transverse section of the FDG-PET image. Calcifying epithelioma was proven by histopathological examination

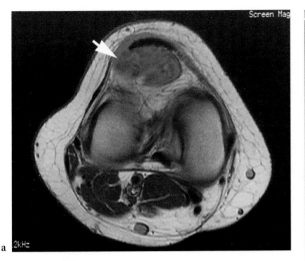
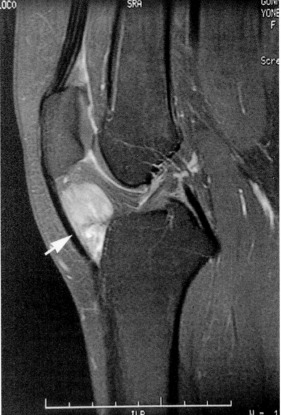
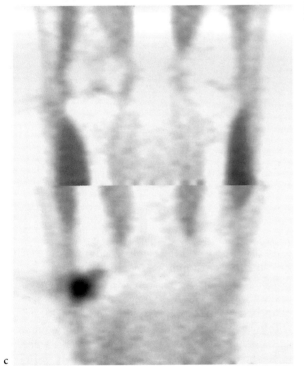

Fig 16.17 a–d. A 24-year-old female with a soft-tissue tumor of the right knee. The patient had complained of right gonalgia for 1 year. **a** Transverse T_1-weighted magnetic resonance (MR) image of the right knee. MR image scan revealed the soft-tissue mass in the infrapatellar fat pad beneath the patellar ligament (*arrow*). **b** Sagittal fat-suppression MR image of the right knee. **c** Two coronal sections of a fluoro-2-deoxy-D-glucose positron-emission-tomography (FDG-PET) image of the right knee. **d** Four contiguous transverse sections of a FDG-PET image of the right knee. A PET scan showed increased uptake of FDG in the lesion (standard uptake value=4.4). Pigmented villonodular synovitis was proven by histopathological examination (see p. 266)

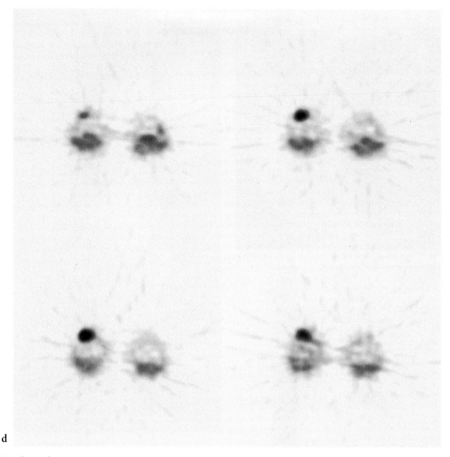

Fig. 16.17 d. For legend see p. 265

Tumor Grading and Staging

Since FDG accumulates in malignant musculoskeletal tumors, the effectiveness of using FDG-PET in musculoskeletal tumors for staging and grading has been evaluated. The first use of FDG for tumor grading was in brain tumors [57]. Regarding the application of FDG-PET for tumor grading in musculoskeletal tumors, Kern et al. reported on five patients with extremity tumors (four soft-tissue tumors and one osteogenic tumor) in which glucose consumptions were measured [58]. Although the sample size was small, they found a positive relationship between glucose utilization and histological grading. Several investigators have reported close correlation between glucose metabolism and histological grading. Adler et al. also reported that FDG uptakes in musculoskeletal tumors in 25 patients showed a significant correlation with histological grade, and all tumors with a standardized uptake value (SUV) of more than 1.6 were classified as high-grade [59].

In order to assess the tumor grading using FDG-PET, the degree of tumor FDG uptake must be evaluated. Visual interpretation using scoring is the easiest way, but not an objective one. For semi-quantitative analysis, a simple ratio of FDG uptake within the suspected tumor to that within comparable normal soft tissue is a convenient and a practical way to evaluate FDG uptake since it is not necessary to measure the injected dose of radioactive compound and perform blood sampling. While the SUV method is now the most popular way to evaluate the tumor uptake of FDG, it requires the measurement of both the total injection dose and body weight, and calibration of a PET scanner for measuring tissue FDG, a well counter for measuring radioactivity in blood and a dosimeter for measuring radioactivity in the injection syringe. The absolute quantification of glucose consumption is the most complex way to measure FDG uptake, since it requires multiple blood sampling and dynamic images. Griffeth et al. pointed out that the SUV method could distinguish ten malignant lesions from ten benign lesions. In contrast, a simple

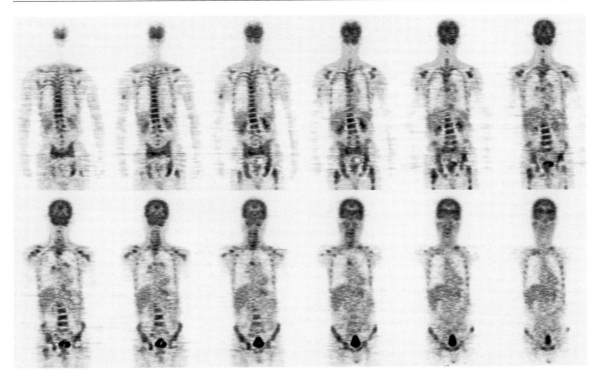

Fig 16.18. Case 7: a 73-year-old male with metastatic osseous disease of prostatic cancer. Contiguous coronal sections of a whole-body positron-emission-tomography scan showed diffuse increased uptake of fluoro-2-deoxy-D-glucose in the systemic skeletal system, including spines, ribs, pelvic bones, humerus and femur

ratio of FDG uptake within tumor to that within comparable normal soft tissue was less successful in helping make this distinction, with overlap in 12 of the 20 cases [60]. Nieweg et al. conducted FDG-PET in 18 patients with soft-tissue sarcoma, including 6 malignant fibrous histiocytomas, 5 liposarcomas and 7 other sarcomas, and 4 patients with benign soft-tissue lesions. In this study, glucose consumption of sarcoma ranged from 2.9 µmol/100 g/min to 41.8 µmol/100 g/min and had a close correlation with the histopathological malignancy grade, but the SUV method did not reveal this close correlation. FDG appears to be unsuitable for discriminating between benign lesions and low- or intermediate-malignancy-grade lesions.

In staging musculoskeletal tumors, the recent development of whole-body PET may contribute to the detection of distant metastasis [61]. Soft-tissue sarcoma tends to disseminate to the lung. FDG-PET has potential clinical value for detecting metastatic lung lesions because of the low physiological lung uptake. The conventional bone scan using ^{99m}Tc-methylene diphosphonate (MDP) is sensitive to metastatic bone lesions. A recent report showed that FDG-PET can help identify osseous and soft tissue metastases with a high positive predictive value (98%) in patients with prostatic cancer (Fig. 16.18), but is less sensitive than bone scan in the identification of osseous metastases [62]. However, whether the detectability of whole-body FDG-PET for osseous metastases is superior to the conventional bone scan is not clear for the other malignant tumors, and further investigation is required. Originally, ^{18}F-fluoride, a positron emitter, was used for bone imaging in the 1970s. Since there was no whole-body PET technology then, ^{18}F-fluoride was replaced by ^{99m}Tc-MDP because of the suitable gamma-ray energy for the scintillation camera. Whole-body PET using ^{18}F-fluoride is now and again mentioned as a useful method for monitoring osseous metastasis or metabolic bone disease [63].

Discrimination of Post-Treatment Changes from Residual or Recurrent Tumors

Approximately 15% of patients with a soft-tissue sarcoma of the extremities develop local recurrence [64]. It is often difficult to differentiate local recurrence of soft-tissue sarcoma from a scar, because the distorted anatomical structure and scar formation by previous surgical and radiation therapies hamper physical examination and morphological diagnosis by CT and MRI. Low metabolic activity and cellularity are characteristic of chronic scar tissue, whereas the recurrent malignant tumor tissues might have high cellularity and high metabolic activity. A dynamic MRI scanning after intravenous administration of contrast improved the capacity to differentiate between recurrent tumor and benign post-operative changes. If the contrast enhancement occurs within 1 min of injection, it suggests high probability of tumor recurrence. Considering the difference in pathological and biochemical conditions between chronic scar and recurrent malignant tumor, PET may be a more suitable diagnostic tool for this differentiation technique. The sensitivity of FDG-PET for the detection of recurrent sarcomas is high (Kole et al. [65] reported 93% sensitivity). Garcia et al. compared diagnostic accuracy of FDG-PET and ^{99m}Tc-sestamibi single-photon-emission computed tomography (MIBI SPECT) in musculoskeletal sarcomas [66]. In their study, the diagnostic sensitivity and specificity were 98% and 90% using FDG and 81.6% and 80% using MIBI, respectively. But in the early phase of post-operative treatment or post-irradiation, the treated region consists of reactive inflammatory cells and young granulation tissue in which FDG accumulates [67]. During this period, FDG-PET seems to show false-positive results for recurrent disease. We compared the diagnostic accuracy of FDG- and CMET-PET in a series of 34 lesions in 24 patients with suspected recurrent tumor, including nine soft-tissue tumors and three bone tumors. In this study, the sensitivity of FDG-PET and CMET-PET were 64.5%, and 61.3%, respectively. PET using FDG and CMET appears to be equally effective in detecting residual or recurrent malignant tumors, but FDG uptakes were slightly higher than CMET uptakes.

Therapeutic Monitoring

The radiotracer reflecting metabolic and proliferative activity of the tumor cells can potentially be used to monitor the response to therapy. PET using FDG and CMET is increasingly widely used.

Nieweg et al. reported FDG-PET results in a patient with liposarcoma of the thigh before and after therapeutic isolated regional limb perfusion with tumor necrosis factor alpha, interferon gamma and melphalan. After perfusion, initial FDG tumor uptake disappeared, which suggested the potential utility of FDG-PET for the evaluation of therapeutic isolated regional limb perfusion in patients with soft-tissue sarcomas [68]. After this report, van Ginkel et al. conducted better-designed clinical trials for evaluating the response to hyperthermic isolated limb perfusion for soft-tissue sarcomas by FDG-PET [69]. PET scans were repeated before, 2 weeks after and 8 weeks after therapy in 20 patients, including 7 pathologically complete remissions, 12 pathologically partial remissions and one patient not evaluated by pathological examination. Since the pretreatment glucose consumption in the group of patients with pathologically complete remission was significantly higher than that in the group of patients with pathologically partial remission, one could estimate the probability of a patient achieving complete remission. FDG-PET after treatment revealed the rim of the increased uptake around the core of absent tracer uptake in 12 patients. In the patients with pathologically complete remission, this rim signal corresponded to a fibrous pseudocapsule with inflammatory tissue, which implies that differentiation between an inflammatory response and the residual tumor tissue was impossible by FDG-PET [69]. Jones et al. also investigated the role of FDG-PET in the monitoring of neoadjuvant therapy (either chemotherapy or combined radiotherapy and hyperthermia) of soft-tissue and musculoskeletal sarcomas [70]. A peripheral rim of FDG uptake was also found to correlate pathologically with the formation of a fibrous pseudocapsule in patients who received combined radiotherapy and hyperthermia. However, FDG accumulation in the tumors which responded to chemotherapy showed more homogeneous reduction throughout the lesions. Garcia et al. showed that four of nine musculoskeletal sarcomas with FDG-positive and ^{99m}Tc-MIBI-negative results did not respond to multidrug therapy [66].

With regard to the monitoring of the gynecological malignancies after radiation therapy, differentiation between recurrent tumors and insufficiency fracture associated with radiation atrophy is important to save the patient from unnecessary treatment, mental anguish and expense. FDG-PET is expected to play some role in making this distinction [71].

In summary, in contrast to morphological diagnostic approaches such as ultrasound, CT, MRI and angiography, PET technology can reveal the biochemical or genetic abnormality in malignant cells, which may occur before the volume of malignant cells becomes large enough to be detected by imaging modalities. FDG-PET is useful in grading tumors, staging tumors and therapeutic monitoring of patients with soft-tissue and bone sarcomas, but with some limitations. Regarding the soft-tissue and bone sarcomas, the clinical application of amino-acid agents, such as ^{11}C-methionine amino acid, still has not been investigated sufficiently for a conclusive report. PET oncology has unlimited potential based on newly developed radiopharmaceuticals such as ^{11}C-choline [72], ^{18}F-labeled fluoroerythronitroimidazole [73], ^{18}F-labeled monoclonal antibody [74] and ^{18}F-labeled alpha-methyl tyrosine [75].

References

1. Landis SH, Murray T, Bolden S, Wingo PA (1998) Cancer statistics, 1998. CA Cancer J Clin 48:6-29
2. Leyvraz S, Costa J (1988) Histological diagnosis and grading of soft-tissue sarcomas. Semin Surg Oncol 4:3-6
3. Sallourn E, Slamant F, Cailland JM (1990) Diagnostic and therapeutic problems of soft tissue tumours other than rhabdomyosarcomas in infants under 1 year of age: a clinicopathological study of 34 cases treated at the Institut Gustave-Roussy. Med Pediatr Oncol 18:37-43
4. Kawai A, Nogushi M, Beppu Y (1994) Nuclear immunoreaction of p53 protein in soft tissue sarcomas. Proc Natl Acad Sci U S A 87:5863-5867
5. Parham DM, Shapiro DN, Downing JR (1994) Solid alveolar rhabdomyosarcomas with the t(2;13): report of two cases with diagnostic implications. Am J Surg Pathol 18:474-478
6. Angervall L, Kindblom LG (1993) Principles for pathologic-anatomic diagnosis and classification of soft tissue sarcomas. Clin Orthop 289:9-18
7. Togushida J, Ishizaki K, Sasaki MS (1989) Preferential mutation of paternally derived RB gene as the initial event in sporadic osteosarcoma. Nature 338:156-158
8. Wadayama B, Togushida J, Shimizu T (1994) Mutation spectrum of the retinoblastoma gene in osteosarcomas. Cancer Res 54:3042-3048
9. Ambros JM, Ambros PF, Strehl S (1991) MIC2 is a specific marker for Ewing's sarcoma and peripheral primitive neuroectodermal tumors. Cancer 67:1886-1893
10. Tur Cavel C, Aurias A, Mugneret F (1988) Chromosomes in Ewing's sarcoma: an evaluation of 85 cases and remarkable consistency of t(11;22)(q24;q12). Cancer Genet Cytogenet 321:229-238
11. Maurer HM, Beltangady M, Gehan EA (1988) The Intergroup Rhabdomyosarcoma Study I. A final report. Cancer 61:209-220
12. Wilner D (1992) Osteogenic sarcoma (osteosarcoma). In: Wilner D (ed) Radiology of bone tumors and allied disorders. Saunders, Philadelphia, pp 1897-2005
13. Fraumeni JF Jr, Boice JD Jr (1982) Bone. In: Schottenfeld D, Fraumeni JF Jr (eds) Cancer epidemiology and prevention. Saunders, Philadelphia, pp 814-826
14. Huros AG, Woodard HQ, Cahan WG (1982) Postradiation osteogenic sarcoma of bone and soft tissues: a clinicopathologic study of 66 patients. Cancer 55:1244-1255
15. Garrison RC, Unni KK, Mcleod RA (1982) Chondrosarcoma arising in osteochondroma. Cancer 49:1890-1897
16. Cavazzana AD, Magnani J, Ross RA (1988) Ewing's sarcoma is an undifferentiated neuroectodermal tumor. In: Evans AC, D'Angio GJ, Knudson AG et al. (eds) Advances in neuroblastoma research II. Liss, New York, pp 487-498
17. Razek A, Perez CA, Tefft M (1980) Intergroup Ewing's sarcoma study: local control related to radiation dose, volume, and site of primary lesion in Ewing's sarcoma. Cancer 46:516-521
18. Ruka W, Enwich LJ, Driscoll DL (1988) Prognostic significance of lymph node metastasis and bone, major vessel, or nerve involvement in adults with high-grade soft tissue sarcomas. Cancer 62:999-1006
19. Pritchard DJ, Reiman HM, Turcotte RE (1993) Malignant fibrous histiocytomas of the soft tissues of the trunk and extremities. Clin Orthop 289:58-65
20. Springfield D (1993) Liposarcoma. Clin Orthop 289:50-57
21. Holden C, Spittle M, Jones E (1987) Angiosarcoma of face and scalp: prognosis and treatment. Cancer 59:1046-1057
22. Costa J, Wesley RA, Glatstein EJ (1984) The grading of soft tissue sarcomas: results of a clinicopathologic correlation in a series of 163 cases. Cancer 53:530-541
23. Kulander BG, Polissar L, Yang CY (1989) Grading of soft tissue sarcomas: necrosis as a determinant of survival. Mod Pathol 2:205-208
24. Enneking WF, Spanier SS, Goodman MA (1980) A system for the surgical staging of musculoskeletal sarcoma. Clin Orthop 153:106-120
25. Ahuja SC, Villacin AB, Smith J (1977) Juxtacortical (parosteal) osteogenic sarcoma. J Bone Joint Surg Am 50:632-647
26. Sanerkin NG (1980) The diagnosis and grading of chondrosarcoma of the bone: a combined cytologic and histologic approach. Cancer 45:582-594
27. Marcove RC (1977) Chondrosarcoma: diagnosis and treatment. Orthop Clin North Am 8:811-819
28. Hadju SI (1987) Benign soft tissue tumors: classification and natural history. CA Cancer J Clin 37:66-70
29. Kubola M, Nagasaki A, Ohgani H (1991) An infantile case of infiltrative lipoma in the buttock. J Pediatr Surg 26:230-233
30. Crim JR, Seeger LL, Yao L (1992) Diagnosis of soft tissue masses with MR imaging: can benign masses be differentiated from malignant ones? Radiology 185:581-586
31. Nelson MC, Stull MA, Teitelbaum GP (1990) Magnetic resonance imaging of peripheral soft tissue hemangiomas. Skeletal Radiol 19:477-482
32. Buetow PC, Kransdorf MJ, Moser RP (1990) Radiologic appearance of intramuscular hemangioma with emphasis on MRI. AJR Am J Roentgenol 154:563-568
33. Quinn SF, Erickson SJ, Dee PM (1991) MR imaging in fibromatosis: results in 26 patients with pathologic correlation. AJR Am J Roentgenol 156:539-544
34. Sundaram M, Chalk D, Merenda J (1989) Pigmented villonodular synovitis (PVNS) of the knee. Skeletal Radiol 18:463-466
35. Binkovitz LA, Berquist T, McLeod RA (1990) Masses of the hand and wrist: detection and characterization with MRI. AJR Am J Roentgenol 154:323-327
36. Peterson KK, Renfrew DL, Feddersen RM (1991) Magnetic resonance imaging of myxoid containing tumors. Skeletal Radiol 20:245-249
37. Varma GK, Moulopoulos A, Sara AS (1992) MR imaging of extracranial nerve sheath tumors. J Comput Assist Tomogr 16:448-453
38. Baran GA, Sundarem M (1991) Accessory soleus muscle. Orthopedics 14:499-502
39. Kneeland JB, Middleton WD, Matloub HS (1987) High-resolution MR imaging of glomus tumors. J Comput Assist Tomogr 11:351-356
40. Hanna SL, Fletcher BD, Parham DM (1991) Muscle edema in musculoskeletal tumors: MR imaging characteristics and clinical significance. J Magn Reson Imaging 1:441-446
41. Fletcher BD, Hanna SL, Fairclough DL (1992) Pediatric musculoskeletal tumors: use of dynamic contrast-enhanced MR imaging to monitor response to chemotherapy. Radiology 184:243-248
42. Bachert P, Bellemann ME, Layer G (1992) In vivo ^{1}H, ^{31}P and ^{13}C magnetic resonance spectroscopy of malig-

nant histiocytoma and skeletal muscle tissue in man. NMR Biomed 5:161–166
43. Negendank W (1992) Studies of human tumors by MRS: a review. NMR Biomed 5:503–508
44. Negendank WG, Crowley MG, Ryan JR (1989) Bone and soft-tissue lesions: diagnosis with combined H-1 MR imaging and P-31 MR spectroscopy. Radiology 173:181–186
45. Ross B, Helsper JT, Cox IJ (1987) Osteosarcoma and other neoplasms of bone: magnetic resonance spectroscopy to monitor therapy. Arch Surg 122:1464–1469
46. Shinkwin MA, Lenkinski RE, Daly JM (1991) Integrated magnetic resonance imaging and phosphorus spectroscopy of soft tissue tumors. Cancer 67:1849–1854
47. Patel SR, Benjamin RS (1994) The role of chemotherapy in soft tissue sarcomas. Cancer Control 194:599–605
48. Koutcher JA, Ballon D, Graham M (1990) ^{31}P NMR spectra of extremity sarcomas: diversity of metabolic profiles and changes in response to chemotherapy. Magn Reson Med 16:19–24
49. Sostman HD, Prescott DM, Dewhirst MW (1994) MR imaging and spectroscopy for prognostic evaluation in soft tissue sarcomas. Radiology 190:269–274
50. Prescott DM, Charles HC, Sostman HD (1993) Therapy monitoring in human and canine soft tissue sarcomas using magnetic resonance imaging and spectroscopy. Int J Radiat Oncol Biol Phys 28:415–421
51. Adler LP, Blair HF, Makley JT, Pathria MN, Miraldi F (1991) Comparison of PET with CT, MRI, and conventional scintigraphy in a benign and in a malignant soft tissue tumor. Orthopedics 14:891–895
52. Hicks RJ (1997) Nuclear medicine techniques provide unique physiologic characterization of suspected and known soft tissue and bone sarcomas. Acta Orthop Scand Suppl 273:25–36
53. Fujimoto T, Itoh M, Kumano H, Tashiro M, Ido T (1996) Whole-body metabolic map with positron emission tomography of a man after running. Lancet 348:266
54. Balm AJM, Coevorden FV, Bos KE et al. (1995) Report of a symposium on diagnosis and treatment of adult soft tissue sarcomas in the head and neck. Eur J Surg Oncol 21:287–289
55. Kubota K, Yamada S, Ishiwata K, Ito M, Fujiwara T, Fukuda H, Tada M, Ido T (1993) Evaluation of the treatment response of lung cancer with positron emission tomography and L-[methyl-^{11}C]methionine: a preliminary study. Eur J Nucl Med 20:495–501
56. Koh WJ, Rasey JS, Evans ML, Grierson JR, Lewellen TK, Graham MM, Krohn KA, Griffin TW (1992) Imaging tumor hypoxia in human tumors with [F-18]fluoromisonidazole. Int J Radiat Oncol Biol Phys 22:199–212
57. di Chiro G (1986) Positron emission tomography using [18F]fluorodeoxyglucose in brain tumors: a powerful diagnostic and prognostic tool. Invest Radiol 22:720–728
58. Kern KA, Brunetti A, Norton JA, Chang AE, Malawer M, Lack E, Finn RD, Rosenberg SA, Larson SM (1988) Metabolic imaging of human extremity musculoskeletal tumors by PET. J Nucl Med 29:181–186
59. Adler LP, Blair HF, Makley JT, Williams RP, Joyce MJ, Leisure G, al-Kaisi N, Miraldi F (1991) Noninvasive grading of musculoskeletal tumors using PET. J Nucl Med 32:1508–1512
60. Griffeth LK, Dehdashti F, McGuire AH, McGuire DJ, Perry DJ, Moerlein SM, Siegel BA (1992) PET evaluation of soft-tissue masses with fluorine-18 fluoro-2-deoxy-D-glucose. Radiology 182:185–194
61. Hoh CK, Hawkins RA, Glaspy JA, Dahlbom M, Tse NY, Hoffman EJ, Schiepers C, Choi Y, Rege S, Nitzsche E, et al. (1993) Cancer detection with whole-body PET using 2-[^{18}F]fluoro-2-deoxy-D-glucose. J Comput Assist Tomogr 17:582–589
62. Shreve PD, Grossman HB, Gross MD, Wahl RL (1996) Metastatic prostate cancer: initial findings of PET with 2-deoxy-2-[F-18]fluoro-D-glucose. Radiology 199:751–756
63. Inoue T, Endo K, Hirano T, et al. (1993) Imaging of bone metabolism with fluorine-18-fluoride ion using a high resolution animal PET. Bioimages 1:27–30
64. Hoekstra HJ, Schraffordt KH, Oldhoff J (1994) Soft tissue sarcoma of the extremity. Eur J Surg Oncol 20:3–6
65. Kole AC, Nieweg OE, van Ginkel RJ, Pruim J, Hoekstra HJ, Paans AM, Vaalburg W, Koops HS (1997) Detection of local recurrence of soft-tissue sarcoma with positron emission tomography using [18F]fluorodeoxyglucose. Ann Surg Oncol 4:57–63
66. Garcia JR, Kim EE, Wong FCL, Korkmaz M, Wong WH, Yang DJ, Podoloff DA (1996) Comparison of fluorine-18-FDG PET and technetium-99m-MIBI SPECT in evaluation of musculoskeletal sarcomas. J Nucl Med 37:1476–1479
67. Kubota R, Yamada S, Kubota K, Ishiwata K, Tamahashi N, Ido T (1992) Intratumoral distribution of fluorine-18-fluorodeoxyglucose in vivo: high accumulation in macrophages and granulation tissues studied by microautoradiography. J Nucl Med 33:1972–1980
68. Nieweg OE, Pruim J, Hoekstra HJ, Paans AM, Vaalburg W, Oldhoff J, Schraffordt Koops H (1994) Positron emission tomography with fluorine-18-fluorodeoxyglucose for the evaluation of therapeutic isolated regional limb perfusion in a patient with soft-tissue sarcoma. J Nucl Med 35:90–92
69. van Ginkel RJ, Hoekstra HJ, Pruim J, Nieweg OE, Molenaar WM, Paans AM, Willemsen AT, Vaalburg W, Koops HS (1996) FDG-PET to evaluate response to hyperthermic isolated limb perfusion for locally advanced soft-tissue sarcoma. J Nucl Med 37:984–990
70. Jones DN, McCowage GB, Sostman HD, Brizel DM, Layfield L, Charles HC, Dewhirst MW, Prescott DM, Friedman HS, Harrelson JM, Scully SP, Coleman RE (1996) Monitoring of neoadjuvant therapy response of soft-tissue and musculoskeletal sarcoma using fluorine-18-FDG PET. J Nucl Med 37:1438–1444
71. Mumber MP, Greven KM, Haygood TM (1997) Pelvic insufficiency fractures associated with radiation atrophy: clinical recognition and diagnostic evaluation. Skeletal Radiol 26:94–99
72. Hara T, Kosaka N, Shinoura N, Kondo T (1997) PET imaging of brain tumor with [methyl-^{11}C]choline. J Nucl Med 38:842–847
73. Yang DJ, Wallace S, Cherif A, Li C, Gretzer MB, Kim EE, Podoloff DA (1995) Development of F-18-labeled fluoroerythronitroimidazole as a PET Agent for imaging tumor hypoxia. Radiology 194:795–800
74. Page RL, Garg PK, Garg S, Archer GE, Bruland OS, Zalutsky MR (1994) PET imaging of osteosarcoma in dogs using a fluorine-18-labeled monoclonal antibody Fab fragment. J Nucl Med 35:1506–1513
75. Tomiyoshi K, Amed K, Muhammad S, Higuchi T, Inoue T, Endo K, Yang D (1997) Synthesis of isomers of ^{18}F-labelled amino acid radiopharmaceutical: positron 2- and 3-L^{18}F-alpha-methyltyrosine using a separation and purification system. Nucl Med Commun 18:169–175

Melanoma, Lymphoma and Myeloma

E. E. Kim

Basic Considerations

Melanoma

Cutaneous malignant melanoma is a common tumor. In the United States, in 1998, an estimated 41,600 new cases will be diagnosed, and 7,300 patients will die of it [1]. Early melanoma is highly curable, but it is nearly always fatal when the cancer becomes disseminated. The overall survival rate has more than doubled in the last three decades, probably due to earlier diagnosis [2]. It is speculated that increased exposure to the sun, especially early in life, has contributed to the rising incidence of melanoma [3].

Some melanomas arise in precursor-pigmented lesions, such as congenital melanocytic nevi and dysplastic nevi or atypical moles [4]. There are several syndromes of Mendelian inheritance of a predisposition to melanoma. These include familial atypical multiple mole melanoma (FAMMM) syndrome, xeroderma pigmentosum, and congenital nevocytic nevus syndrome [5]. Patients shared an abnormal genetic locus at the 9p13–p22 chromosomal region. The locus has also been mapped to the 9p21 area, cloned and given the name multiple tumor-supressor 1 (MTS1) gene, which appears to be the same locus as tumor-suppressor gene, p16 [6]. Melanocytes in the basal layer of the epidermis synthesize the melanin, which is a protective factor against the damaging effects of B-range ultraviolet light. Melanocyte-stimulating hormone supports the growth of melanocytes, while melatonin suppresses melanocyte function. Malignant melanocytes produce growth factors to stimulate melanoma growth [7]. It has been demonstrated that normal melanocytes require four mitogens which grow the following: insulin or insulin-like growth factor, fibroblast growth factor-alpha, melanocyte-stimulating hormone, and phorbol esters [8]. Albelda et al. [9] showed expression of the beta-3-integrin subunit by metastatic melanomas, but not by benign melanocytes. It has been suggested that urokinase and tissue-type plasminogen activators also play a role in malignant melanoma invasion [10]. Histopathologic examination of melanoma often reveals an active mononuclear inflammatory infiltrate and fibrosis. When these cells are invading within the melanoma mass, they are called tumor-infiltrating lymphocytes (TIL), and the infiltrating phenomenon is called pathologic regression. The presence of TIL may be a favorable prognostic factor in melanoma [11]. The role of cytotoxic T lymphocytes and natural killer (NK) cells in preventing the establishment of metastatic disease has been well defined in animal models [12]. NK cells seem to be present in metastatic melanoma more frequently than in primary lesions. The ability of NK cells to kill melanoma is enhanced when downregulation of class-I antigens is induced by c-myc overexpression in melanoma cell lines [13].

Lymphomas

Although there have been many advances in the treatment of Hodgkin's disease (HD), its diagnosis still rests on the identification of the Reed-Sternberg cell, which accounts for only 1% of the cells present, with the remainder consisting of lymphocytes, granulocytes, histiocytes, plasma cells, and fibroblasts [14]. HD is uncommon, and 7500 new cases will occur in the United States during 1998 [1]. It occurs more frequently in developed than in underdeveloped countries and, for unknown reasons, in underdeveloped countries the first peak occurs at an earlier age. The nodular sclerosing subtype has a female predominance, with the remaining subtypes occurring more commonly in males. Carbone et al. [15] found that CD-40 antigen is strongly represented on the surface of Reed-Sternberg cells and can help in the differentiation between nodular sclerosing HD and other lymphoid malignancies. Epstein-Barr virus (EBV) has been implicated as a causative agent, and immunodeficiency induced by the human immunodeficiency virus type 1 has also been associated with the mixed-cellular subtype of HD [16].

The indolent non-Hodgkin's lymphomas (NHLs) are usually associated with relatively prolonged survival, and they are almost exclusively of B-cell origin and mostly low-grade. Lymphocytes arise in the bone marrow from a hematopoietic stem cell, and early B-cells undergo differentiation in the bone marrow, while early phases of T-cell differentiation occur in the thymus. The earliest sign of B-lineage commitment is the rearrangement of the immunoglobulin (Ig) heavy-chain locus on chromosome 14p32. A failed rearrangement is the case with the t(14,18) translocation. The production of the μ chain in the cytoplasm is the hallmark of the pre-B-cell. Once the heavy-chain locus rearranges, kappa light-chain gene rearrangement follows on chromosome 22(p11). A complete Ig molecule will be produced and expressed on the cell surface after binding to the μ heavy chain; the hallmark of a mature B-cell is the expression of surface immunoglobulin (sIg). Most mature B-cells will undergo apoptosis and dual signaling via sIg receptors, and CD 40 rescues B-cells from apoptosis [17].

Follicular lymphoma cells carry the characteristics of mature B-cells and express CD19, CD20, CD22, and sIg (mostly IgM/IgD). T-cells commonly seen in infiltrating follicular lymphomas may contribute to B-cell proliferation, but T-cell infiltration is also associated with spontaneous regression. About 85% of all follicular lymphomas are shown to have t(14;18)(q32;q21) translocation, juxtaposing the *bcl-2* gene from 18q21.3 with the Ig heavy-chain locus on 14q32.2 [18].

A wide variety of lymphomas of both B- and T-cell origin, as well as normal mantle zone lymphocytes overexpress the Bcl-2 protein, while follicular hyperplasia and normal germinal centers do not [19]. The overexpression of Bcl-2 plays a critical role in blocking apoptosis [20]. Most investigators found no clear difference in long-term survival among the different subtypes of low-grade lymphoma [21]. Tumor burden, host factors, and response to initial therapy has been clinically shown to correlate with survival in follicular lymphoma. Adverse host factors include advanced age, male gender, low hemoglobin level, and poor performance with B symptoms [22].

The overall 10-year survival rate was about 75% for the low-risk group and 0% for the high risk group. More than 80% of complete responders were alive at 7 years compared with a median survival of 2 years among those failing to achieve a complete response to initial therapy [21]. Laboratory criteria correlating with poor prognosis include: elevation of serum lactate dehydrogenase (LDH) and β-2-microglobulin levels, as well as increased expression of the nuclear proliferation antigen Ki-67, and the increased percentage of cells in S-phase [23]. Breaks in the short or long arm of chromosome 17 were shown to be a predictor of poor outcome [24]. Several studies reported a higher incidence of clonal excess (CE) by sIg staining with fluorescent monoclonal antibody (mAb) against human kappa or lambda chains in patients with low-grade lymphoma [25]. Intermediate- and high-grade tumors comprise nearly 55% of NHLs, with a proportionately higher number of high-grade tumors in children and young adults [26]. Hereditary factors, childhood lymphomas, and high-grade tumors are closely associated. Three factors appear common to the etiology of lymphomas: host defects including autoimmune diseases, specific infections such as HIV and EBV, and specific mutations or chromosome translocations.

Myeloma

Multiple myeloma is a malignant proliferation of plasma cells which produces a monoclonal globulin, and results from a mutation of terminally differentiated B-cells or even from early but committed B-cells [27]. In 1998, approximately 12500 new patients will be diagnosed in the United States [1]. The median age of patients is approximately 70 years, and the incidence increases with age. The doubled frequency among African Americans, with a 10.2 to 6.7 male-to-female ratio is due to unknown genetic factors. The *ras* mutation correlates with a low treatment-response rate, and the *p53* gene mutation has been noted in patients with extramedullary proliferation of plasma cells [28]. Interleukin-6 (IL-6), considered the most important myeloma growth factor, binds to the IL-6 receptor or plasma cells [29]. The increased expression of *p*-glycoprotein, the multidrug resistance (MDR) gene product, has been recently noted after ingestion of high cumulative doses of vincristine and doxorubicin [30]. The level of serum β-2-microglobulin, a catabolic product of the histocompatibility leukocyte antigen on lymphoid and plasma cells, was the single most important prognostic indicator [31]. Shortened survival with poor response to chemotherapy has been noted in patients with high serum LDH level, DNA hypodiploidy, low plasma-cell RNA level, high plasma-cell labeling index, plasmablastic histology, and the expression of common acute lymphoblastic leukemia antigen (CALLA) [32].

Pathology, Diagnosis and Staging

Malignant *melanoma* has four major subtypes with unique clinical features: superficial spreading, nodular, lentigo and acral lentiginous. Superficial spreading melanoma constitutes 70% of melanomas, generally arising in a pre-existing nevus. It is a flat lesion with mixtures of deeply pigmented areas and amelanotic foci. The second most common (15–30%) subtype is nodular melanoma, which is typically blue-black and raised or dome shaped. It generally begins in uninvolved skin on the trunk and head and neck areas; it is more aggressive and develops more rapidly than superficial melanoma. Lentigo malignant melanoma constitutes 4–10% of melanomas and is typically located on the faces of older white women. It is generally large, tan, flat and always associated with sun-related changes in the dermis and epidermis. The fourth subtype is acral lentiginous melanoma, which occurs on the palms of the hands, soles of the feet or beneath the nail beds; it represents only 2–8% of melanomas in whites, but accounts for 35–60% in dark-skinned patients, and is primarily seen with ulceration in older patients.

Three less-common types of melanomas are desmoplastic, uveal, and mucosal. The desmoplastic type involves the epidermis and is frequently amelanotic. It has a tendency to track along the peripheral nerve sheath with early dissemination [33]. Uveal (ocular) melanoma is rare and has a propensity to metastasize to the liver [34]. Mucosal melanoma can arise in the mouth, anus, genital tract, upper respiratory or gastrointestinal tract. It tends to present as advanced local disease. Malignant melanoma should be suspected in any pigmented skin or mucosal lesion that changes in color or size, begins to itch, or bleeds spontaneously. An elliptical excisional biopsy with a 2-mm margin of normal-appearing tissue is usually indicated for diagnostic purposes. Tumor thickness is the most important prognostic factor. In Breslow's microstaging system, the thickness of the lesion is measured with an ocular micrometer to determine the maximal vertical thickness of the melanoma [35]. Less accurate Clark's levels of microinvasion reflect increasing depth of tumor penetration into the dermis layers and the subcutaneous fat. Clark's level I indicates in situ; level II, invasion of the papillary dermis; level III, invasion of the papillary-reticular dermal interface; level IV, invasions of reticular dermis; and level V, invasion of the subcutaneous tissue [36]. Table 17.1 compares the American Joint Committee on Cancer (AJCC) and World Health Organization (WHO) staging systems for malignant melanoma [37].

When the survival rates were adjusted for tumor thickness, there was no difference in the 10-year-survival rates between superficial and nodular melanomas [38].

The Rye modification divides *HD* into four histologic types: lymphocyte-predominant, nodular sclerosis, mixed cellularity, and lymphocyte depletion. Two variants (nodular and diffuse) of lymphocyte-predominant type have been identified. Nodular lymphocyte-predominant subtype is now widely regarded as a B-cell lymphoma [39], and the nodular sclerosis type may be difficult to distinguish from large-cell lymphoma. MacLennan et al. [40] have divided nodular sclerosing types into grade-I and grade-II histology. Mixed cellularity types have rare Reed-Sternberg cells and may be confused with peripheral T-cell lymphoma. The lymphocyte-depleted type is rare, partly because many reported cases were mistaken for large cell lymphoma.

The initial evaluation of patients with HD has both prognostic and therapeutic significance. Bilateral bone marrow biopsy should be routinely performed, and lymphangiography remains a valuable procedure. Modal status can easily be serially evaluated on X-ray films to assess a therapeutic response. Staging by laparotomy remains a

Table 17.1. Staging for melanoma

AJCC		WHO	
IA	<0.75 mm	I	Skin
IB	0.76–1.5 mm		
IIA	1.6–4.0 mm	II	Regional nodes
IIB	>4.0 mm		
III	Regional nodes or intransit metastasis	III	Distant metastasis
IV	Distant metastasis		

Table 17.2. Ann Arbor staging for Hodgkin's disease

Stage I	Single lymph-node region (I) or single extralymphatic organ or site (I_E)
Stage II	Two or more lymph-node regions on the same side of diaphragm (II) or local involvement of extralymphatic organ or site (II_E)
Stage III	Lymph-node regions on both sides of diaphragm (III) or local involvement of extralymphatic organ or site (III_E), spleen (III_S), or both (III_{SE})
Stage IV	Diffuse, one or more extralymphatic organs with or without lymph node involvement; (P) pulmonary; (O) osseous; (H) hepatic. (A) indicates asymptomatic patient; (B) indicates fever, night sweats or weight loss >10% of body weight

controversial subject. Glatstein et al. [41] found that the presence of "B" symptoms (unexplained fever above 38 °C, night sweats and weight loss exceeding 10% of body weight) was predictive of abdominal disease. Gallium scans may be used to detect therapeutic response. In untreated HD, the sensitivity of gallium scan was 64%, with a specificity of 95% [42].

The Ann Arbor staging system (Table 17.2) has been used for HD; its modifications were developed at the Cotswalds Conference in 1989. Masses larger than 10 cm or greater than one-third the chest-wall diameter have a stage designated with the suffix "X", and greater than 90% partial response with stable adenopathy is designated as "CRU" (complete response uncertain). Stage III$_1$ has splenic involvement or involves splenic hilar, celiac or portal nodes, while stage III$_2$ involves the para-aortic, iliac, or mesenteric nodes identified by computed tomography (CT).

B symptoms occur in no more than 15% of patients with indolent lymphomas. Splenomegaly may be the only sign in patients with primary splenic lymphoma. The occurrence of direct-pressure symptoms by mediastinal-lymph-node involvement is extremely unlikely, and symptoms of gastrointestinal-tract involvement are nonspecific. Excisional lymph-node biopsy is crucial to establish the diagnosis. Fine-needle aspiration (FNA) is inadequate since it does not preserve the nodal architecture. Bilateral bone-marrow biopsies are necessary for accurate staging. Laboratory data may show anemia or thrombocytopenia. Platelet-associated antibodies may be positive in immune thrombocytopenia. The serum LDH and β-23-microglobulin levels may be elevated. Imaging studies should include a chest X-ray, and chest CT if the X-ray shows a suspicious lesion. Abdominal and pelvic CT scans are essential with high sensitivity in detecting mesenteric lymphadenopathy. A baseline gallium scan is not usually indicated for the diagnosis, but is obtained for the evaluation of therapeutic response.

The Ann Arbor staging system has drawbacks when applied to NHLs, which often spread discontiguously. Most patients with indolent NHL have advanced (stage III or IV) disease at presentation, and even those with limited disease will have tumor cells detected in marrow and peripheral blood. The National Cancer Institute (NCI)

Table 17.3. Working formulation for non-Hodgkin's lymphomas

Classifiable non-Hodgkin's lymphoma (NHL)	Unaccounted-for NHL
Low grade	
Small lymphocytic chronic lymphocytic leukemia (CLL)	Mucosa-associated lymphomas CD5-, CD10-
Follicular; small-cleaved cell	
Follicular, mixed small and large cell	
Intermediate grade	
Follicular, large cell	
Diffuse mixed small and large cell	Mantle-cell lymphoma. CD5+, CD23-, t11;14 PRAD 1
Diffuse mixed small and large cell	Lennert's lymphoma. T-cell+
Diffuse large cleaved and noncleaved cell	T-cell variants: t14;18+. Transformed from low grade NHL
High-grade	
Large cell, immunoblastic, plasmacytoid, clear cell	Anaplastic large cell lymphoma, T-cell; Ki-1 (CD 30)+, t2;5
Small noncleaved cell Burkitt's; Follicular areas	
Miscellaneous	Other T-cell NHL
Composite	Human T-lymphotropic virus-1 lymphoma, T-cell CLL
Mycosis fungoides	Angioimmunoblastic lymphadenopathy
Histiocytic	Lymphomatoid granulomatosis
Unclassifiable	

Table 17.4. Staging for multiple myeloma

Stage I	Hemoglobin (Hb) >10 g/dl, Ca 12 mg/dl. Normal bone or plasmacytoma on X-ray. Low M-component product rates. Immunoglobin G (IgG) <5 g/dl, IgA<3 g/dl Urine light-chain M-component <4 g/24 h	<0.6×10^{12} (low) myeloma cell/m^2
Stage II	Not fitting Stage I or III	0.6–1.2×10^{12} (med) myeloma cells/m^2
Stage III	Hb <8.5 g/dl, Ca >12 mg/dl. Multiple lytic bone lesions on X-ray. High M-component product rates IgG<7 g/dl, IgA >5 g/dl Urine light chain M-component >12 g/24 h	>1.2×10^{12} (high) myeloma cells/m^2

initiated the NHL pathologic classification project through a Working Formulation (Table 17.3).

A diagnosis of NHL should be made based on the pathologic examinations of a lymph node. Lymphomas were diagnosed using FNA in 86% of cases and were accurately categorized into low, intermediate, or high grade in 68% of the cases [43]. In some instances, it may be necessary to establish clonality to confirm malignancy. In B-cell NHL, monotype immunohistochemical staining for kappa or lambda light chain is often all that is needed to confirm clonality. Gene-rearrangement studies are diagnostic and reliable in more than 96% of NHL cases [44]. For some time NHL was staged anatomically; however, NHL cannot be reliably staged solely by anatomic methods.

The clinical presentation of *multiple myeloma* is quite variable. Bone pain, especially from compression fractures of vertebrae or ribs, is the most common symptom. Bone lesions are due to accelerated osteoclast formation, and IL-1-β induces and is synergistic with the bone-resorbing activity of IL-6 [45]. Nearly 70% of patients with myeloma have lytic bone lesions, and MRI provides greater detail of bone disease, paraspinal involvement, and epidural components [46]. Hypercalcemia (serum Ca level >11.5 mg/dl) occurs in approximately 20% of myeloma patients. Approximately 20% of patients also present with renal insufficiency. A normocytic, normochromic anemia is present in 60% of patients at the time of diagnosis. Many patients with myeloma develop bacterial infections, probably related to impaired host defense mechanisms. A diagnosis of multiple myeloma requires the presence of bone-marrow plasmacytosis and monoclonal protein. Biclonal elevations of myeloma protein levels occur in less than 1% of cases. The types of monoclonal protein are IgG (60%), IgA (20%), IgD (2%), IgE (<0.1%), and light-chain kappa or lambda (18%) [47]. Different criteria have been used to stage myeloma at different institutions (Table 17.4).

Magnetic Resonance Imaging

Melanomas are usually a mixture of high- and low-signal-intensity lesions on T_1- and T_2-weighted images due to hemorrhage or a paramagnetic property of melanin, which is present at various concentrations (Fig. 17.1) [48]. Intense thick ring enhancement is usually seen in the immediate postgadolinium-injection T_1-weighted images, reflecting hypervascularity. The lung, liver, brain and lymph nodes are the most common sites of metastasis. Essentially every visceral or-

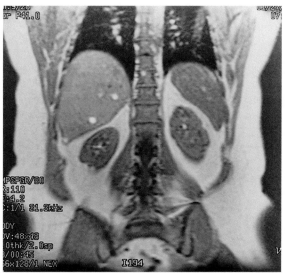
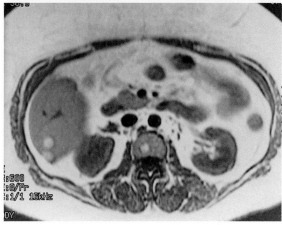

Fig. 17.1 Coronal (*upper*) and axial (*lower*) T_1-weighted images of the abdomen show multiple small nodular metastatic melanoma lesions in the liver with high signal intensity

gan, including heart, adrenals, spleen, pancreas, gastrointestinal tract, bone, thyroid, bone marrow, pleura, diaphragm, ovaries, prostate and genitourinary tract, may be involved.

Magnetic resonance imaging (MRI) has been shown to be as accurate as CT in the assessment of mediastinal and hilar lymphadenopathy. Lymphoma invasion of chest wall, cardiac and paracardiac structures are better evaluated with MRI than with CT [49]. An important problem in the management of lymphoma is the presence of incomplete tumor regression after adequate therapy. This problem can occur in up to 88% of patients with HD and up to 40% of patients with NHL [50]. A partially regressed mass represents residual fibrotic tissue with no viable tumor and has been defined as sterilized lymphoma [51]. CT cannot distinguish active tumor from sterilized

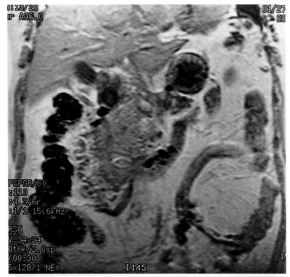

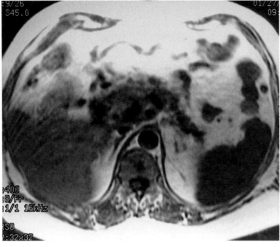

Fig. 17.2. T_1-weighted coronal (*upper*) and axial (*lower*) images of the abdomen show an ill-defined lymphoma mass in the pancreatic head with intermediate signal intensity

mass because of identical densities, representing a serious clinical dilemma. Because MRI signal intensity is related to the proportion of water and proteins, it is conceivable that MRI signal intensity may vary between fibrotic residual masses and active tumor. Lymphomatous masses contain a larger amount of free water, whereas inactive masses of sterilized lymphoma are composed of stable fibrosis containing less water [51]. It has been observed that islands of high signal intensity on T_2-weighted images may reappear in the residual mass, preceding clinical symptoms of relapse by 8–12 weeks [52].

There are four signal patterns characteristic of lymphomas that have been observed in various organs [52]. The homogeneous active pattern, consisting of a homogeneous low signal intensity on T_1-weighted images and a homogeneous high signal intensity on T_2-weighted images, is usually found in untreated lymphoma (Fig. 17.2). The heterogeneous active pattern, consisting of low signal intensity on T_1-weighted images and a mixture of low and high signal intensity on T_2-weighted images, can be seen in untreated sclerosing HD and also during the response phase of lymphomas after therapy (Fig. 17.3). In the early post-therapeutic phase, high signal intensity on T_2-weighted images suggesting active disease may be caused by inflammation, necrosis, or early developing fibrosis [53]. Radiation pneumonitis producing impaired bronchial mucociliary function can also result in a high signal intensity on T_2-weighted images. The heterogeneous inactive pattern, consisting of mixed low and high signal intensity on T_1- and T_2-weighted images, is seen in mediastinal lymphomas regressing with distortion or the reappearance of surrounding fat. The residual tumor shows low signal intensity. The homogeneous hypointense pattern is characteristic of inactive residual fibrotic masses after successful therapy of lymphoma. A favorable therapeutic response is characterized by a decrease in tumor size and a homogeneous decrease in signal intensity. A decrease in size with a persistent active heterogeneous hyperintense pattern suggests a partial response. Persistent high signal in a regressing tumor may indicate active disease, cystic degeneration, or necrosis. MRI of bone lymphoma is indistinguishable from metastatic carcinoma. Focal areas of low signal intensity on T_1-weighted images and high signal intensity on T_2-weighted images will be noted. Lymphoma is almost always a focal, rather than diffuse, bone marrow process (Fig. 17.4) [54].

MRI may be the most valuable imaging technique for establishing the presence and precise location of malignant marrow proliferative disorders or guiding a biopsy, because the disease may be focal or diffuse, and blind marrow aspirates in the pelvis may not accurately reflect the nature of the lesion. Multiple myeloma has a variable MRI appearance, but the distribution usually involves the axial skeleton or proximal humeri or femora, where rich vascular red marrow exists. Plasma cell infiltration may be diffuse, focal, or inhomogeneous with a nonuniform variegated appearance. Myeloma almost always has signal intensity equal to or lower than skeletal muscle or disk on T_1-weighted images (Fig. 17.5). High signal intensity on T_2-weighted images is seen in 50% of untreated myeloma patients (Fig. 17.6) [55]. Low signal intensity on T_1- and T_2-weighted images

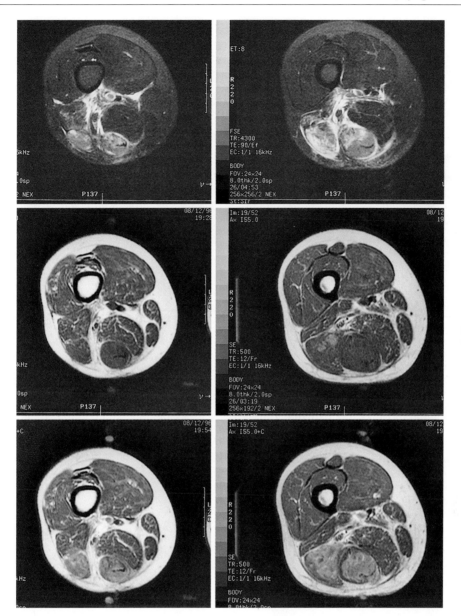

Fig. 17.3. Residual lymphoma in the posterior compartment of the right thigh after chemotherapy shows small focal areas of hemorrhage in the biceps femoris muscle as high signal intensity in the T_1-weighted axial image (*middle right*) and heterogeneous contrast enhancement in the biceps femoris and semitendinous muscles in the post-gadolinium-injection T_1-weighted axial image. Note diffuse heterogeneous high signal intensity in the T_2-weighted axial image (*top right*)

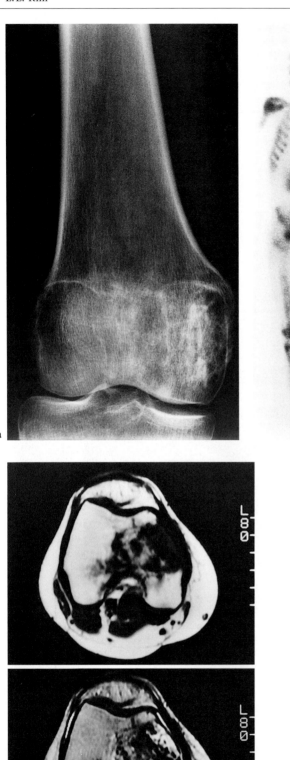

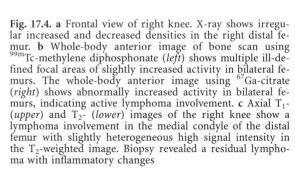

Fig. 17.4. a Frontal view of right knee. X-ray shows irregular increased and decreased densities in the right distal femur. b Whole-body anterior image of bone scan using ^{99m}Tc-methylene diphosphonate (*left*) shows multiple ill-defined focal areas of slightly increased activity in bilateral femurs. The whole-body anterior image using ^{67}Ga-citrate (*right*) shows abnormally increased activity in bilateral femurs, indicating active lymphoma involvement. c Axial T_1- (*upper*) and T_2- (*lower*) images of the right knee show a lymphoma involvement in the medial condyle of the distal femur with slightly heterogeneous high signal intensity in the T_2-weighted image. Biopsy revealed a residual lymphoma with inflammatory changes

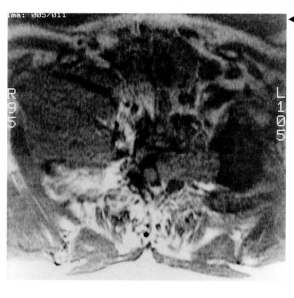

◀ **Fig. 17.5.** Axial T_1-weighted image of the upper chest shows a myeloma lesion in the left pedicle of T_1 spine with intermediate signal intensity, extending into the thecal sac as well as the left lung apex

Fig. 17.6. a Frontal view of the pelvic X-ray shows osteolytic myeloma lesions in the right pubic bone and right acetabulum. Note also questionable lesions in the bilateral sacral wings. **b** T_1- (*upper*) and T_2- (*lower*) axial images of the lower pelvis show an expansile myeloma lesion involving the right pubic bone with slightly heterogeneous intermediate signal intensity in the T_1-weighted image and high signal intensity in the T_2-weighted image. **c** Axial T_2-weighted image of the upper pelvis shows a myeloma involvement in the right sacrum and right posterior ilium with high signal intensity

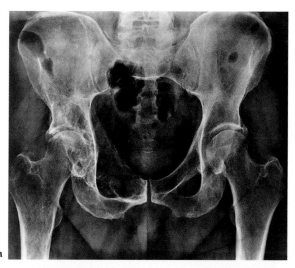

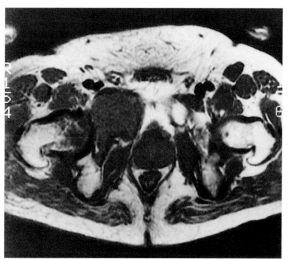

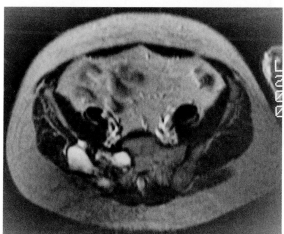

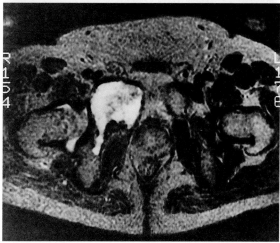

can be seen in successfully treated lesions or some untreated lesions. Complete response to chemotherapy can demonstrate a complete resolution of abnormality, persistent abnormality with no contrast enhancement or peripheral rim enhancement only [56].

MRI can establish the presence of disease process, extent and location with great sensitivity. The therapeutic response can be monitored with follow-up MRI scans, obviating the need for repeat or misdirected marrow biopsies.

Magnetic Resonance Spectroscopy

Clinical magnetic resonance spectroscopy (MRS) can no longer be confined to research laboratories or to late-night sessions on borrowed instruments. As in the early days of MRI, cancer dominates the interest of spectroscopists. Our knowledge of human cancer has been augmented by information derived directly from MRS. A fingerprint of large tumors has emerged from studies with phosphorus-31. An excess of phosphomonoesters (PMEs) and phosphodiesters (PDEs), a group of unusual but universal compounds, characterizes cancers, including lymphoid cancers and lymphoma. MRS is limited only by the difficulty of access to deep or small tumors. The ^{31}P MRS of B-cell lymphoma (Fig. 17.7) before chemotherapy showed only a marginally increased PME peak in the whole-volume spectrum, although the PME level had actually risen at least threefold in the appropriate region of the tumor. Subsequent examinations 3 days after chemotherapy showed a return toward normal spectra [57]. Activation of lymphocytes with IL-2 dramatically switches its metabolism as monitored by MR. This gives hope that immunotherapy may be especially well monitored with MRS.

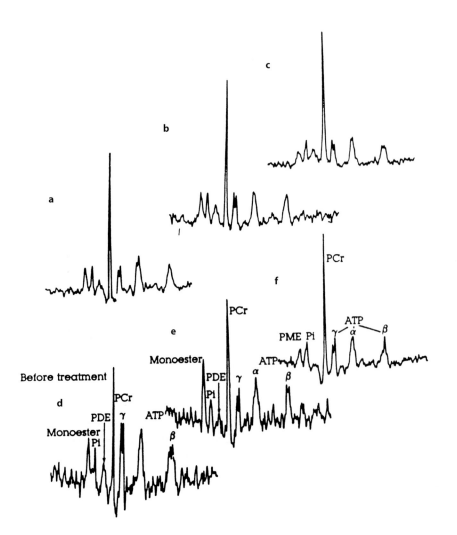

Fig. 17.7 a–f. ^{31}P magnetic resonance spectra of B-cell lymphoma of bone. Whole-volume (*upper*) and localized (*lower*) spectroscopy were performed before (**a** and **d**) and 3 days (**b** and **e**) after chemotherapy. Phosphomonoester (PME), which rose only marginally in the whole-volume spectrum, actually rose at least threefold in the appropriate region of tumor. Subsequent examinations (**c** and **f**) show a return toward the normal spectra (reprinted with permission from [57])

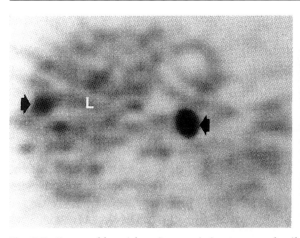 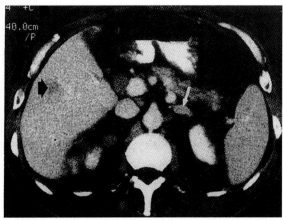

Fig. 17.8. Comparable axial positron-emission-tomography (*left*) and contrast-computed-tomography (*right*) images show metastatic melanomas in the right hepatic lobe and left adrenal gland (reprinted with permission from [58])

Positron Emission Tomography

In a small study for staging of metastatic melanoma, positron emission tomography (PET) imaging had an overall accuracy of 100%, detecting 7 of 7 metastatic lesions and predicting 13 of 13 negative lymph-node regions (Fig. 17.8) [58]. For intra-abdominal, visceral, and lymph-node metastases, fluoro-2-deoxy-D-glucose (FDG)-PET sensitivity for lesions detection was 100% (15 of 15). PET revealed three metastatic foci which were later found on CT. Two metastatic foci were seen only on follow-up CT several months later. The sensitivity of PET for detecting small lung metastases was lower than CT and was attributed to respiratory motion or prior cancer therapy.

Quantification of biologic processes with PET imaging provides a means for directly measuring metabolic and biochemical abnormalities as well as assessing treatment responses. Hematopoietic cytokines, such as granulocyte-macrophage-colony-stimulating factor (GMCSF) and macrophage-colony-stimulating factor (MCSF), are a family of glycoprotein growth factors that have been used for preventing patients from developing the myelosuppressive effects of chemotherapy and radiation. Yao et al. [59] have evaluated the effects of cytokines on bone-marrow glucose metabolism by serial quantitative FDG-PET images in 18 patients with metastatic melanoma. In both GMCSF and GMCSF with monoclonal antibody, rapid increases in bone-marrow glucose metabolic rates were observed during therapy, whereas MCSF had only a slight effect. After GMCSF exposure was stopped, bone-marrow glucose metabolic rates rapidly decreased in both groups.

The accuracy of FDG-PET in thoraco-abdominal lymphomas compared with that in CT was studied in 11 patients with NHL and 5 patients with HD (Fig. 17.9) [60]. In this study, FDG-PET detected 54 lesions, whereas CT detected 49 lesions. There was no lesion missed by PET. In addition, PET detected five lesions that were not seen on CT. There was also no difference between PET detection of low- and intermediate-grade lymphomas (Fig. 17.10).

In a more recent study comparing whole-body PET with that of conventional staging in 18 patients, both imaging algorithms detected 33 of 37 lesions, although not all lesions detected were the same [61]. Staging using whole-body PET was concordant with conventional staging in 14 of 17 patients, better than conventional staging in three patients and worse in one patient. The actual total cost for the conventional staging was $66292, whereas the cost for a whole-body PET-based staging was almost half ($36250). The lesions not detected by whole-body PET were small lesions in the lung parenchyma in a patient with NHL and 1-cm nodes in the mediastinum and periaortic areas in another NHL patient. A whole-body FDG-PET-based staging algorithm may be an accurate and cost-effective method for staging or restaging HD and NHL [62]. The use of simultaneous transmission and emission scans may allow more semiquantitative criteria for tumor uptake and more specificity in differentiating between tumor and non-tumor uptake and estimated tumor response to therapy. FDG-PET scanning proved to be capable of delivering important additional information for diagnosis of untreated lymphoma. FDG-PET is a particularly promising method for the evaluation of spleen, liver, and bone marrow,

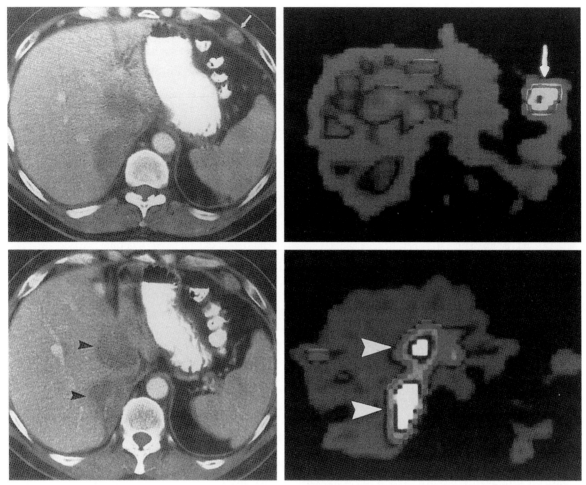

Fig. 17.9. Comparable contrast-computed-tomography (*left*) and ^{18}F-fluoro-2-deoxy-D-glucose positron-emission-tomography (*right*) axial image of the upper abdomen show low-grade non-Hodgkin's lymphoma lesions abutting the left-hemidiaphragm (*arrows*) and right adrenal gland and caudal hepatic segment (*arrowheads*) (reprinted with permission from [60])

which to date require invasive biopsy methods (Fig. 17.11). PET not only allowed recognition of all but one case of extranodal involvement seen in CT, but also allowed detection of additional lesions and changes in staging levels in 16% of 43 NHL and 38 HD patients [63].

Multiple myeloma is characterized by malignant proliferation of clonal plasma cells and excessive formation of Ig. Detection of bone lesions in the early phase of the disease and evaluation of changes during treatment are often difficult. Quantitative analysis of serum and urine M-protein is useful after the general progression of the disease, but does not reflect the status of developing or existing bone lesions. Radiographic changes are not reliable indicators of prognosis, and bone scan with ^{99m}Tc-MDP is relatively insensitive [64]. There was a case of intense ^{99m}Tc-sestamibi uptake in bone marrow correlating with the extent of the disease, while ^{18}F-FDG-PET showed focal increased activity only in areas of active disease progression associated with pain [65].

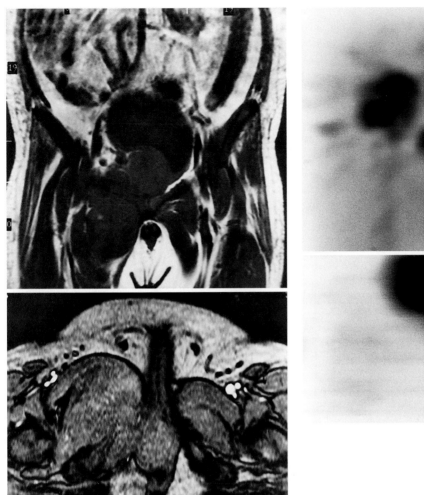

Fig. 17.10. a T$_1$-weighted coronal (*upper*) and T$_2$-weighted axial (*lower*) images of the pelvis show low-grade lymphoma masses in the right inguinal region extending into the prostatic gland. **b** Selected coronal (*upper*) and sagittal positron-emission-tomography (*lower*) images of the lower pelvis show a markedly increased uptake of ^{18}F-fluoro-2-deoxy-D-glucose in the lymphoma masses, indicating active malignant lesions

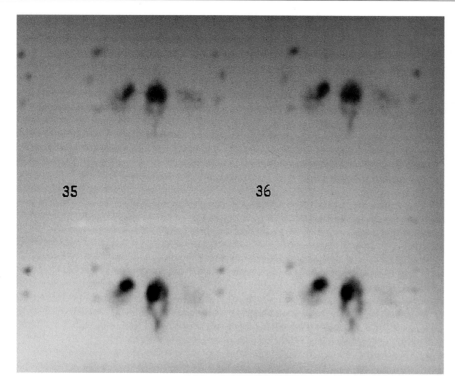

Fig. 17.11. Selected axial positron-emission-tomography images of the upper abdomen show a markedly increased uptake of ^{18}F-fluoro-2-deoxy-D-glucose-FDG in the right side of L2 vertebral body, corresponding to lymphoma involvement. A bone scan using ^{99m}Tc-methylene diphosphonate was positive (not shown), and the biopsy confirmed the lymphoma involvement

References

1. Landis SH, Murray T, Bolden S, Wingo PA (1998) Cancer statistics, 1988. CA Cancer J Clin 48:6–29
2. Sober A (1991) Cutaneous melanoma: opportunity for cure. CA Cancer J Clin 41:1997–1999
3. Lew R, Sober A, Cook N (1983) Sun exposure habits in patients with cutaneous melanoma: a case control study. J Dermatol Surg Oncol 9:981–986
4. Rhodes A, Wood W, Sober A (1981) Non-epidermal origin of malignant melanoma associated with a giant congenital nevocellular nevus. Plast Reconstr Surg 67:782–790
5. Lynch H, Fusaro R (1986) Hereditary malignant melanoma: a unifying etiologic hypothesis. Cancer Genet Cytogenet 20:301–304
6. Hussussain C, Struewing J, Goldstein A (1994) Germline p16 mutations in familial melanoma. Nat Genet 8:15–21
7. Rodeck U, Herlyn M (1991) Growth factors in melanoma. Cancer Metastasis Rev 10:89–101
8. Menrad A, Herlyn M (1992) Tumor progression, biology and host response in melanoma. Curr Opin Oncol 4:351–356
9. Albelda S, Mette S, Elder D (1990) Integrin distribution in malignant melanoma: association of the beta-3 subunit with tumor progression. Cancer Res 50:6757–6764
10. Meissauer A, Kramer M, Hofmann M (1991) Urokinase-type and tissue-type plasminogen activators are essential for in vitro invasion of human melanoma cells. Exp Cell Res 192:453–459
11. Mackensen A, Carcelain G, Viel S (1994) Direct evidence to support the immunosurveillance concept in a human regressive melanoma. J Clin Invest 93:1397–1402
12. Markovic S, Murasko D (1991) Role of natural killer and T-cells in interferon induced inhibition of spontaneous metastases of the B16F10L, murine melanoma. Cancer Res 51:1124–1128
13. Peltenburg L, Steegenga W, Kruse K (1992) C-myc-induced natural killer cell sensitivity of human melanoma cells is reversed by HLA-B27 transfection. Eur J Immunol 22:2737–2740
14. Banks PM (1990) The pathology of Hodgkin's disease. Semin Oncol 17:683–689
15. Carbone A, Gloghini A, Gattei V (1994) Expression of the CD-40 receptor on Reed-Sternberg cells: a highly reliable tool and a new clue for understanding the pathophysiology of Hodgkin's disease (abstract). Proc Am Soc Clin Oncol 13:373
16. Ree HJ, Strauhen JA, Khan AA (1991) Human immunodeficiency virus-associated Hodgkin's disease: clinicopathologic studies of 24 cases and preponderance of mixed cellularity type characterized by the occurrence of fibrohistiocytid stromal cells. Cancer 67:1614–1619
17. Tsubata T, Wu J, Hongo T (1993) B-cell apoptosis induced by antigen receptor crosslinking is blocked by a T-cell signal through CD40. Nature 364:645–648
18. Yumis J, Oken M, Kaplan (1982) Distinctive chromosomal abnormalities in histologic subtypes of non-Hodgkin's lymphoma. N Engl J Med 307:1231–1236
19. Zutter (1991) Immunolocalization of the bcl-2 protein with hematopoietic neoplasms. Blood 78:1062–1066
20. Hockenberry D, Nunez G, Korsmeyer J (1991) Bcl-2 is an inner mitochondrial membrane protein that blocks programmed cell death. Nature 348:334–339
21. Gallagher C (1986) Follicular lymphoma: prognostic factors for response and survival. J Clin Oncol 4:1470–1480
22. Vuckovic J, Stula N, Capkun V (1994) Prognostic value of B-symptoms in low grade non-Hodgkin's lymphoma. Leuk Lymphoma 13:357–358
23. Macartney JC (1991) DNA flow cytometry of follicular non-Hodgkin's lymphoma. J Clin Pathol 44:215–219
24. Cabanilles F, Grant G, Hagemeister F (1989) Refractoriness to chemotherapy and poor survival related to ab-

normalities of chromosome 17 and 7 in lymphoma. Am J Med 87:167–172
25. Johnson A, Cavallin-Stahl E (1991) Incidence and prognostic significant of blood lymphocyte clonal excess in localized non-Hodgkin's lymphoma. Ann Oncol 2:739–743
26. National Cancer Institute (1982) National Cancer Institute sponsored study of classifications of non-Hodgkin's lymphomas: summary and description of a working formation for clinical usage. The Non-Hodgkin's Lymphoma Pathological Classification Project. Cancer 49:2112–2135
27. Epstein J (1992) Myeloma phenotype: clues to disease origin and manifestation. Hematol Oncol Clin North Am 6:249–256
28. Neri A, Baldini L, Trecca D (1993) p53 gene mutations in multiple myeloma are associated with advanced forms of the malignancy. Blood 81:128–135
29. Gearing DP, Comeau MR, Friend DJ (1992) The IL-6 signal transducer gp130: an oncostatin M receptor and affinity converter for the L1F receptor. Science 255:1434–1437
30. Grogan TM, Spier CM, Salmon SE (1993) p-Glycoprotein expression in human plasma cell myeloma: correlation with prior chemotherapy. Blood 81:490–495
31. Bataille R, Durie BF, Grenier J (1986) Prognostic factors and staging in multiple myeloma: a reappraisal. J Clin Oncol 4:80–87
32. Kyle RA (1988) Prognostic factors in multiple myeloma. Hematol Oncol 6:125–130
33. Jain S, Allen P (1989) Desmoplastic malignant melanoma and its variants. Am J Surg Pathol 13:358–373
34. Shields J (1993) Management of uveal melanoma: a continuing dilemma. Cancer 72:2067–2068
35. Breslow A (1975) Thickness, cross-sectional areas and depth of invasion in the prognosis of cutaneous melanoma. Ann Surg 182:572–575
36. Clark WJ, From L, Bernadin E (1969) The histogenesis and biologic behavior of primary human malignant melanomas of the skin. Cancer Res 29:705–726
37. Goldsmith H (1979) Melanoma: an overview. CA Cancer J Clin 29:194–199
38. Urist M, Balch C, Soong S-J (1984) Head and neck melanoma in 536 clinical stage I patients: a prognostic factors analysis and results of surgical treatment. Ann Surg 200:769–775
39. Hagemeister FB (1991) Controversies in management of Hodgkin's disease. In: Freireich EJ, Kantajian H (eds) Therapy of hematopoietic neoplasia. Dekker, New York, pp 249–264
40. MacLennan KA, Bennett MH, Tu A (1989) Relationship of histopathologic features to survival and relapse in nodular sclerosing Hodgkin's disease. Cancer 64:1686–1693
41. Glatstein E, Guernsey JM, Rosenberg SA (1969) The value of laparotomy and splenectomy in the staging of Hodgkin's disease. Cancer 24:704–709
42. Hagemeister FB, Fesus SM, Lamki LM (1990) Role of the gallium scan in Hodgkin's disease. Cancer 65:1090–1095
43. Das DK, Gupta SK, Datta BN (1991) FNA cytodiagnosis of non-Hodgkin's lymphomas and its subtyping under working formulation of 175 cases. Diagn Cytopathol 7:487–498
44. Cossman J, Zehnbauer B, Garrett CT (1991) Gene rearrangements in the diagnosis of lymphoma/leukemia guidelines for use based on a multi-institutional study. Hematopathology 95:347–354
45. Bataille R, Jourdan M, Zhang X (12992) Mechanisms of bone lesions in multiple myeloma. Hematol Oncol Clin North Am 6:285–295
46. Ludwig H, Fruhwald F, Tscholakoff D, Rasoul S, Neuhold A, Fritz E (1987) Magnetic resonance imaging of the spine in multiple myeloma (abstract). Lancet 177:364–366
47. Pruzanski W, Ogryzlo MA (1970) Abnormal proteinuria in malignant disease. Adv Clin Chem 13:335–382
48. Outwater E, Tomaszewski JE, Daly JM, Kressel HY (1991) Hepatic colorectal metastases: correlation of MRI and pathologic appearance. Radiology 180:327–332
49. Bergin CJ, Carlsen SE, Healy MV, Castellino RA (1990) MR imaging evaluation of chest wall lymphoma (abstract). Radiology 177:97p
50. North LB, Fuller, LM, Sullivan-Halley JA, Hagemeister FB (1987) Regression of mediastinal Hodgkin's disease after therapy: evaluation of time interval. Radiology 159:305–310
51. Chen JL, Osborne BM, Butler JJ (1987) Residual fibrous masses in treated Hodgkin's disease. Cancer 60:407–413
52. Rahmourni A, Tempany C, Jone R, Mann R, Yang A, Zerhouni E (1993) Lymphoma: monitoring tumor size and signal intensity with MRI. Radiology 188:445–451
53. Lee JK, Glazer HS (1990) Controversy in the MRI appearance of fibrosis. Radiology 177:21–22
54. Smith SR, Williams CE, Davies JM, Edwards RHT (1989) Bone marrow disorders: characterization with quantitative MRI. Radiol 172:805–810
55. Steiner RM, Mitchell DG, Rao VM, Schweitzer ME (1992) MRI of diffuse bone marrow disease. Radiol Clin North Am 31:383–409
56. Mouloupoulos LA, Dimopoulos MA, Alexanian R, Leeds NE, Libshitz HI (1994) Multiple myeloma: MR patterns of response to treatment. Radiology 192:441–446
57. Ross B (1988) Clinical uses broaden for MR spectroscopy. J Diagn Imaging (November) 258–263
58. Gritters LS, Francis IR, Zasadny KR (1993) Initial assessment of positron emission tomography using 2-fluorine-18-fluoro-2-deoxy-D-glucose in the imaging of malignant melanoma. J Nucl Med 34:1420–1427
59. Yao W-J, Hoh CK, Hawkins RA, Glaspy JA, Weid JA, Lee SJ, Maddahi J, Phelps ME (1995) Quantitative PET imaging of bone marrow glucose metabolic response to hematopoietic cytokines. J Nucl Med 36:794–799
60. Newman JS, Francis IR, Kaminski MS (1994) Imaging of lymphoma with PET with 2-[F-18]-fluoro-2-deoxy-D-glucose: correlation with CT. Radiology 190:111–116
61. Hoh CK, Schiepers C, Seltzer MA, Gambhir SS, Silverman DHS, Czernin J, Maddahi J, Phelps ME (1997) PET in oncology: will it replace the other modalities? Semin Nucl Med 27:94–106
62. Hoh CK, Glaspy J, Rosen P, Dahlborn M, Lee SJ, Kunkel L, Hawkin RA, Maddahi J, Phelps ME (1997) Whole-body FDG-PET imaging for staging of Hodgkin's disease and lymphoma. J Nucl Med 38:343–348
63. Moog F, Bangerter M, Diederichs CG, Guhlmann A, Merkle E, Frickhofen N, Reske SN (1998) Extranodal malignant lymphoma: detection with FDG PET versus CT. Radiology 206:475–481
64. Scutellari PN, Spanedda R, Feggi LM, Cervi PM (1985) The value and limitations of total bone scan in the diagnosis of multiple myeloma: a comparison with conventional skeletal radiography. Haematologica 70:136–142
65. El-Shirbing AM, Yeung H, Imbriaco M, Michaeli J, Macapinlac H, Larson SM (1997) Technetium-99m-MIBI versus fluorine-18-FDG in diffuse multiple myeloma. J Nucl Med 38:1208–1210

Subject Index

A
abscess 250
acetonenitride 84
ACTH 5, 125
activation 40
ADC 7, 217–218
adenoacanthoma 10
adenocarcinoma 124
adenoma 10, 98, 164, 235
adenomyosis 205
adenosquamous cancer 201
adenosine diphosphate 64
adenosine monophosphate 64
adenosine 82, 85, 222
ADP 4, 152
adrenal 126, 135
affinity 101
AFP 5, 160, 184
aldotamoxifen 83
aliasing 114
analogue 81
aneuploidy 199, 233
angiogenesis 14, 147, 182, 217
angiomyolipoma 185
angiosarcoma 245
Ann Arbor staging 273–274
annihilation 72
anthracosis 135
antiangiogenesis 82
antibody 7, 8, 97, 98, 269
anti-CEA 162
antiestrogen 82
antigen 7, 8, 97, 124
antioxidant 82, 83
apoptosis 5, 6, 123, 272
apparent diffusion coefficient 35
arterial input 112
artifact 107, 113, 114, 115
asialoglycoprotein 98
aspiration 132
Astler-Coller system 162
Astrocytoma 211
ATP 5, 152, 190
attenuation 137
autoradiogram 82, 83

B
B cells 7, 272
back projection 72
Baker's cyst 247
bandwidth 21, 29, 114, 115
bcl-2 182, 272
benzamide 102
benzodiazepine 119
beta symbol-hCG 183–184
BGO detector 74, 75
binding 101
biochemistry 3

biology 3
bioreduction 82
blood-brain barrier 24, 36
bladder cancer 181, 189, 194
blood flow 112, 257
blood volume 36, 217–218
blotting 3, 4
Blumer's rectal shelf 161
BOLD 39
bond 101
bone scan 125, 135
Botyroid sarcoma 245
breast 145
breast cancer 81
Broder's system 162, 200
bromodeoxyuridine 82
bromotamoxifen 82

C
^{11}C acetate 172
^{11}C methionine 175
^{13}C 48, 65
CA15-3 147
CA-125 199
cachectin 5
cachexia 5
CALLA 272
camera 73
cAMP 5
cancer 3, 159, 181
carcinogen 7, 123
carcinoid 162
carcinoma 10
carcinomatosis 212
cat scratch disease 248
catabolism 4
cathepsin D 147
CD antigen 271
CEA 5, 8, 124, 147, 172
Cell death 217, 219
cervical cancer 200
chemical shift 107, 109, 114
– c. s. imaging 152
CHESS 49, 219
cholangiopancreatography 26
cholecystokinin 98
choline 62, 191–192, 219
chondroitin 6
chondrosarcoma 244, 246
choriocarcinoma 184
chromosome 163, 182
CIN 202
cirrhosis 163, 167
CIS 146, 183
cisplatin 84
citrate 191–192
clear cell carcinoma 201
clear cell sarcoma 245

cloning 3
CMET 268
CO 111
CO_2 111
coil 115, 233
coincidence 72, 73
collagen 9
collagenase 6
collimator 73
colorectal cancer 160, 162
compartment 78
computed tomography 13
contrast agent 95, 97, 149
contrast enhancement 95
core biopsy 145, 161
coregistration 224
cost effectiveness 14
Courvoisier's sign 162
cross-excitation 115
CSI_{31} 109
Cyclin D1 gene 231
cyclotron 71
cysteinate 227
cytidine 82
cytokine 7
cytology 145
cytosarcoma 146
cytotoxicity 7

D
DCIS 146
DEA 3
decision 14
dedifferentiation 4
deoxyglucose 109
deoxyhemoglobin 39
dephasing 20, 107, 110, 116
desmoid 247
desmoplasia 10
detection 74
detector 73, 76
dextran 98
differential absorption
  ratio 133
differential uptake ratio 78, 133
diffusion 34, 216–218
dipole 95
dissociation constant 102
Dixon 32
DNA ploidy 146
dopamine 102, 103, 222
DRESS 49
ductal carcinoma 146
Dukes' system 162
DUR 238
dynamic imaging 37, 77
– d. MRI 149, 163, 166, 189
dysplasia 202, 231, 243

E

echo
- e. time 107
- e. train 26

echo-planar imaging 27
ECM 6
eddy current 116
edema 213–214, 217
EGF 123
EGFR 182, 199, 231
elastin 6
elastofibroma 247
electron 71, 95, 96
electrophoresis 3, 4
embryonal carcinoma 184
encephalomalacia 214
enchondroma 262
enchondromatosis 244
encoding 113, 114, 115
endocytosis 98
endometrial cancer 199
endometriosis 81, 83
ependymoma 212, 215
EPI 110
epidermal growth factor 182
epithelioma 264
Epstein-Barr virus 231, 271
equilibrium 95
ERCP 162
estradiol 81, 103, 200
estrogen 81, 82, 146, 199
Ewing's sarcoma 243–244
excitation 110
exostoses 243

F

^{18}F-fluoride 267
^{19}F 48, 65
FAMMM 271
fasciitis 247
fat supression 29, 149, 166, 185
FATS 149
fatty acid 117
FDG 111, 112, 116, 117, 118, 133, 135
- brain tumor 222, 227
- breast cancer 153
- gastric cancer 172
- gynecologic cancer 207–208
- hepatoma 168
- lymphoma 281
- pancreatic cancer 176
- pheochromocytoma 194
- renal cancer 193
FDG-6-phosphate 117
Feridex 96
ferromagnetic 95, 116
fibrin 9
fibrinolysis 6
fibrolamellar HCC 160
fibromatosis 247
fibronectin 6, 9
fibrosis 235, 276
FID 56
FIGO 201, 202
film 13
filter 56, 114
fine needle aspiration (see FNA)
FISP 110
FLAIR 32
FLASH 111
flip angle 18
flow cytometry 146
fluoromisonidazole 82
fluorotamoxifen 82, 92, 93, 155
fluorouracil 82, 171
FMISO 236, 257
f MRI 39
FNA 125, 145, 161, 232, 274
FNH 165
Fourier-transform 22, 48, 113, 218
free induction decay 19, 48, 95, 107
frequency-encoding 21, 22
FSE 26, 110
functional image 216

G

gadolinium 24, 96
gallium scan 274
ganglioside 6
gas 111, 112
gastric cancer 159
gastroenteropancreatic tumor 172
gastrointestinal cancer 159
gating 113
GCSF 8
gene 3
germ cell tumor 160, 184–185, 202
ghost 113
glassy-cell carcinoma 202
Gleason grade 182, 184
glioblastoma multiforme 211, 213
glioma 211
gliomatosis 214
gliosis 214, 225
glomus tumor 248
glottic tumor 234
glucokinase 4
gluconeogenesis 5
glucose 112, 222
glycogen-storage disease 167
glycolipid 6
glycolysis 4, 118, 219, 257
GMCSF 281
goiter 235
gradient echo 24, 109
gradient 110, 113
granulomatosis 274
GRASS 110
Graves' disease 102, 119, 235
growth 5
gyncologic cancer 199
gyromagnetic ratio 17, 47

H

^{1}H 48
hamartoma 185
HCC 159, 163
Helicobacter pylori 159
hemangioma 163, 164, 246
hemangiosarcoma 245
hematometria 204
hemorrhage 213, 217, 246
hemosiderin 185, 213, 246
heparanase 6
hepatitis 9
hepatocarcinogenesis 4
hepatocellular carcinoma 159
HER-2/neu 8, 147, 182, 199, 200
hexokinase 4, 117
histocompatibility 7
HMPAO 227
Hodgkin's disease 271, 273
homozygosity 4
hormone 81
Horner's syndrome 124
hybridization 1
hydrocarbon 123
hypercalcemia 125
hyperemia 217
hyperestrinism 199
hyperkeratosis 231
hyperplasia 201, 235
hypersensitivity 8
hyperthermia 41
hypoglycemia
hypoxia 82, 84, 90, 94, 142, 219

I

idotamoxifen 83, 86, 88
IGF 124
image-contrast 23
image-pixel-value 77
imaging time 110
imaging 13
immunity 7, 8, 9
immunization 9
immunoglobulin 7, 231
immunology 7
immunomodulator 8
immunotherapy 8
in situ carcinoma 145
infarct 217
influx 112
inhomogeneity 20, 115, 116
inorganic phosphate 63
in-phase 26, 109
interferon 7, 8
interleukin 5, 7, 272
intervention 41
inversion recovery 29, 107
inversion time 107
iododeoxyuridine 227
iron oxide 96
ischemia 217
ISIS 50, 52, 218
IUDR 227

J

J-coupling modulation 52
Jewett-Marshall staging 183
junctional zone 205

K

keratin 232
k-space 54

L

lactate 60, 109, 219
LAK cell 9
Larmor frequency 18, 19, 21, 95
laryngeal tumor 232–233
lattice 95
LCIS 145
LDH 272, 274
leiomyoma 205
leiomyosarcoma 245
leptomeningeal disease 212, 215
leukopladia 232
Leydig cell tumor 184
ligand 81, 101
ligand-protein 101
lipid 62, 63
lipid peroxidase 82, 90
lipoma 258
lipomatosis 246
liposarcoma 243, 245
liposome 98
lobular carcinoma 145
location 20, 21, 48, 50
LSO detector 76
lump constant 153

lung cancer   123, 130
lymphangiosarcoma   245
lymphocyte   7
lymphoepithelioma   232
lymphoma   212, 215, 271, 276
lymphoscintigraphy   147

M
MAC system   162
macromolecule   81, 96
macrophage   8, 119, 222
Madelung's disease   246
magnetization transfer   33, 149, 253
magnetization   17, 18, 19, 30, 95, 107, 110
magnevist   96
mammography   145
mangafodipir   96
matrix   6
MCSF   281
MDR   272
mdr-1   124
mediastinal node   130, 134
mediastinal staging   134
mediastinoscopy   125
medullary carcinoma   146
Medulloblastoma   212
melanocyte   271
melanoma   271, 273
meningioma   212, 214
mesothelioma   123
metabolism   64
metabolite   218
metastasis   163–164, 182, 212, 215, 245, 267
methionine   131, 222, 226, 239, 257, 268
methyluridine   86
MFH   190, 244, 250
MIBG   193
MIBI   155, 268
microcalcification   145
microsphere   84
microvessel density   147
misonidazole   82, 85, 142
mitomycin   82
Mn-DPDP   164
modeling   77
monocyte   7
monokine   7
motion   113
M-protein   282
MRA   25, 27, 110
MRCP   166
MRI technique   107
MRI   13, 17
mRNA   3, 4
MRS   47
– breast   150
– liver   167
– prostate   190
– sarcoma   255
MTC   7
MTR   253
mucinous carcinoma
– breast   150
– colon   162
– ovary   200
– prostate   190
multidrug resistance   124
multidrug-related protein   124
musculoskeletal tumor   243
mutagen   231
mutation   4, 7, 8, 231
myasthenia   102

myc oncogene   123
myeloma   271–272, 275
myocardium   117
myositis   248
myxoma   248

N
^{13}N-ammonia   257
N-acetylaspartate (NAA)   59, 60
NaI detector   74
nasopharyngeal cancer   231
nature killer   7
necrosis   5, 10, 214, 221, 245
nephrotoxicity   192
neruofibroma   248
neurilemoma   212
neuroblastoma   192-193
neuroendocrine tumor   172
neurofibromatosis   212
neurofibrosarcoma   245
neuroma   212, 247
neuropathy   82
neurotransmitter   102, 103
neutron   71
nevus syndrome   271
nicotinamide adenosine dinucleotide   64
nicotine   124
nitroimidazole   85, 94
nitrosamine   123
NK cell   271
NMSP   226
node   134
nodule   132
NOE   255
Non-Hodgkin's lymphoma   272
NSCLC   123
nucleoside   82
nucleotide   82, 222, 227
nucleus   48, 71
null point   107

O
^{15}O CO   112
^{15}O O$_2$ 112
^{15}O water   112, 171
octreotide   104, 241
ODC   5
Oligodendroglioma   212
Omniscan   96
oncogen   8, 231
opposed image   109
osteoarthropathy   124
osteogenesis   244
osteosarcoma   243, 245, 246
otitis   232
out-of-phase   26, 109
ovarian cancer   199
Overhauser effect   255
oxygen free radical   217
oxyhemoglobin   40

P
p^{53} 4, 5, 8, 123, 181, 182, 199, 200, 211, 231, 243
p^{97} 9
^{31}p   48
PAGE   3
Paget's disease   119, 146, 243
Pancoast's syndrome   124
pancreas cancer   159, 166
panendoscopy   232
Papanicolaou smear   201
papillary carcinoma

– breast   146
– endometrium   201
papilloma   10, 215
– p. virus   200, 231
paramagnetic   24, 95, 96, 97
parametry   38, 77
paraneoplastic syndrome   200
parathyroid   235
pasammoma   200
Pasteur effect   4
pathology   9
Patlak plot method   78
PCNA   231
PCR   3, 231
peptide   8, 103, 123, 124, 125
perfluorocarbon   95
perfusion   36, 216, 227
permeability   38, 81
pernicious anemia   159
peroxidase   82
peroxidation   83
perspective   15
PET   14
p-glycoprotein   117
phase-contrast   27
phase-encoding   21, 11
phenylalamine   227
pheochromocytoma   181, 185
phosphocreatine   60, 152, 167
phosphodiester   63, 152, 167, 190
phosphofructokinase   4
phospholipase   5
phosphomonoester   63, 152, 167, 190
phosphosotidylcholine   63
piriformis sinus tumor   233
pitfall   116
plasminogen   6, 271
ploidy   10
PNET   243
PNST   248pO$_2$ 85
polyanthanide   97
polycystic ovarina syndrome   200
polylysine   98
polymer   98
polymorphism   3
polypeptide   7
polyposis   160
positron   71
predictive value   15
PRESS   50, 51, 218
probe   3, 85
PROBE/SV   59, 220
Prohance   96
prostaglandin   7, 160
prostate   190
prostatitis   190
protease   6
protein kinase   160
proteoglycan   6, 9
proton   104, 114
PSA   183, 184
pseudocapsule   164
pseudogating   113
pseudomyxoma   200
putrescine   5
PVNS   247
pyridine   85

Q
quantitation   77

R
Radiation change   219
radical   82

radiofrequency pulse 107
radiography 13
radioimmunodetection 9, 13
radioimmunoimaging 13
radioimmunotherapy 9
radiopharmaceutical 81
radiosensitization 82
radon 123
ras 8
RASE 110
receptor 81, 97, 101, 103
- dopamine 222
- estrogen 146
- somatostatin 172
Recklinghausen's disease 245
reconstruction 118
Reed-Sternberg cell 271, 273
refocusing pulse 110
relaxation time 19, 218
relaxation 17, 95, 107
renal cell cancer 181, 185, 193
reperfusion 217
repetition time 107
rephasing 107
retinal 82, 86, 94
retinoblastoma gene 181, 243
retinoic acid 82
retinol 82
retrodifferentiation 4
RF
- coil 19
- energy 115
- noise 115
- pulse 21. 109, 110
- shield 115
RFLP 3
rhabdomyosarcoma 184, 243, 244, 250
rim enhancement 216
RNA 3
Robson's staging 183
RODEO 149
Rye classification 273

S
Santorini's plexus 190
sarcoid 131
sarcoma 10, 243
scar 171
schwannoma 212, 248, 260
SCLC 123
screening 14
SD5 4
selenium 82
seminal vesicle 190
seminoma 184
sensitivity 15, 97
sensitizer 82
sentinel node 147
serotonin 5
serous tumor 200
sestamibi 241, 268

shimming 115
SI-SV method 54
signal 8, 114
- s. drop-out 114
- s. overlap 114
signaling 8
signal-to-noise 13, 17, 102, 103, 110, 218
Signet-ring cell 162
silicone 31
small cell carcinoma 202
sodium 109
somatostatin 102, 104, 124
specific activity 102
specificity 15, 97
SPECT 72
spectral process 54
spectroscopic imaging 49, 53, 190
spectroscopy 47
spermidine 5
spermine 5
S-phase fraction 146, 147, 184
spin echo 107
spin-spin interaction 107
spiperone 102, 226
squamous cell carcinoma 124, 232
staging 134
standard uptake value 78, 83, 86, 112, 133
Stauffer's syndrome 181
STEAM 50, 51, 219
STIR 30, 107, 250
stroke 35
stroma 9
superior sulcus tumor 126
superoxide 82
superparamagnetic 95, 96, 97
suppression 49
susceptibility 20, 36, 39, 110, 116
SUV
- brain tumor 224
- breast cancer 153
- musculoskeletal tumor 266
SVC syndrome 124
Synovial sarcoma 245
Synovitis 247, 265

T
T cell 7, 272
T1 24, 95, 107
T2 24, 95, 107
T2* 25, 36, 40, 95, 107, 110
tamoxifen 81, 82, 83, 200
target 97
taxol 95
TCR 7
TdT 4
technique 107
teratoma 184
testicular cancer 182
testosterone 182
TGF 8, 82, 199, 232

thrombus 185
thymidine 227, 239
thymocyte 7
thyroid cancer 172
thyrosine 227, 269
TIL 9, 271
time-of-flight 27
TNM staging for cancer
- bladder 183
- breast 147
- kidney 183
- liver 161
- pancreas 162
- prostate 184
- stomach 161
- testis 185
tomography 72
topoisomerase 124
transcriptase 4
transfection 7
transformation 7, 8
transforming growth factor 199
transitional carcinoma 182, 183
transplant 192
trophoblastic disease 205
Trousseau's sign 162
truncation 113, 114
tumor
- t. growth 14
- t. necrosis factor 199
- t. size 14
- t. volume 14
tumorigenesis 4, 231

U
urologic cancer 181

V
vaccination 9
vaccine 8
variant 117, 119
vasoactive intestinal peptide 103
VENC value 28
Verrucous carcinoma 202
virus 8
vitamin 82, 83
vocal cord 234
von Hippel-Lindau disease 181

W
water suppress 49
Wilms' tumor 10
wrap-around 114

Y
yolk-sac carcinoma 184

Z
zebra-stripe 113
zero-line 115
zipper 115